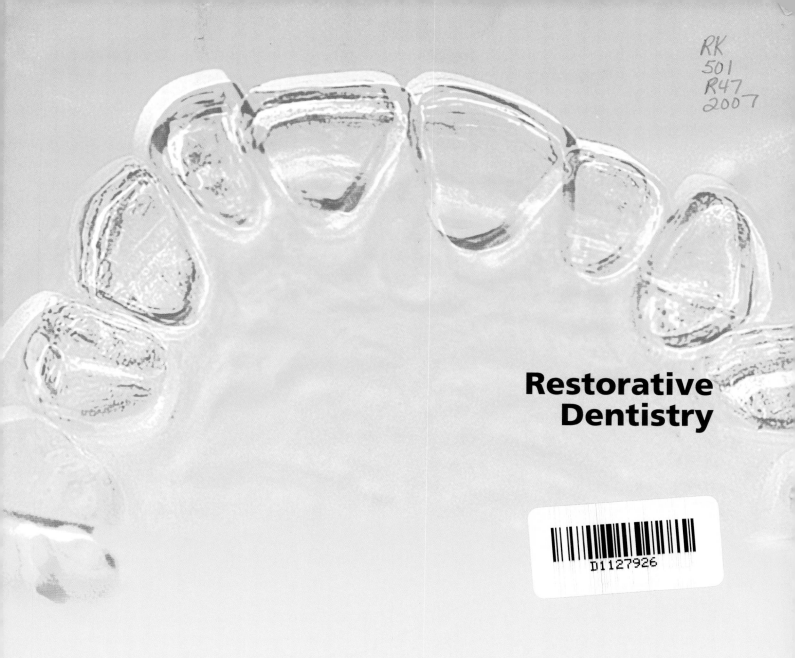

Restorative Dentistry

Commissioning Editor: Michael Parkinson
Project Development Manager: Lulu Stader
Project Manager: Joannah Duncan
Design Direction: George Ajayi
Illustrator: Ian Ramsden

Restorative Dentistry

Second Edition

A. Damien Walmsley BDS MSc PhD FDSRCPS
Professor of Restorative Dentistry,
The University of Birmingham
Consultant in Restorative Dentistry,
South Birmingham Primary Care Trust,
Birmingham, UK

Trevor F. Walsh BDS MSc DDS FDSRCS
Professor of Restorative Dentistry,
The University of Sheffield
Consultant in Restorative Dentistry,
Sheffield Teaching Hospitals NHS Trust, Sheffield, UK

Philip J. Lumley BDS MDentSc PhD FDSRCPS
Professor of Endodontology,
The University of Birmingham
Consultant in Restorative Dentistry,
South Birmingham Primary Care Trust,
Birmingham, UK

F. J. Trevor Burke DDS MSc MDS FDS MGDS RCS
(Edin) FDSRCPS (Glas) FFGDP (UK)
Professor of Primary Dental Care,
The University of Birmingham
Consultant in Restorative Dentistry,
South Birmingham Primary Care Trust,
Birmingham, UK

Adrian C. C. Shortall BDS DDS FDSRCPS FFDRCS
Reader in Restorative Dentistry,
The University of Birmingham
Consultant in Restorative Dentistry,
South Birmingham Primary Care Trust,
Birmingham, UK

Richard Hayes-Hall BDS DGDP (UK)
Lecturer in Conservative Dentistry,
The University of Birmingham
Associate Specialist in Restorative Dentistry,
South Birmingham Primary Care Trust,
Birmingham, UK

Iain A. Pretty BDS (Hons) MSc PhD MFDS RCS (Edin)
Senior Lecturer in Restorative Dentistry,
Dental School and Hospital Manchester, Manchester, UK

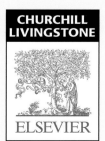

CHURCHILL LIVINGSTONE

ELSEVIER

Edinburgh London New York Oxford Philadelphia St Louis Sydney Toronto 2007

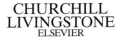

© Harcourt Publishers Limited 2002
© Elsevier Limited 2007

Second edition 2007

ISBN (13) 9780-443-10246-2

British Library Cataloguing in Publication Data
A catalogue record for this book is available from the British Library

Library of Congress Cataloging in Publication Data
A catalog record for this book is available from the Library of Congress

Notice

Neither the Publisher nor the Authors assume any responsibility for any loss or injury and/or damage to persons or property arising out of or related to any use of the material contained in this book. It is the responsibility of the treating practitioner, relying on independent expertise and knowledge of the patient, to determine the best treatment and method of application for the patient.

The Publisher

Working together to grow
libraries in developing countries

www.elsevier.com | www.bookaid.org | www.sabre.org

ELSEVIER   BOOK AID
             International   Sabre Foundation

 ELSEVIER   your source for books,
journals and multimedia
in the health sciences

www.elsevierhealth.com

The
publisher's
policy is to use
**paper manufactured
from sustainable forests**

Printed in China

Contents

Contributors

Fixed and removable prosthodontics
A. Damien Walmsley BDS MSc PhD FDSRCPS
Professor of Restorative Dentistry, The University of Birmingham
Consultant in Restorative Dentistry, South Birmingham Primary Care Trust, Birmingham, UK

Periodontology
Trevor F. Walsh BDS MSc DDS FDSRCS
Professor of Restorative Dentistry, The University of Sheffield
Consultant in Restorative Dentistry, Sheffield Teaching Hospitals NHS Trust, Sheffield, UK

Endodontics
Philip J. Lumley BDS MDentSc PhD FDSRCPS
Professor of Endodontology, The University of Birmingham
Consultant in Restorative Dentistry, South Birmingham Primary Care Trust, Birmingham, UK

Operative and adhesive dentistry
F. J. Trevor Burke DDS MSc MDS FDS MGDS RCS (Edin) FDSRCPS (Glas) FFGDP (UK)
Professor of Primary Dental Care, The University of Birmingham
Consultant in Restorative Dentistry, South Birmingham Primary Care Trust, Birmingham, UK

Operative and adhesive dentistry, fixed prosthodontics
Adrian C. C. Shortall BDS DDS FDSRCPS FFDRCS
Reader in Restorative Dentistry, The University of Birmingham
Consultant in Restorative Dentistry, South Birmingham Primary Care Trust, Birmingham, UK

Occlusion
Richard Hayes-Hall BDS DGDP (UK)
Lecturer in Conservative Dentistry, The University of Birmingham
Associate Specialist in Restorative Dentistry, South Birmingham Primary Care Trust, Birmingham, UK

Caries and preventative dentistry
Iain A. Pretty BDS (Hons) MSc PhD MFDS RCS (Edin)
Senior Lecturer in Restorative Dentistry, Dental School and Hospital Manchester, Manchester, UK

Preface

In 2002, the first edition of *Restorative Dentistry* was launched on an unsuspecting dental profession. It was an attempt to bring together all aspects of restorative dentistry and allow an understanding on how they interacted with each other. Whilst the book was well received, there were some useful comments suggesting where the content could be further improved. Therefore in this new edition, many of the chapters have been updated and new material has been included. We welcome the contribution from our new co-author, Iain Pretty. Iain is clinical lecturer and honorary specialist registrar in restorative dentistry at Manchester Dental School. He has added a new chapter on 'Caries and Other Reasons for Restoring Teeth' and also rewritten the introduction to the chapter on simple restoration of teeth. We welcome his contribution as it provides a bridging link between the basic science and the clinical application of caries management. The provision of immediate and complete dentures was not included in the original edition and after feedback from our readers this has been added as a new section in the chapter 'The Principles of Tooth Replacement'. All these new changes reflect the wide range of procedures and techniques that are involved in restorative dentistry.

Covering the whole subject of restorative dentistry is a difficult task, and this book does not pretend that it can be done in a single text. However, what it does aim to do is generate enthusiasm for this subject, which is at the essential core of dentistry. It is hoped that it will introduce readers to restorative dentistry and encourage them to learn more by using it as an introductory text. Therefore, whilst it will be of interest to the junior undergraduate student first entering the clinic, it also contains areas of interest to more senior students coming towards the end of their studies. Informal feedback from the first edition has also shown that the book is useful to the young clinician who wishes to obtain an overview of restorative dentistry. There are sections where the depth may extend beyond the undergraduate level but it is hoped that by doing so it provides an insight into the more varied work that can be done when specialising in this area. There are many texts available which will allow the subject areas contained within the book to be followed up, and these are listed in the further reading section at the end of the book.

Once again I am indebted to the work of my co-authors and I thank them for once again assisting me in the preparation of the material. The publishers have been immensely helpful, and this second edition would not have been possible without the constant help and encouragement of Mr Michael Parkinson and Dr Lulu Stader from Elsevier.

Finally I am grateful for the many comments and other feedback that I have received from readers of the first edition. It is my wish that the book acts as a guide to the care of restorative patients and will lead to further reading and debate around this important area of dentistry. Such feedback makes such projects worthwhile and on behalf of all the authors I wish to extend a big thank you for taking the time to read and learn from *Restorative Dentistry*.

A.D.W.
Birmingham 2007

Acknowledgements

In the age of clinical photography, both digital and conventional, the authors themselves took many of the photographs displayed in the text. However, we would like to express our gratitude to Mr M. Sharland and Miss M. Tipton of the School of Dentistry at the University of Birmingham for their assistance in the reprinting and duplication of many of the clinical photographs. There are many examples of excellent technical work contained within the book and it would be impossible to name everybody's work, but the authors would like to thank in particular Mr P. Browning, Mr S. Smith, Mr D. Spence, Mr P. Murphy and Mr W. B. Hullah. All were involved in the vast majority of the technical work seen in the text. The authors would also like to thank the Conservation Laboratory for assistance in the fixed restorations illustrated in the book.

The authors wish to thank all our colleagues at the Universities of Sheffield, Birmingham and Manchester who gave helpful advice during preparation of the text. Those colleagues who allowed us to include their clinical photographs have been acknowledged in the text.

1 Introduction to restorative dentistry

Keeping teeth is important for many functions, such as eating and speech, whilst in our present society good aesthetics are a high priority for the majority of people. A realistic outcome of dentistry must be a healthy comfortable mouth with sound intact teeth. Dental care must also be designed to prevent any future problems and to help to maintain this healthy environment. Restorative dentistry involves the care of patients who require restoration of the oral and dental tissues. This area of dentistry crosses many of the traditional departments that exist in teaching hospitals throughout the world and includes the disciplines of periodontology, operative dentistry, endodontics, and fixed and removable prosthodontics. Other specialities, such as oral surgery and orthodontics, are often involved in the planning of restorative care.

Although the restoration of the oral tissues requires technical skills, the clinician is intimately involved in the decision-making process. A patient should receive investigations that lead to a correct diagnosis. The clinician reaches the diagnosis after careful history-taking and examination of the patient. Only then can a treatment plan be drawn up which helps to achieve oral stability. The clinician should be an expert in all the disciplines that make up restorative dentistry, but should also be able to integrate them in a sensible order and not as compartmentalised procedures.

The subject areas in the book are arranged in a traditional order with periodontology at the start, and fixed and removable prosthodontics towards the end. The last chapter hopes to show, with the use of case studies, that the progress of patient care often does not follow such steps. Patients often require intervention with an immediate partial denture towards the beginning of treatment prior to the instigation of periodontal care. A patient with irreversible pulpitis requires pain relief, which involves the use of endodontic care. The fracture of a tooth needs temporising or, when occurring to the anterior teeth, a temporary crown or other restoration is required. The list of interactivity between the traditional disciplines is long and shows the diverse nature of treatment planning that will take place.

Prevention of damage to the tooth is a fundamental part of restorative care. This will range from motivating patients to clean their teeth effectively, to monitoring their diet and giving appropriate advice. An increase in the demand for more advanced treatment reflects changes in patient expectation, with a reluctance to accept tooth loss and an increasing demand for advanced restorative treatment. There is often a need for comprehensive periodontal assessment and for advice and treatment of periodontal problems, which in the past have received insufficient attention. Tooth wear is an increasing problem that causes sufferers concern, requiring careful assessment and sometimes complex reconstructive techniques to avoid future treatment and failure.

The restorative dentist is the leader of the dental team and is responsible for the management of nursing and hygiene care and laboratory support. Such a dentist must be active in the field of clinical audit, establishing indices of treatment need and measures to assess the outcome of treatment procedures. Clinical governance is defined as corporate accountability for clinical performance and is about standards of quality. The restorative dentist should take part in continuing professional development programmes and offer leadership to develop and improve the quality of restorative dentistry care.

2 The healthy mouth

The mouth is a highly specialised organ whose complex topographical anatomy reflects the diverse activities that it must perform.

LIPS AND CHEEKS

The lips are muscular structures surrounding the opening of the mouth. Externally they are covered with skin which is tightly bound down to the underlying connective tissue and muscle, and which contains sweat glands, hair follicles and sebaceous glands.

The inner surface of the lips is covered with stratified squamous epithelium, tightly attached to the underlying connective tissue and muscle. The epithelium is thin, and through it the underlying blood vessels are visible. The surface is irregular with slight prominences caused by the presence of large numbers of small mixed salivary glands.

The mucous membrane of the cheeks is also tightly bound down to the underlying connective tissue and muscle. To allow for stretching, and accommodation to the movements of the mouth and cheeks, the mucous membrane has a finely wrinkled form in the resting state. Superiorly and inferiorly, the boundaries of the inner surface of the cheek are the buccal sulci of the maxillary and mandibular alveolar processes. Posteriorly, the ptery-gomandibular raphe – a fibrous tissue band – stretches from the pterygoid process to the retromolar pad of the mandible (Fig. 2.1). Anteriorly the mucous membrane is continuous with that of the lips.

In the maxillary second molar region, the mucous membrane of the cheeks is pierced by a duct – the parotid duct – which ends as a papilla of variable size. Further down in the cheek, level with the occlusal surfaces of the teeth, there is often a slightly raised, horizontal whitish band (Fig. 2.2). This is a band of keratinisation produced by chronic trauma from the teeth. While often barely noticeable, it can be pronounced and lead to confusion with other, pathological, types of white lesion.

Posteriorly and in line with the corners of the mouth there are often a small number of ectopic sebaceous glands. These are of no significance but can be alarming when present in large numbers. At times a large area may be covered by such sebaceous glands which appear as yellowish spots – Fordyce's spots – and these can cause anxiety when noticed for the first time.

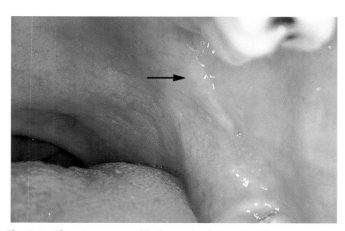

Fig. 2.1 The pterygomandibular raphe (arrow), a fibrous tissue band which stretches from the pterygoid process to the retromolar pad of the mandible.

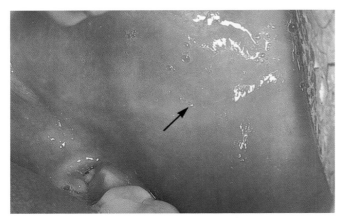

Fig. 2.2 The occlusal line (arrow), a slightly raised, horizontal whitish band of keratinisation produced by chronic trauma from the teeth.

Superiorly and inferiorly, the mucous membrane which is bound down to the underlying muscle loses its attachment and is reflected onto the bone of the alveolar processes. The zone of reflection – the sulcus – must allow for the mobility of the cheeks and the mucous membrane is attached to the underlying structures only by loose connective tissue. The sulci are horseshoe-shaped and are divided into buccal and labial sections related to the cheeks and lips, respectively. Where the sections join, their continuity is interrupted by a variable number of sickle-shaped fraenal attachments. The most consistently present of these are in the upper midline (Fig. 2.3), which is usually well developed, and the lower midline, which is less so. Smaller fraenal attachments are usually found in the upper and lower sulci in the canine/premolar region. Fraenal attachments do not contain muscle and consist only of mucous membrane separated by a little thin fibrous tissue.

The upper midline fraenal attachment may be enlarged and have a fibrous insertion into the maxilla which, if it is associated with lack of bony fusion, may be an orthodontic

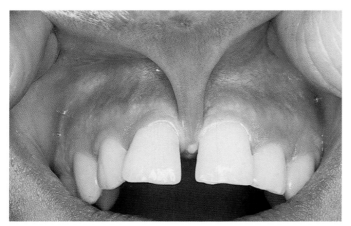

Fig. 2.3 A well developed fraenal attachment in the upper midline. This may interfere with oral hygiene.

problem. Fraena may also be a contributory factor in periodontal disease by interfering with plaque removal, and in the edentulous patient where the denture base may need to be deeply notched to provide relief over the fraenum. The fraenal attachment may then require surgical removal.

ALVEOLAR PROCESSES

The mucous membrane covering the alveolar processes is of two types. That part which is continuous with the sulcus, the alveolar mucosa, is thin and loosely attached to the underlying bone by thin connective tissue. This allows it to accommodate to the free movement of the lips and cheeks and permits the painless deposition of local anaesthetic into the underlying connective tissue. The thinness and the plentiful blood supply give it a red colour.

In health, the alveolar mucosa is separated by a scalloped line, the mucogingival junction, from a band of thicker tissue – the gingiva – which are keratinised and which surround the teeth in a band approximately 5 mm thick.

FLOOR OF THE MOUTH AND TONGUE

On the lingual side of the mandibular alveolar process, the attached mucosa surrounding the teeth changes to loosely attached alveolar mucosa which is reflected from the bone onto the ventral surface of the tongue, so forming the lingual sulcus and the floor of the mouth. The lingual sulcus is horseshoe-shaped.

From its most distal point, the lingual sulcus runs forwards as a channel bounded medially by the hyoglossus muscle and laterally by the origin of the mylohyoid muscle, widens to form the floor of the mouth and ends at the midline lingual fraenum. In the floor of the mouth runs a fold which increases in size postero/anteriorly and contains the submandibular duct. The fold runs over a slight mound in the premolar region which marks the site of the sublingual gland. The ducts of the sublingual gland mostly enter the submandibular duct as it passes over its surface. The submandibular duct, and its overlying fold of mucosa, passes further forwards until it ends close to the midline in a papilla, in the centre of which is the duct orifice. With the tongue raised, the midline fraenum is tensed and the right and left papillae can be seen as swellings on either side of the midline (Fig. 2.4). Sometimes the midline fraenum is short and tight, binding down the tip of the tongue and giving rise to a 'tongue tie'. The condition does not often give rise to functional difficulties, although at one time surgical removal was a common recommendation. Occasionally it makes cleaning the lingual surfaces of the mandibular anterior teeth difficult, causing periodontal problems, and in these cases its removal may be indicated.

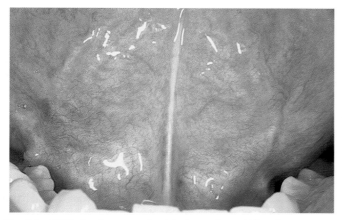

Fig. 2.4 With the tongue raised to tense the midline fraenum, the right and left papillae can be seen as swellings on either side of the midline.

The undersurface of the tongue is marked by several fimbriae or folds and is covered by squamous epithelium. Beneath the thin mucosa, tortuous, bluish veins are often visible. The marked tortuosity allows for accommodation to the movements of the tongue.

The dorsal surface of the tongue is divided into two zones. The anterior two-thirds is separated from the posterior third by a V-shaped groove – the terminal sulcus – the apex pointing backwards. Several types of papillae are visible. Immediately anterior to the terminal sulcus is a line of large, mushroom-shaped circumvallate papillae, the larger nearer the midline. Each is surrounded by a trough containing taste buds. Much of the remainder of the anterior dorsal surface is covered with filiform and fungiform papillae. The filiform are the more numerous (Fig. 2.5), each being hair-like, keratinised and surrounding the shorter, mushroom-like fungiform papillae. The fungiform papillae have a thinner coating of epithelium and are correspondingly more red in colour. They contain variable numbers of taste buds. On the lateral border of

the tongue, posteriorly, can be found a few foliate papillae containing numerous taste buds.

A marked central fissure is often characteristic of the anterior two-thirds of the dorsum of the tongue. The posterior third of the tongue is pale pink and faces back into the pharynx. It is covered with lingual follicles, which are low prominences containing lymphoid tissue and surrounded by shallow furrows. The sum total of the lymphoid tissue in the posterior third of the tongue is called the lingual tonsil.

HARD PALATE, SOFT PALATE AND PHARYNX

The hard palate forms the roof of the mouth and, having an accessory part to play in mastication, is covered with keratinised epithelium. Peripherally it is covered with mucoperiosteum continuous with the attached gingiva, and attached firmly to the underlying bone. More centrally, in the angle between the palatine and alveolar processes of the maxilla, it is separated from the bone by intervening connective tissue containing blood vessels and nerves. The presence of connective tissue between the epithelium and bone allows anaesthetic to be infiltrated without causing pain. Further centrally and in the midline, the epithelium is again tightly bound down to the underlying bone, which is sometimes raised in the midline as a midline palatal torus of variable size.

In the midline, behind the central incisor teeth lies the incisive papilla, an oval prominence covering the incisal fossa and marking the entry into the mouth of the naso-palatine nerves. The incisive papilla serves as a useful landmark when attempting to anaesthetise the nerve supply to the soft tissues lingual to the maxillary central incisor teeth. Just distal to the incisive papilla there are a variable number of roughly parallel irregular raised folds of muco-periosteum, the palatal rugae (Fig. 2.6). Even further posteriorly, marking the junction of hard and soft palate,

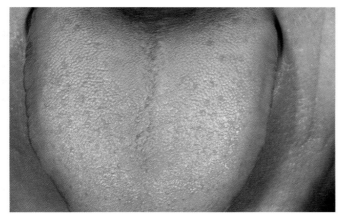

Fig. 2.5 The dorsal surface of the tongue showing filiform and fungiform papillae; the filiform are the more numerous.

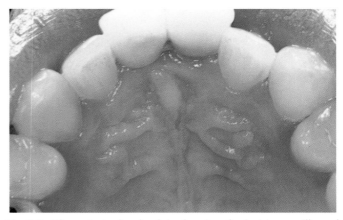

Fig. 2.6 The anterior hard palate showing the incisive papilla and rugae.

lie two small indentations, one on either side of the midline. These are the foveae palatini, where the ducts of two small clusters of salivary glands open into the mouth.

The soft palate is covered with stratified squamous epithelium and divides the oropharynx from the nasopharynx. It terminates distally in a short muscular projection, the uvula, and by its contact with the posterior wall of the pharynx regulates the flow of air through the mouth and nose when breathing and speaking. At this point on the posterior wall of the pharynx, a functional thickening of the superior constrictor muscle, called the ridge of Passavant, aids production of an airtight seal.

Laterally the side of the pharynx is marked by two arches. The anterior is produced by the presence of the palatoglossus muscle. It is separated by the pharyngeal tonsil from the distal arch, which is formed by the palatopharyngeus muscle (Fig. 2.7). The pharyngeal tonsil is a collection of lymph tissue and in young patients is frequently red and swollen in response to infection. In later life, it atrophies and even shows calcification, which can be a source of diagnostic confusion on panoramic radiographs. The pharyngeal tonsil is part of a ring of lymphoid tissue, the other parts of which are the lingual tonsil, found on the posterior third of the tongue, and the adenoids, a collection of lymph tissue found in the midline of the posterior wall of the nasopharynx.

THE TEETH

A tooth may be divided into crown and root, the crown being covered by enamel and the root by cementum. The two surfaces meet at the cement–enamel junction which is visible as the cervical line on the neck of the tooth. In the healthy mouth of a young adult, the level of gingival attachment will be coronal to the cervical line. The anatomical crown ends at the cervical line, in contrast to the clinical crown which is the amount of tooth protruding

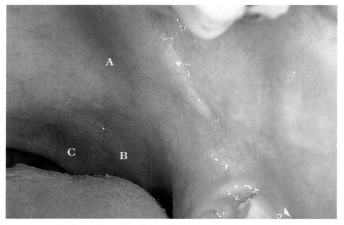

Fig. 2.7 The lateral wall of the pharynx: A, palatoglossal arch; B, pharyngeal tonsil; C, palatopharyngeal arch.

beyond the gingival margin into the patient's mouth. Variations in clinical crown length are often produced by different levels of gingival attachment to the tooth and are seen in patients suffering from gingival recession and hence showing increased clinical crown length. Short clinical crowns are seen in teeth that have worn excessively, commonly due to bruxism, or where teeth have been worn down by attrition.

Incisors and canines have four axial surfaces converging in an incisal edge. Premolars and molars have five surfaces, the incisal edge being replaced by an occlusal surface. The surface of the crown shows many elevations and depressions which make up the typical appearance of the tooth. The following terms are used in the description of crown anatomy:

Cusp: an elevation or mound on the occlusal surface.

Cingulum: the lingual convex bulge on an anterior tooth.

Tubercle: a small elevation on some part of the crown produced by an extra formation of enamel and dentine. These are quite frequently seen buccally on deciduous first molars (the tubercle of Zuckerkandl) and lingually on upper first molars (the cusp of Carabelli).

Ridge: a linear elevation on the surface of a tooth. A good example is the marginal ridge found on the mesial and distal surfaces of molars and premolars.

Fissure: an irregular linear depression in the tooth surface. A pit is a small pinpoint depression.

Developmental groove: a developmental deformity in the crown and/or root of a tooth. This type of defect will encourage the formation of a periodontal pocket, particularly when it involves the root, because dental plaque will collect there undisturbed. Grooves are sometimes seen on permanent upper lateral incisors, especially on palatal surfaces.

Mamelon: any one of the three rounded protuberances found on the incisal edges of recently erupted anterior teeth. Mamelons wear away quickly, usually within two years of eruption.

Facet: a small, smooth, flat surface seen on the occlusal aspect of the crown indicating an abnormal pattern of wear on the enamel.

Perikymata: seen commonly on recently erupted incisors as a series of horizontal ridges running parallel to the incisal edge and quite often affecting the whole of the labial surface of the crown.

The primary dentition

The eruption of the primary teeth begins at about 6 months of age with the mandibular incisors. All primary teeth have usually erupted by the age of 2 years, although there is considerable individual variation, with some children not exhibiting their first teeth until they are over 1 year old. There do not appear to be any ethnic differences in the dates of eruption, but severe malnutrition may cause delayed eruption as well as seriously affecting other aspects of the child's growth.

The usual order of appearance of the primary teeth in the mouth is:

1. central incisors
2. lateral incisors
3. first molars
4. canines
5. second molars.

Mandibular teeth usually erupt before maxillary teeth. As the child approaches the age of 5 years, spacing will appear between the primary teeth as a result of the jaw growth required to accommodate the developing permanent teeth.

Permanent dentition

Eruption of the mandibular permanent teeth tends to occur slightly ahead of the maxillary, by a few months. Some studies have shown boys to have delayed eruption compared with girls. Interestingly, black children in the USA show slightly earlier eruption dates compared with Caucasians. This has also been shown to be true when African Blacks are compared with European Caucasian subjects. Only the permanent molars erupt without displacing a primary predecessor, and the first permanent molar appears at the age of 6 years.

PULP DENTINE COMPLEX

The pulp dentine complex consists of pulp tissue, odontoblasts and dentine. The dental pulp is a soft tissue containing nerves, blood vessels, cells and ground substance. The young pulp has numerous cells and few fibres, whereas the older pulp has relatively few cells and more fibrous tissue. The dental pulp is contained within a rigid chamber of dentine, which limits its ability to expand during episodes of vasodilation such as an inflammatory response to noxious stimuli. The response produces a rise in intrapulpal pressure and it has been suggested that this rise in pressure may result in compression of blood vessels and reduction in blood supply. The amount of damage is dependent upon the severity and length of insult, with local feedback mechanisms limiting damage by increasing the rate of fluid removal. Thus pulpal damage may be localised in a specific area of the tooth rather than throughout.

The main function of the dental pulp is to produce dentine (Box 2.1), the major structural part of the tooth; however, it also has a sensory role.

Dentine is produced by odontoblasts, columnar-shaped cells which differentiate during the bell stage of tooth

---

Box 2.1   Dentine

- Dentine is permeable
- This permeable structure allows noxious stimuli to reach the pulp
- Noxious stimuli may result in the production of sclerotic dentine, which limits diffusion

---

development. Odontoblasts have a process around which dentine tubules are formed. These tubules make up approximately 20–30% of the total volume of human dentine, which, as a result, is permeable and can allow noxious stimuli through to the pulp. Thus odontoblasts link dentine and pulp and are the first cells to encounter irritation. Partial or complete occlusion of dentine tubules may occur with age or in response to noxious stimuli. When tubules become filled with mineral deposits the dentine is termed sclerotic and limits diffusion of noxious stimuli; the decreased permeability of dentine protects the pulp from irritation.

Radiographs give some idea of basic root canal anatomy although the reality is far more complex. The variations in internal root canal anatomy are infinite. Single roots may contain more than one canal, which may remain separate or join along their length. Studies of cleared extracted teeth have shown that all roots enclose a minimum of one root canal system, which frequently consists of a network of branches. The apical anatomy is usually described as there being a narrowing (constriction) and a wider foramen on the side of the root (Fig. 2.8). This classical anatomical arrangement, however, does not always exist, especially in cases where there is apical pathology or frank evidence of root resorption. In such situations the apical constriction may be absent.

Communications with the periodontal ligament exist either in the furcation (furcal canals) or laterally (lateral canals). In addition, the root canal may frequently terminate as more than one opening (as opposed to the single exit described above) with an array of accessory canals forming an apical delta. These furcal, lateral and apical communications have been termed 'portals of exit' from the root canal system. Furcal, lateral and accessory canals

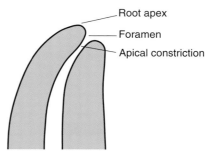

Fig. 2.8   The apical anatomy as classically described.

are created during tooth formation either when there is a break in the sheath of Hertwig or when the sheath grows around an existing blood vessel. On occasions, such canals can be as large as the apical foramen. Their significance is not fully understood, but it would seem sensible to use a preparation technique that aims to clean as much of the root canal system as possible.

The pulp chamber and root canal orifices may be reduced in size as a result of deposition of secondary and tertiary dentine. If the irritation is severe, with extensive destruction of pulpal cells, then further inflammatory changes involving the rest of the pulp will take place and could lead to pulp necrosis. Such pulpal degeneration starts coronally and progresses apically. Necrotic pulpal break-down products may leach out of the root canal system to form lesions of endodontic origin around the portals of exit. Frequently these changes in the periodontium will be visible lateral to the root before they are apparent apically. It is therefore extremely important to examine roots periradicularly as opposed to periapically, as such examination may provide an early indication of pulp degeneration (Fig. 2.9).

Some general considerations on pulpal anatomy are given in Box 2.2.

Sensory nerves of the pulp arise from the trigeminal and enter via foramina in close association with blood vessels. They pass upwards through the radicular pulp and fan out to form the plexus of Raschow. The two types of sensory nerve fibres principally found in the pulp are A (myelinated) and C (unmyelinated). Ninety per cent of the A fibres are A-delta, located in the region of the pulp dentine junction. They have a relatively low threshold and produce sharp responses. C fibres are distributed through-out the pulp, have a high threshold and are usually asso-ciated with tissue injury; the response is more severe than that of A-delta fibres. Nerve fibres of the pulp are relatively

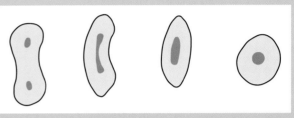

Box 2.2 General considerations on pulpal anatomy

- The shape of the coronal pulp and the outline of the canals are a reflection of the outline of the crown and root surfaces (Fig. 2.10)
- Root canal anatomy is frequently more complex than radiographs suggest
- Pulp morphology is altered by age, irritants, attrition, caries, abrasion and periodontal disease
- Most roots are curved; however, many curvatures are towards or away from the two-dimensional radiographic film

Fig. 2.10 Cross-sections of root canal anatomy showing the relationship between pulpal and radicular shape.

resistant to necrosis and C fibres may still be able to respond to stimulation in the degenerating pulp.

Dentine sensitivity is thought to be due to the move-ment of fluid in the tubules and is referred to as the hydro-dynamic theory of sensitivity. This movement is thought to be translated by sensory receptors into a pain stimulus, usually of short duration, which is responded to principally by A fibres.

Painful pulpitis is more associated with C fibre stimu-lation and results in a dull aching and poorly localised response.

PERIODONTAL TISSUES

The periodontal tissues consist of the *gingiva*, covering the alveolar processes, and the *periodontal ligament*, with dense bundles of fibres which run from the *cementum* lining the root surface to the *alveolar bone* to which the fibres are attached (Fig. 2.11).

Gingiva

The gingiva line the external surface of the periodontium (Fig. 2.12, Box 2.3). The gingival tissue runs from the mucogingival line, which marks the boundary with the non-keratinised buccal mucosa, and covers the coronal aspect of the alveolar process. On the palatal aspect, the mucogingival line is absent as the gingiva here is con-tinuous with the keratinised, non-mobile palatal mucosa.

The gingiva ends at the cervix of each tooth, surrounds it and attaches to it by a ring of specialised epithelial tissue

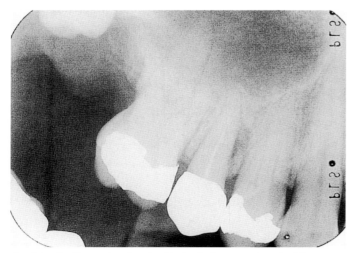

Fig. 2.9 Radiograph of periradicular lesion associated with a lateral canal.

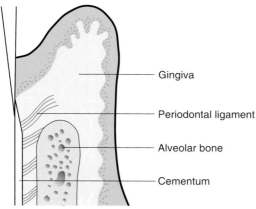

Fig. 2.11 The periodontal tissues.

– the junctional epithelium. This epithelial attachment provides continuity of the epithelial lining of the oral cavity with the surface of the teeth.

Healthy gingiva is described as '*salmon*' or '*coral pink*'. It may be pigmented, which reflects the ethnic origin of the subject. The gingiva is firm in consistency and firmly attached to the underlying alveolar bone. The surface of gingiva is keratinised and may exhibit an orange peel appearance, called 'stippling'. The width of attached gingiva can vary dramatically between patients and within an individual's mouth, from as little as 1 mm to over 10 mm.

Figure 2.12 shows healthy gingiva. The free gingival margin covers the cemento-enamel junction (CEJ) and the gingival papillae fill the embrasures. A shallow linear depression, the gingival groove, can be observed in some areas, distinguishing the free gingival margin from the attached gingiva. Microscopically, gingiva consists of stratified squamous epithelium supported by a thin layer of dense fibrous connective tissue (Box 2.4). The gingival epithelium may be divided into the oral epithelium cover-

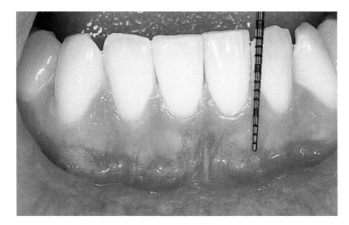

Fig. 2.12 Labial view of lower incisor teeth showing features of the gingiva: adjacent to the teeth is the free gingiva, and below this the attached gingiva which merges into the lining mucosa at the mucogingival junction.

Box 2.3   The gingiva

The gingiva may be divided into the following areas:
- *free marginal gingiva*, about 1.5 mm wide in health
- *the attached gingiva*, of variable width
- *the interdental gingiva*, occupying the embrasure space between adjacent teeth
- *the gingival crevice or sulcus* leading from the marginal gingiva to the junctional epithelium

ing the external surface of the gingiva, the crevicular epithelium lining the gingival crevice, and the non-keratinised junctional epithelium (Fig. 2.13). The crevicular epithelium resembles the oral gingiva coronally and the junctional epithelium apically. The degree of keratinisation varies, therefore, according to relationship to the tooth. Underneath the gingiva is the dense gingival connective tissue.

Junctional epithelium

The junctional epithelium (JE) adjacent to the tooth is that part of the gingiva which attaches the connective tissue to the tooth surface (Fig. 2.14). It forms a band 2–3 mm

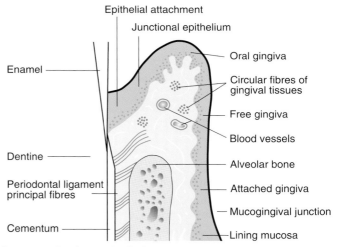

Fig. 2.13 The dento-gingival area.

Box 2.4   Fibres of the free gingiva

The collagen fibres of the free gingiva are arranged in three main groups:
- circular fibres – these form a collar around the neck of the tooth holding the free gingiva tightly against it
- gingival fibres – these originate from the cementum of the cervical part of the root and fan outwards into the free gingiva
- transeptal fibres – these run from the cervical cementum on the distal side of one root to the cementum on the mesial aspect of the next tooth

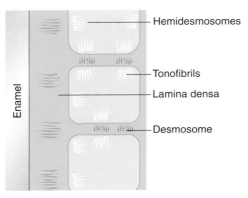

Fig. 2.14 The junctional epithelium and its relationship to the tooth surface.

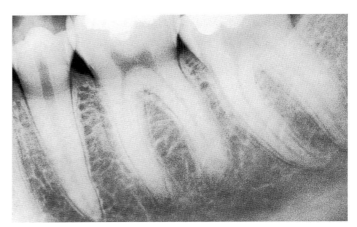

Fig. 2.15 A radiograph of teeth with surrounding periodontally healthy tissues.

wide around the tooth, and is approximately 15–30 cells thick coronally and tapers to a single cell apically. This attachment is continuously being renewed throughout life. JE turnover rate is high (4–6 days) compared with oral epithelium (6–12 days). The cells are non-keratinised and have wide intercellular spaces. The JE attaches to enamel (in a patient without recession) by a basal lamina and intercellular hemidesmosomes.

The JE has a key role in the maintenance of periodontal health: it creates the firm attachment of the soft gingival tissue to hard tooth tissue. However, as it is permeable, it serves as a pathway for diffusion of the metabolic products of plaque bacteria such as toxins, chemotactic agents and antigens.

Even when the gingiva do not appear inflamed clinically, the JE has many polymorphonuclear leucocytes (PMNs) moving through it towards the sulcus. These form an important part of the defence mechanism.

Periodontal ligament

The periodontal ligament is the connective tissue attachment between the root and the alveolar bone. It consists of collagen fibrils arranged in dense fibre groups and their supporting cells, blood vessels, nerves and ground substance. The fibres are almost entirely collagenous and are of two main types:

- *Interstitial fibres* – these are randomly arranged throughout the periodontal ligament, supporting the blood vessels and nerves
- *Principal fibres* – these are much more dense than interstitial fibres and are the fibre bundles which run from cementum to bone, holding the tooth firmly in its socket.

These fibre groups, known as Sharpey's fibres, are inserted into the alveolar bone at one end and run across into the cementum lining the root. The fibres are named according to the direction in which they run: crestal, horizontal, oblique, interradicular and apical. Figure 2.15 is a radiograph of periodontally healthy teeth. There is no

reduction seen in the height of the alveolar bone and the crest of this is located about 1 mm apical to the CEJ. The lamina dura is seen as a white line around the teeth, indicating that the rate of bone turnover is low.

Cementum

The thin layer of cementum which covers the whole surface of the root is an important tissue for the maintenance of periodontal health as it attaches the fibres of the periodontal ligament to the tooth. Two types of cementum are recognised: cellular cementum, which contains cells called cementocytes, and acellular, which does not. The first formed cementum is usually of the acellular type and that formed later is cellular. Therefore, acellular cementum is found covering the cervical two-thirds of the root, and cellular cementum tends to cover the apical third and normally overlaps the acellular type.

Cementum is softer than dentine and is similar in many ways to bone. Just over 55% is a thin organic matrix of collagen fibres lying parallel to the root surface and mucopolysaccharide ground substance. As well as the thin fibres of the matrix, there are larger Sharpey's fibres, which are the embedded portions of periodontal fibres. Cementum is not a static tissue, but alters in response to the functional requirements of the tooth. Throughout life there is a threefold increase in thickness of cementum as more is deposited on the root surface by the cementoblasts (Box 2.5).

Alveolar bone

Like all bones, the alveolar bone consists of outer and inner cortical plates, between which lies the cancellous bone. Between the two cortical plates are the tooth sockets which are lined by a thin plate of bone, termed the *lamina dura*. This is visible on dental radiographs (Fig. 2.15) and is often of diagnostic importance. Into the alveolar lamina dura are inserted the ends of the periodontal fibres which,

---

Box 2.5 Important changes facilitated by the continual deposition of cementum

- Newly formed periodontal fibres can be embedded in the cementum, replacing those which have aged
- Alteration of the inserted fibres allows the tooth to move bodily through the alveolar bone. This occurs during eruption, growth and orthodontic treatment
- The deposition of more cementum at the apex of the root helps to compensate for wear of the occlusal surface or incisal edge during the functional life of the tooth

---

like those inserted into the cementum, are called Sharpey's fibres. The lamina dura is also pierced by large numbers of bony canals called Volkmann's canals and, for this reason, it is often referred to as the cribriform plate.

The rim of the tooth socket is termed the alveolar crest and it may be seen from a dried specimen of the maxilla or mandible that the alveolar crest is scalloped in outline, matching the gingival contour. The thickness of the labial and lingual alveolar cortical plates varies considerably from one area to another and from person to person and this has a significance when inflammatory periodontal disease affects the tissues. It tends to be thin on the labial aspect of the anterior teeth and may even be completely missing in places, which is termed a dehiscence. Dehiscences are of some importance with regard to the progress of periodontal disease and they may be a leading factor in the occurrence of localised severe gingival recession.

The bone of the alveolar process is not static but is being continually remodelled by osteoblasts and osteoclasts. Osteoblasts deposit bone and osteoclasts resorb it. Both these cells are present in the tooth socket and it is by their action that teeth can move bodily through the bone, either during growth or during orthodontic treatment. The bone of the socket on the side towards which the tooth is moving is resorbed by osteoclasts, while more bone is deposited on the opposite side by osteoblasts.

3 Examination of the patient and treatment planning

OVERVIEW

A patient attending for treatment of a restorative nature may present for a variety of reasons. Many patients will be returning for their regular half yearly or annual recall. Others will be attending with a problem, which may be related to their gums, the hard tissues of the teeth or to the restorative work that has been undertaken on previous visits. As the clinician you possess the skills to intervene and rectify problems and to undertake requests for dental treatment. Patients may present with a problem or a clinical situation which is not immediately apparent to them but which requires intervention. It cannot be overstressed that the outcome of this first visit is vital to the success of any subsequent treatment undertaken.

This success is built upon *careful history-taking* coupled with a logical progression to *diagnosis of the problem* that has been presented to you. Each stage follows on from the preceding one. A description of the *patient's complaint* should be carefully recorded in the notes. This written record is based on accurate questioning which is carefully structured but which does not necessarily lead the patient. *A medical history* is taken at this stage in order to ascertain whether the patient has any conditions of relevance to the dental treatment. Certain medical conditions may affect the management of the patient and these should be identified when the treatment plan is being drawn up. Once this is completed, *the clinical examination*, which includes both the *extraoral* and *intraoral* examinations, can be started. The extraoral examination includes observation and investigation of the patient and structures around the mouth. The intraoral examination includes the *soft and hard tissues* and a *restorative assessment*.

This chapter aims to help the reader undertake a good history and examination with guidance to the *formulation of a treatment plan*. The plan should involve a holistic approach to what is required. It is important that the patient's mouth is not seen merely as a long list of items each of which requires completion before the next one can be started. Furthermore, the patient should not be classed as a 'perio' or 'cons' patient. All dental disciplines, from prosthetics to oral surgery, may need to be considered and integrated into the patient's subsequent care.

PHASE 1: HISTORY AND EXAMINATION

Greeting patients in a friendly manner during the initial introductions goes a long way to establishing personal contact and allows them to familiarise themselves with both yourself and the surroundings. When seating patients in the chair, the ideal arrangement for conducting the history is to be facing them while maintaining eye contact. A simple, but effective and necessary, method to initiate the proceedings is to confirm that the patient's details are correct. Talking about the weather, travel, holidays, news topics, sports and the like will quickly initiate a two-way discussion and often relaxes the patient. A few minutes spent in this way can often gain a patient's confidence and establish a rapport that will bring rewards in the latter treatment stages.

Reason for attendance

Patients should be asked why they made this appointment, and their response should be recorded as a simple statement, including why they have come to you, from whom and from where.

Complains of

At this stage, patients are simply asked if they have any problems with their mouth. This is important in order to establish the nature of the problem, and a few simple sentences paraphrasing the patient's own description of it should be recorded in the notes. The final treatment plan must consider how to solve this problem or the patient may well not be happy with the outcome of this initial consultation.

History of present complaint

This often proves to be the most important aspect of the history-taking and, with experience, can be developed into a sensitive clinical tool. Encourage the patient to articulate worries or complaints and record these findings in your notes. The skill at this stage is to use carefully structured questions which help to establish the problem. Often, listening to the approaches of other clinicians will help you to identify both good and bad techniques of history-taking. Patients will have different complaints. The most obvious complaint will be of a *'painful tooth or gum'*. However, complaints may also be related to *loose restorations* such as bridges or dentures; there may even be uncemented or missing crowns. Another important complaint that is often high on the patient's agenda concerns the *aesthetics* of the teeth and restorations. There may be dissatisfaction with previous treatment. Any complaints about previous dental treatment should be entered into the notes, but you should not take sides in any dispute. The aim is to listen and to learn about the patient's concerns and problems.

When patients present with pain in or around the mouth, clinicians must use their skill to discover the cause of the discomfort. *Pain histories* are obtained (Table 3.1). These will include the *location* and the type of pain. Its character may be described as sharp or dull. In addition, the *intensity* can be estimated with the aid of simple questions; for example, does it interfere with sleep or eating? Asking the patient when the pain began will reveal the *onset*. A chronic pain will have been present for many weeks, whilst an acute episode will require rapid action to ensure relief. The *duration* is recorded as the time that the pain is present. Questions related to the *previous history* may reveal that this pain has occurred before, and an indication of how it was treated may offer a possible explanation for the recent episode. The pain may have only occurred once or it may come on many times during the day and this will indicate its *frequency*. There may be *initiating factors* such as thermal stimuli or discomfort on biting on the tooth. There may be certain *relieving factors* such as pressure on the tooth.

All these factors will build up a picture of the pain and will assist during the examination of the patient (Table 3.1). They will allow you to begin to formulate the different possibilities of what might be producing the pain. Pain should not immediately be seen as necessarily tooth-related. The pain history may be related to the periodontal tissues, partially erupted teeth or removable prostheses. It is a common mistake to look for a pulpal cause immediately and to dismiss other common causes such as painful gums or problems with wisdom teeth.

A history may not only be of specific pain but may also relate to a problem that has occurred over a lengthy time period. For instance, a presenting periodontal problem may have started several years ago with bleeding of the gums followed by localised abscesses.

Another problem that may arise is looseness of a bridge or denture. The questions will then include how and when the restoration became loose. The patient is asked when bridges were placed and how many have been constructed

Table 3.1 Questions to help build a pain history

Aspect of pain	Questions to ask
Location of pain	Where is the pain? Is it localised or does it radiate?
Intensity	How severe is the pain? Does it keep you awake at night?
Onset	When did the pain start and how long has it been present?
Duration	Does it last a few seconds or a couple of hours?
Previous history	Has this pain occurred before?
Frequency	How often do you get the pain?
Initiating factors	Is the pain spontaneous or does it require a stimulus? Is it affected by hot or cold, sweet things, biting or postural position?
Relieving factors	What relieves the pain? Is it helped by analgesics, biting or the application of cold?

previously. Problems related to denture-wearing may include a history of previous denture-wearing. This should include the age of the denture, how many have been constructed in the past and how successful these previous dentures were. Any alteration of shade or appearance of the teeth that has been noted by the patient is recorded. Wear of the teeth may only have been noticed at a recent examination and brought to the patient's attention by his or her own dentist. Patients will first become aware of loss of tooth substance when their teeth are starting to become smaller in length. Tooth wear may be associated with sensitivity of the teeth and this symptom may highlight an erosive diet or the possibility of parafunction during sleep.

It is impossible to cover all the different histories that may arise. No history is the same and, often, histories taken of the same patient by different dentists are different.

Listen to and observe other clinicians and always be prepared for the unexpected. History-taking is an art form and it has only been possible to provide the basic building bricks in this account, but the clinician should always be prepared to learn and be aware of the patient's presenting symptoms.

Medical history

This is an essential part of any examination and will have an important bearing on all aspects of the diagnosis and subsequent treatment planning. *Any relevant medical history is required, for the protection of a patient, other patients and the dental team.* A simple way to avoid missing any relevant aspects of a patient's history is to use a medical history sheet, an example of which is given in Box 3.1.

Box 3.1 Example of a medical history questionnaire. The form is designed as an aide-memoire and it is essential that relevant details of positive medical history information are sought and recorded.

FOR COMPLETION BY THE CLINICIAN			
Are you:	**Yes**	**No**	**Details**
1. Receiving medical or hospital treatment at present?			
2. Taking any tablets, medicines or any other substance, e.g. inhalers?			Please list on separate page
3. Allergic to any tablets, medicines or any other substance, e.g. penicillin/latex (rubber)?			
4. Pregnant (if appropriate)?			
Have you:			
5. Ever had a heart murmur, rheumatic fever (e.g. chorea, St Vitus' dance) or any other problem with your heart?			
6. Ever had raised blood pressure, angina, a heart attack or thrombosis, e.g. CVA, DVT?			
7. Ever had hepatitis, jaundice or been diagnosed with HIV disease?			
8. Ever had any chest problems, e.g. asthma/bronchitis or tuberculosis?			
9. Ever had an operation or illness treated in hospital?			
10. Been diagnosed with epilepsy?			
11. Been diagnosed with diabetes?			
12. A family member or close relative with Creutzfeldt–Jakob disease (CJD)?			
13. Ever had prolonged bleeding following a tooth extraction or other surgery?			
14. Ever had a problem with local or general anaesthetic			
15. Any other problems that may be relevant?			

Date   Signature ....
Medical history form updated and checked
Date   Signature ....
Date   Signature ....
Date   Signature ....

The first questions ask patients whether they are receiving medical treatment, and this includes medicines, tablets or injections. It is often useful to ask patients to bring any medication they are taking along to the next visit, so that the precise drugs and dosages can be identified. Some aspects highlighted in the form may need to be clarified by contacting the patient's doctor. Many patients are taking a concoction of drugs and an up-to-date version of the *British National Formulary* (BNF) will help to identify their use and, more importantly, any known interactions. This is important for dental procedures, which often involve the use of drugs, ranging from local anaesthetics to sedatives. Penicillin and related drugs are commonly given prophylactically or to treat infections, and allergies to them should be recorded to avoid the occurrence of any anaphylactic reactions. Furthermore, the increased use of latex gloves and rubber dam for operative and endodontic procedures has led to an increased incidence of contact dermatitis. Such potential allergic reactions to rubber should be noted. Females of child-bearing age are asked if they are pregnant.

The next set of questions cover the cardiac and respiratory systems together with other important conditions of immediate relevance to dentistry. Patients who have had the following conditions may require some form of antibiotic cover: rheumatic fever, chorea, heart defect, heart murmur or heart valve replacement. Up-to-date antibiotic regimes are covered in the BNF. The need for antibiotic cover may well influence the subsequent treatment planning. For instance, lengthy treatment plans over many visits may not be feasible and simplification may well be required. Patients who have suffered angina or heart attacks must be closely monitored and their appropriate medication should be on hand if problems arise. Patients with raised blood pressure may be on medication that will interact with local anaesthetics and other drugs. The risk of cross-infection is high in patients suffering from hepatitis or those with a history of jaundice. Simple questioning will reveal whether it was hepatitis A or the more infectious B, C etc. conditions. Details of other infectious diseases such as HIV are checked at this stage.

Patients may also reveal relevant medical details when asked about operations and other illnesses they may have had. Chest conditions may limit the tolerance of a patient to certain procedures of long duration, and consideration should be given to this in the treatment plan. Asthma is a condition that is rising in prevalence. Patients may be taking corticosteroids with inhalers and these should be present in case patients become distressed and suffer an asthma attack during treatment. Tuberculosis (TB) is an infectious disease that is increasing in prevalence. Patients identified as suffering from TB will often require special cross-infection control procedures, and contact must be made with their doctor. Epileptics are identified and the clinician should be prepared for an attack. Advanced restorative procedures such as bridges and removable partial dentures may need careful planning with such

patients. Diabetics will range from those whose diabetes is diet- or tablet-controlled to those who are insulin-dependent. Dental procedures may be influenced according to when they last ate. Their diabetes may also have direct relevance to their periodontal status (see p. 29).

Transmissible spongiform encephalopathies are rare, fatal degenerative brain diseases which may affect humans. Any patient with such a disease (e.g. Creutzfeldt–Jakob disease) would require the clinician to undertake the highest standard of cross-infection control with the use of disposable instrumentation. Likewise, serious problems with bleeding must be recognised and will necessitate contact with the patient's medical practitioner. Patients are also asked whether they have had problems with local or general anaesthesia and any positive responses are recorded.

The final question of the medical history is to enquire whether there is any other health matter or other problems that are of relevance and that have not been mentioned earlier. Any relevant history may be discussed with the patient's GP, either by letter or by telephone, who will always be happy to help and give advice.

A patient's medical history is not static and it is prudent to ensure that changes are regularly checked and updated and that this is clearly recorded as a dated entry in the patient's clinical notes. It is useful to have an agreed marker on the patient's notes (such as a red sticker) that immediately flags up, at a glance, an important aspect of the medical history to other clinicians who may be involved with the patient's treatment. A list of those conditions which justify such a marker is given in Box 3.2.

A well-structured medical history, completed, signed and dated and subsequently updated on a regular basis, is a key part of the essential duty of care owed by a dentist to his or her patient.

Dental history

Careful questioning at this stage can quickly reveal the patient's approach to dentistry. Such questioning includes the frequency of visits to the dentist and details of the last sequence of treatment. This may often reveal differing attitudes to dentistry that will assist in later planning. Any difficulties patients have previously experienced with dental treatment may well influence your treatment plan. Also at this stage, a patient presenting with complex dental problems may express a reluctance to undertake a series of lengthy visits.

Personal/social history

The clinician can gain an insight into the patient's dietary habits and approach to oral hygiene measures by careful questioning. The frequency, amount and diversity of sugar intake are recorded. Any erosive eating or drinking preferences need to be identified and noted for further discussion. This requires some sensible questioning as

---

Box 3.2 Conditions that justify a hazard sticker attached to the front of the hospital record

- Cardiac surgery
- Pacemaker
- Cardiac murmur (other than functional)
- Organ transplant
- Rheumatic fever
- Infective endocarditis
- Hypertension
- Warfarin therapy
- Bleeding disorder
- Drug allergies

- Systemic steroid therapy
- Intravenous drug user
- Hepatitis B/C
- HIV/AIDS
- Chronic renal failure
- Severe asthma
- Active tuberculosis
- Epilepsy
- Diabetes
- History of head and neck radiotherapy

---

patients may not attach importance to such details in their diet, but they may be highly relevant to their dental condition. For instance, many patients link fruit consumption with health and are therefore unlikely to associate this with their dental problems. An initial idea of a patient's oral hygiene can be obtained from the frequency of toothbrushing and the use of interdental aids such as dental floss or brushes. If the patient wears dentures, the prosthetic hygiene regime should be recorded.

Smoking and alcohol intake should be enquired about and, where necessary, as a health professional, it is your duty to advise on such matters. Smoking habits will have a direct influence on periodontal treatment; for example, wound healing is delayed following surgery in smokers. This may well, once again, dictate the level of dental care that is given to the patient.

Enquiry into a patient's personal/social history is often covered in a superficial manner, but with careful questioning, a patient's attitude towards and motivation in respect of dentistry will be revealed and these may provide clues to the presenting problem that may not have been immediately apparent in the earlier history-taking. Furthermore, the subsequent treatment process may be influenced by the patient's ability to cope with the treatment. This could affect your decision on whether to embark on a short simple course of visits or a complicated treatment plan of an advanced nature.

PHASE 2: EXAMINATION

During the examination process, only what is seen is recorded and any formal diagnosis should be left until the end. It is easy to become diverted and go immediately to the patient's problem. The whole mouth should be examined in a systematic manner before the main area of complaint is considered.

Extraoral

A general impression of the overall appearance of the patient is a useful indicator and any abnormalities should be recorded. An assessment is made on the vertical dimension as to whether it is normal or if there is overclosure. Gross skeletal discrepancies in the relationship of the mandible to the maxilla are recorded during the examination. Other problems such as swellings or generalised asymmetry to the overall face are noted. Muscular hypertrophy may be evident and is a useful empirical indicator of parafunctional activity. The muscles of mastication should be palpated to check for any tenderness. Assessment of the temporomandibular joints is made by palpation, looking for the presence of clicks and observing any unnatural movements on opening and closing of the jaw. Deviation may relate to a number of conditions or may be a normal observation. The submandibular lymph nodes are palpated. Good access to the lymph nodes is obtained by asking the patient to bring the head forwards and drop the chin. The lymph nodes can then be located by dragging them over the lower border of the mandible and feeling their subsequent recoil to the soft tissue. Any palpable nodes may be indicative of a recent infection.

Intraoral

Soft tissues

A thorough inspection should be made of the surfaces of the tongue, palate, floor of mouth, buccal and lingual mucosa (including the lips), looking for any abnormalities such as ulcers, erosive areas and colour changes of the mucosa. The cheeks and tongue may show markings and indentations which may be an indication of tongue or cheek biting. This will be the result of some form of parafunctional activity of the teeth.

Periodontal assessment

An examination of the periodontal tissues should be made. The aim is to provide a basic screening of the tissues and to obtain an indication of the treatment requirements of the patient.

Basic periodontal examination (BPE). This is performed clinically using the CPITN (community 17 periodontal index of treatment needs) periodontal probe. It is a simple and effective method which provides a rapid overview of the periodontal status (Fig. 3.1). The mouth is divided into six sextants and the worst score in each sextant is recorded (Table 3.2).

Plaque assessment. Further to the BPE it is useful to record the plaque control status, which can simply be noted as poor, fair or good control. A simple plaque and bleeding index using four surfaces of the following teeth may be used to give a baseline on tooth cleaning: UR6 & 1, UL4, LL1 & 6, and LR4. The tooth surfaces are identified as shown in Figure 3.2 and the presence or absence of bleeding or plaque is noted. This is recorded in the patient's notes and used for further reference.

Recession. Any recession or loss of attachment around the teeth should be noted and recorded in the patient's notes. This is most likely to occur around those teeth that are prominent either buccally or lingually in the arch.

Mobility. The mobility of the teeth is simply recorded as grade I to III, where I indicates slight movement, II excessive side-to-side movement in the socket, and III both lateral and vertical movement.

Conservative assessment (including endodontic and fixed prosthodontics)

The teeth that are present are recorded and displayed in the patient's notes. A full dental charting may be included, especially if this is the patient's first visit to your practice (Fig. 3.3). On subsequent visits, unless there have been major changes, a detailed charting is not required.

Dental caries. As well as marking the dental chart, a brief written note should be made of those teeth that have active and arrested caries. Good illumination is required and a

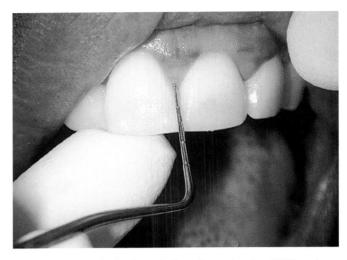

Fig. 3.1 Picture of a basic periodontal examination (BPE) probe.

dental probe is only used to remove debris in order to get better visual access to the tooth.

Restorations. The standard of the restorations can be simply recorded as either satisfactory or unsatisfactory, with the latter being highlighted in the notes. Any decementation of cast restorations should be recorded. The margins of crowns are probed for any gaps or recurrent caries. The clinician should look for any possible uncementation of the crown that has not been noticed by the patient.

Tooth surface loss. Many patients are now presenting with some form of tooth surface loss and this can simply be recorded as present or absent. If present, an indication of the severity is written down. The appearance of the teeth is noted and also where the tooth surface loss is occurring. Wear may not be found on the occlusal surfaces

Table 3.2	Scoring for basic periodontal examination	
Score	Indicates	Treatment required
0	Health	
1	Bleeding on probing only	OHI
2	Plaque retentive factor (calculus/overhang)	Removal of retentive factor
3	Probing depth 3.5–5.5 mm	OHI
	Black band is partially visible	Scale and polish Review need for root planing
4	Probing depth is greater than 5.5 mm Black band disappears	Radiographs indicated Detailed probing depth and attachment charting Plus OHI, scale and polish, root planing
—	Used when no teeth present in sextant	

OHI, oral hygiene instruction.

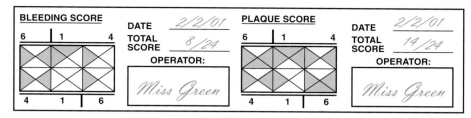

Fig. 3.2   Simple plaque and bleeding index chart.

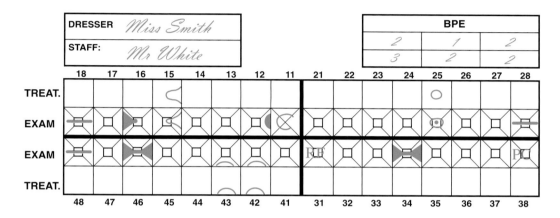

Fig. 3.3   Dental chart including basic periodontal examination (BPE) scores.

alone, but may also be taking place on buccal and palatal surfaces. Recording tooth surface loss is a difficult procedure and a number of indices have been used. One of the more commonly accepted scoring systems is the Smith and Knight index, which is shown in Table 3.3. This index records the degree of wear on all tooth surfaces, regardless of cause, and allows monitoring of the effectiveness of preventive measures, even when the aetiology is obscure.

Tooth fracture. Any trauma or fracture of the teeth is recorded, together with an indication of any looseness of the tooth in its socket.

Table 3.3   The Smith and Knight index. This requires the surface of each tooth to be given a score between 0 and 4 according to its appearance

Score	Surface	Criterion
0	BLOI C	No loss of enamel characteristics No change of contour
1	BLOI C	Loss of enamel surface characteristics Minimal loss of contour
2	BLO I C	Enamel loss just exposing dentine < 1/3 of the surface Enamel loss just exposing dentine Defect less than 1 mm deep
3	BLO I C	Enamel loss just exposing dentine > 1/3 of the surface Enamel loss and substantial dentine loss but no pulp exposure Defect 1–2 mm deep
4	BLO I C	Complete enamel loss, or pulp exposure or 2° dentine exposure Pulp exposure, or 2° dentine exposure Defect more than 2 mm deep, or pulp exposure or 2° dentine exposure

B, buccal or labial; L, lingual or palatal; O, occlusal; I, incisal; C, cervical.

Discoloration. Alteration in the colour or any other similar problems related to the natural teeth are noted. Any alteration to the shade and appearance of any fixed restorations is entered into the notes.

Removable prosthodontic assessment

The following information gives a simple overview of any removable prosthesis that the patient is wearing. It can also be modified for an assessment of the load-bearing structures prior to the decision to construct a prosthesis.

Partially dentate/edentulous. The nature of the support given to the prosthesis is recorded. This may be simply recorded as either tooth or mucosa, or a combination of the two, i.e. tooth/mucosa. This latter situation is encountered with the free end saddle.

Edentulous areas. The quality of the mucosa and bone support is evaluated. The ridge may be palpated to determine its firmness. Any bony irregularities or structures that may interfere with the design of the removable partial denture (RPD) should be examined.

Condition of existing dentures. If existing dentures are present they should be examined and an assessment made of their stability, the base extension and the retention of the prosthesis.

Static/dynamic occlusion of teeth/prosthesis

All teeth are examined for tilting rotation, overeruption, malalignment, wear faceting and burnished areas on restorations. The patient is asked to close the teeth together and an assessment is made of the occlusal relationship. The occlusion is assessed as canine protected or group function, and any non-working side contacts are noted.

The intercuspal position is the relation of the mandible to the maxillae when the teeth are together in maximum intercuspation. The majority of patients have a habitual intercuspal position (i.e. a comfortable position that they close into without any guidance).

Lateral excursions are guided commonly by the canine and the premolar teeth. In canine guidance, the posterior teeth will disclude in lateral excursions. In group function, a group of teeth, such as the canines and premolar teeth, are contacting on the working side (i.e. the side to which the mandible moves). In protrusive movements, the anterior teeth move over each other with the posterior teeth discluding. However, in tooth wear, the posterior teeth may be in function due to excessive wear of the anterior teeth. The retruded contact position of the mandible is where it is in its furthest distal position when contacting the upper teeth. Generally the patient can be guided into this position, which is usually 1–2 mm further

posterior to the intercuspal position. Interferences are abnormal contacts that interfere with the smooth movements of the mandible and may be the cause of tooth fracture or cementation failure of a crown etc., or may lead to tooth mobility. Such deviations from the normal movements are recorded in the notes.

Special investigations

Having reached this part of the examination, the clinician will have identified any problems that may be present. If the patient has a specific problem then it will have become evident during the examination. The clinician may now wish to examine in more detail the area of complaint. It is useful to make a provisional diagnosis of the condition prior to these tests. This hypothesis will then be either proved or disproved during these stages leading to a final diagnosis. However, to confirm such a judgement, further investigations must be undertaken, such as those described below.

Vitality testing of the pulp

Vitality of the tooth may be tested using either electrical or thermal stimulation. Electrical testing will require a small charge to be applied to the tooth. The charge is generated by a machine and the patient becomes part of the circuit when the tip is applied to the tooth. Good electrical contact is achieved by the use of prophylactic paste. The present machines do not require clinician contact, as the use of rubber gloves often prevents a good electrical circuit being formed. Thermal stimulation may be through either cold or heat, but cold stimulation is preferred. This is done using an ice stick or a pledget of cotton wool soaked in ethyl chloride, which will give a quick response. However, a more intense cold stimulus can be provided by the use of dry ice (CO_2).

Study casts

Study casts of the teeth may be required and these may be poured from preliminary alginate impressions taken in a stock try. A more accurate determination of the occlusal relationship will require alginate impressions in individual trays made from the preliminary casts. Registration of the occlusion together with a face bow recording may be necessary. This will be incorporated in the provisional treatment plan prior to the finalised treatment.

Other tests

These include the use of a diet sheet to investigate for high caries/erosive nature. Any suspicious alteration to the mucosa within the mouth will require the opinion of an oral medicine or oral surgery specialist, who may wish to obtain a biopsy of the area to confirm the diagnosis from a histological specimen. This may also include blood tests if an underlying disorder is suspected.

Radiographic examination

The most common special investigation performed is the radiographic examination. This will provide further evidence that may confirm your provisional diagnosis. The most useful technique is long cone radiography, in order to produce bite wings or periapical views of the hard dental tissues together with the immediate supporting tissues. Bite wings are indicated where there are multiple contacts between the teeth and they are the only reliable method for detecting approximal caries. They should be taken on a 2-yearly basis unless there are indications of a rapid carious process taking place, in which case they should be taken more frequently. If the patient is new to your practice then a set of bite wings should be taken. Information gained from such radiographs includes the presence of caries (new or recurrent), bone levels around the teeth and the marginal contour of the restorations.

When there is apical involvement, as indicated by the history, a long cone periapical is taken. This will provide information over and above that obtained from the bite wing radiograph and will reveal any problems related to the pulpal chamber, such as internal resorption, status of previous root canal therapy (if present) or the surrounding periapical tissues (i.e. bone loss due to periapical infection or cyst formation). It will also provide more detailed information relating to alveolar bone loss between the teeth or furcation involvement.

Where indicated, further radiographic examination may be required to examine larger structures, e.g. orthopantomographs (OPG) for the mandible, occipital mental (OM) for the sinuses and temporomandibular joint (TMJ) views. Where there are areas of concern that are not immediately apparent, the views of a consultant radiologist should be sought.

PHASE 3: DIAGNOSIS

You are now in a position to formulate a definitive diagnosis concerning the nature of the problem. A brief summary of the findings should be written down and the diagnosis stated. Many individuals find this statement difficult to articulate and it is often left open. The diagnosis must be stated in the notes. For example, it may be caries caused by high sugar consumption, or chronic adult periodontitis; there may be reversible or irreversible pulpitis. It is important to be precise and to write down your diagnosis clearly. It can be modified in the light of further contact with the patient but it is the key to your treatment planning.

TREATMENT PLAN

Once a firm diagnosis has been made, a treatment plan is drawn up which is aimed at correcting the patient's presenting problem. This plan may be provisional or final and should not be changed without good reason. It is often tempting, if one has not seen the patient at the examination stage, to change another clinician's plan. If this is to be done, any changes should only be made following discussion with the person who instigated the treatment. A treatment plan should be drawn up with the patient's consent and should take into consideration the patient's commitment to the work involved and the number of visits required to complete it.

SIGNATURE

A patient's history is a legal document and should be signed clearly. Although written records are still kept, there is a trend towards the computerisation of data. This can still be held as a legal document but there must be safeguards regarding access to the information, and back-up files need to be made in case of disk failure.

Box 3.3 Aide-Memoire*	
Referred by:	Reason for referral:
Date of referral:	Date seen:

1. Reason for attendance		RFA
2. Complains of		CO
3. History of present complaint		HPC
4. Medical history		MH
5. Dental history		DH
6. Personal/social history		PH/SH
7. Examination		
(a) *Extraoral*		EO
(b) *Intraoral*		IO
Soft tissue exam		
Hard tissue exam		
Periodontal assessment		
BPE screen		
Assessment of edentulous areas		
Assessment of removeable/fixed appliances		
Static/dynamic occlusion of teeth/prosthesis		
8. Special investigations		
9. Diagnosis		
10. Treatment plan		
11. Signature		

*An 11-point structure to history-taking, examination, diagnosis and treatment planning with appropriate abbreviations (these may differ between teaching institutions but the general approach will be similar).

SUMMARY

The legal nature of the notes cannot be stressed enough and it is important that entries into patients' records are neat and legible. Untidy or inaccurate records often lead to difficulties, misunderstandings or mistakes at later clinical visits. Finally, as an assistance to taking a good history the aide-memoire shown in Box 3.3 may be used to assist with the basics of patient note taking.

4 Inflammatory periodontal diseases

Recent epidemiological evidence indicates that between 10 and 20% of the world's population is highly susceptible to some form of destructive periodontal disease; 40% are likely to suffer from milder forms of plaque-induced periodontal diseases. These inflammatory diseases will vary from early forms of gingivitis, frequently seen in children and adolescents, to advanced periodontitis, more prevalent in the fourth and fifth decades of life. It has been shown by clinical and epidemiological studies that the majority of inflammatory periodontal diseases are initiated by microbial plaque deposits on the teeth and the adjacent tissues. However, they may be complicated by the presence of systemic diseases or the taking of medication, as well as other restorative factors.

GINGIVITIS

Gingivitis is characterised by superficial inflammation of the gums, shown by the classic signs of redness, swelling and loss of stippling. There is no clinical bone loss or mobility. Any pocketing is of the 'false' variety, caused by gingival swelling, which may be oedematous or fibrous in nature.

Types of gingivitis

There are a number of different types of gingivitis including both acute and chronic forms.

Acute traumatic gingivitis

This condition may be caused by physical, thermal or chemical factors. Diagnosis will usually be apparent from the history, together with the appearance of the lesions. Physical causes include toothbrush trauma, especially when a new brush has recently been purchased, and damage from sharp items inserted into the mouth, an activity particularly common in children. One type of damage may be caused deliberately by the patient – a condition termed 'gingivitis artefacta'. When this condition is associated with a psychiatric disorder, it is termed 'gingivitis artefacta major' and when it is an innocent habit it may be termed 'minor'. Despite its innocent background, severe damage may be caused to the gingiva, even leading to tooth loss, as shown in Figure 4.1. This problem is particularly seen in young children.

Other causes of acute traumatic gingivitis are damage from hard food and iatrogenic damage from dental treatment. Many dental procedures have the ability to cause transient acute gingivitis. These include cavity preparation adjacent to the gingiva and gingival abrasion by brushes and burs. In all such situations, the gingiva will be eroded to some degree, often with a ragged margin with visible tags of damaged epithelium. Long-standing cases will have a surrounding area of keratosis where the stimulus has been less acute.

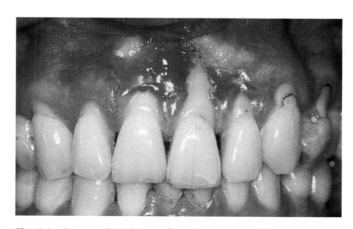

Fig. 4.1   Severe gingivitis artefacta in a young child.

Thermal causes are principally related to eating hot food. The classic history of hot, melted cheese on French onion soup or fondues sticking to and burning the gingiva is well known. Dental cautery or overheated ultrasonic scalers may produce similar damage. The history of the condition will usually identify the cause.

Chemical trauma may be caused by a number of substances. Burns caused by the application of aspirin to the gingiva alongside a tooth that is a source of pain, in the belief that this will have a local or topical effect, are still occasionally seen (Fig. 4.2). As well as a relevant history, the early chemical lesion will have a white covering where the epithelium has been damaged, but this is rapidly lost to leave a tender area of acute gingivitis.

Acute non-specific gingivitis

This condition is most commonly seen as an acute exacerbation of pre-existing chronic gingivitis (Fig. 4.3). The diagnosis is made by excluding other causes of acute gingivitis, including acute necrotising and herpetic gingivitis. It may be associated with a lowering of host resistance, such as occurs with systemic illnesses. There may also be local causes such as lack of lip seal in the upper incisor area or mouth breathing, which may cause palatal acute gingivitis.

Acute hypersensitivity reactions

Hypersensitivity reactions to the constituents of toothpastes and occasionally cosmetics are sometimes seen as an 'allergic gingivitis' (Fig. 4.4). The symptoms reported may vary considerably but a common feature is a widespread diffuse granular gingivitis involving the full width of the attached gingiva. Other features may include oral ulceration, glossitis and cheilitis. The commonest hypersensitivity reaction is to the cinnamonaldehyde constituent of toothpastes. This flavouring is currently used in tartar

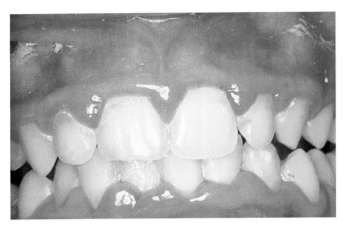

Fig. 4.3 Acute non-specific gingivitis: an exacerbation of pre-existing chronic gingivitis.

control toothpastes to hide the unpleasant taste of the pyrophosphate active agent. The histological features of gingival biopsies are generally non-specific, although the presence of a plasma cell infiltration may sometimes be seen.

Acute necrotising ulcerative gingivitis

This is an acute gingivitis characterised by necrotising interdental ulcers which rapidly spread to the other areas of the gingiva. Characteristically, the ulcers are covered by a yellowish pseudomembrane which is composed of sloughed epithelial cells, polymorphs, fusiforms and spirochaetes in a fibrinous exudate. The condition is usually very painful and the gingivae are very sore to touch and bleed easily on manipulation. There is a characteristic halitosis and the sufferer may report spontaneous haemorrhage from the ulcers (Fig. 4.5). There may be swelling and tenderness of the regional lymph nodes together with systemic fever and malaise. Although the condition starts

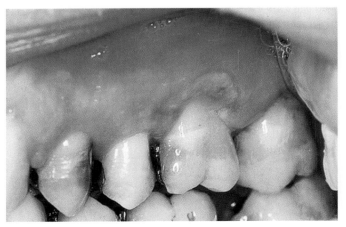

Fig. 4.2 A burn produced by applying aspirin directly to the soft tissues.

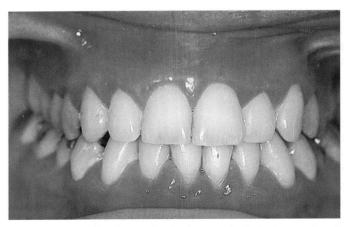

Fig. 4.4 Acute allergic reaction in the marginal gingiva produced by a reaction to a toothpaste.

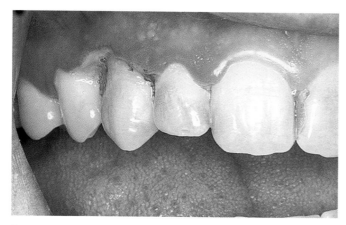

Fig. 4.5 Acute necrotising ulcerative gingivitis in a young patient with a smoking habit.

as an acute condition, it often subsides into a chronic state which is identical to adult-type periodontitis, except for the presence of typical tissue deformities. The American Academy of Periodontology has recently adopted the term 'acute necrotising ulcerative periodontitis', which relates to the loss of attachment that is an invariable consequence of this stage of the disorder.

The aetiology of the condition is unclear but certain common predisposing conditions may be observed. The patient, who is frequently aged between 18 and 30 years, usually has a pre-existing inflammatory periodontal disorder, either gingivitis or periodontitis, and is often a smoker. There may be a history of a recent systemic illness such as the common cold, which lowers the tissue resistance, or the disease may follow a stressful episode in the patient's life, such as bereavement, divorce or redundancy. Recently the disease has been found to have a high occurrence in HIV-infected individuals.

The microbiology of the condition is interesting. Vincent (1898) first described the fusospirochaetal complex consisting of the microorganisms *Bacillus fusiformis* and *Borrelia vincentii*. Since that time, a variety of other organisms have been shown to be usually present, including *Vibrio*, *Bacteroides* and *Selenomonas* species. The part played by these organisms in the development of the condition is unclear.

HIV-associated gingivitis

Recently an acute form of gingivitis has been described that is seen in sufferers of acquired immune deficiency syndrome (AIDS); this has been categorised as a definitive form of gingivitis. It is most probable that this condition is only an exaggerated or unusual response to dental plaque due to the immune deficits that occur in these patients.

The commonest symptom is an intense marginal gingivitis in a patient who has been diagnosed as infected with the human immunodeficiency virus (HIV). In the

more severe cases, there may be ulceration similar to that seen in acute necrotising ulcerative gingivitis.

Acute herpetic gingivostomatitis

The oral cavity may be involved in infection with herpes simplex viruses, types I and II. Infection with type I usually occurs in childhood, but because infection is increasingly avoided in childhood it is becoming more common in both adolescents and adults (Fig. 4.6). Type II infection, which is usually sexually transmitted, is more commonly seen in adults. Clinically, both types have similar oral manifestations. The oral signs are soreness of the oral mucosa, with small vesicles which form and rapidly burst to form ulcers surrounded by a bright red halo. There may also be a concomitant marginal herpetic gingivitis. Systemically, there is often malaise, fever and lymphadenitis. Children will be irritable, salivate excessively and may have difficulty in eating. Dehydration may occur within a short period of time.

Chronic marginal gingivitis

Gingivitis has been shown by epidemiological, clinical and research investigations to be initiated and maintained by the presence of mature plaque deposits around the teeth. Dental plaque has been shown to develop a complex gram-negative anaerobic flora with time which releases a variety of irritant metabolites, destructive enzymes and antigens that stimulate the inflammatory and immune systems. These cause local damage in the gingival tissues which bring about breakdown and the classic signs of gingivitis.

The severity of chronic gingivitis may vary from a slight change in texture and colour of the gingival margin to a severe erythema with a tendency to spontaneous bleeding following minor trauma. Hyperplastic swelling of the gingiva may also be a feature of the disorder. Although

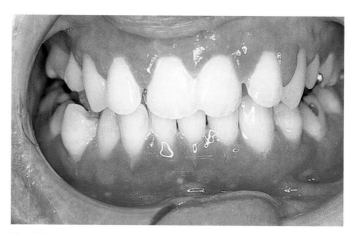

Fig. 4.6 Acute herpetic gingivostomatitis: vesicles can be seen scattered throughout the oral mucosa.

the underlying disease is usually a chronic inflammatory process, acute exacerbations are common.

Chronic gingivitis is largely symptomless and most people suffering from it are totally unaware of the fact. On occasions, however, one of the following may be noted:

- bleeding from the gums, especially after toothbrushing
- colour change with varying degrees of redness
- change of texture with loss of gingival stippling
- alteration in consistency as the gingivae lose their firmness and become soft and spongy
- alteration in form with loss of the knife-edge gingival margins.

Chronic desquamative gingivitis

This is a chronic gingival condition characterised by red, sore gingiva with thin, poorly keratinised gingiva (Fig. 4.7). It is more common in females of 40 or 50 years of age. Chronic desquamative gingivitis presents many of the features of chronic gingivitis, overlaid with superficial acute erythema of the surface epithelium. The epithelium can be rubbed off easily with slight physical pressure. On occasions, small vesicles may form which, when they rupture, leave raw, painful areas. Patients may complain of sore gums which are aggravated by hot or spicy foods. The sore patches may persist for long periods of time and then gradually clear, only to recur at a later date. Recurrent episodes may continue for several years and, in some cases, may then stop completely.

Most cases of desquamative gingivitis have a background of dermatological problems, the commonest of which are lichen planus or lichenoid reactions and occasionally benign mucous membrane pemphigoid. It is thought that these conditions lower the tissue resistance and alter the character of the gingivitis.

PERIODONTITIS

Periodontitis typically is revealed by loss of attachment, either pocketing and/or recession which, together with bone loss, are all historical signs of past disease. Present activity may be indicated by bleeding on gentle probing from the base of the pocket, pus formation or other signs of active inflammation, as well as progressive loss of attachment.

Unlike gingivitis, where the inflammation is confined to the superficial gingival tissues, periodontitis affects all of the periodontal tissues, especially the ligament or membrane. It may be accompanied by a variable amount of gingivitis, which may differ not only from patient to patient, but also from one site to another in the mouth. The characteristics of periodontitis (Box 4.1) are loss of attachment caused by the apical migration of the junctional epithelium, which may present as pocketing and/or recession, together with bone loss. In the later stages of the

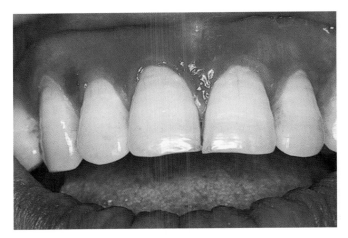

Fig. 4.7 Chronic desquamative gingivitis.

disease, mobility and drifting of the affected teeth may occur. Other symptoms may include halitosis and pus formation in walls of the pockets, some of which progress to lateral periodontal abscesses.

Adult periodontitis

This is the commonest type of periodontitis. It usually occurs in older patients, whose tissues respond well to plaque-induced damage and break down slowly over a long period of time. Although there may be periods of rapid breakdown, as with any type of inflammatory disease, generally the increase in probing depths is slow (Box 4.2). There may be a large amount of reparative fibrosis in the inflamed gingiva (Fig. 4.8).

Aggressive forms of periodontal disease

There are a number of other types of periodontal disease which may be considered to be aggressive inflammatory conditions, either because they occur in younger age groups than adult-type periodontitis, or because they

---

Box 4.1   Clinical characteristics of periodontitis

- Variable degree of gingivitis
- Loss of attachment shown by:
  - pocketing
  - recession
  - combination of both
- Pocket activity demonstrated by:
  - bleeding on deep probing
  - suppuration
  - deepening of pocket
- Bone loss
- Mobility

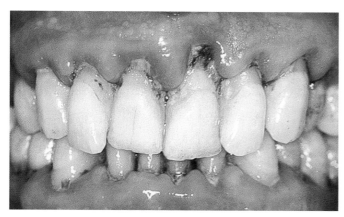

Fig. 4.8 A patient with adult periodontitis showing large amounts of dental plaque deposits but a low-grade inflammatory response.

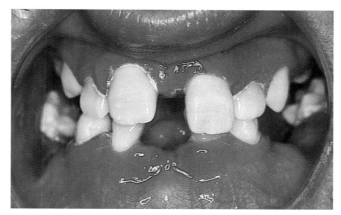

Fig. 4.9 A young patient with prepubertal periodontitis. A lower incisor has already fallen out.

Box 4.2   Clinical features of adult periodontitis

These are very varied but will always include the following features:

- Loss of attachment, which will present as periodontal pocketing or gingival recession, or a combination of both
- Bone resorption
- Tooth mobility
- Drifting
- Suppuration from the active sites

Box 4.3   Systemic diseases associated with prepubertal periodontitis

- Papillon–Lefèvre syndrome
- Insulin-dependent diabetes
- Primary or acquired immunodeficiency
- Leukaemias
- Hypophosphatasia
- Histiocytosis X
- Neutropenia
- Chediak–Higashi syndrome
- Agranulocytosis

---

progress at a more rapid rate, and for this reason they are often termed 'aggressive or progressive disease'.

Prepubertal periodontitis

As can be judged from its name, prepubertal periodontitis occurs in children before adolescence (Fig. 4.9). The greatest incidence occurs during the eruption of the permanent dentition, although the primary teeth are not exempt from its ravages. The occurrence of true pocketing and progressive periodontitis in children is rare and, when it occurs, is often a sign of a systemic defect (Box 4.3), although in some children no underlying predisposing disease can be demonstrated.

The characteristics of this disease are not well known, although localised and generalised forms have been described. The gingival inflammation is extremely acute, and granulation or proliferation from the active sites may occur, giving rise to gingival swellings termed epulides which are often of the pyogenic variety. There is often very rapid destruction of alveolar bone and sometimes gingival recession. Immune system defects, including functional defects of peripheral blood leucocytes and monocytes, may be found in these patients and a lack of neutrophils

has been described in the affected gingival tissues. The patients may also have a history of other problems, including respiratory and middle-ear infections. Little is known about the microbiology of this disease.

Juvenile periodontitis

Juvenile periodontitis is an unusual form of periodontitis which occurs around the permanent teeth of adolescents. Classically, the periodontal lesions occur around the first molars and the incisors (Fig. 4.10), although, as with prepubertal periodontitis, localised and generalised forms

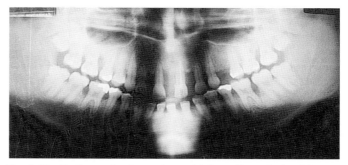

Fig. 4.10 Radiograph of a patient with juvenile periodontitis. Note the bone loss around the molars and incisors.

have been described. The disease has its onset at puberty, although it may present at any time between 11 and 13 years of age. More females than males are seen with this problem in treatment clinics, but epidemiological investigations in the community have shown that the prevalence is equal in both males and females.

The amount of gingival inflammation seen in these patients is frequently low and the oral hygiene may vary from excellent (Fig. 4.11) to appalling. In all patients, however, the degree of breakdown is excessive for the amount of local irritants. There is some evidence that this disease may be subject to remission or burn-out.

The defects occur in siblings and the familial distribution is consistent with an autosomal recessive genetic trait. It is thought that all affected individuals probably have functional defects of neutrophils or monocytes. The microbiology has been studied in some depth and two endotoxin-producing organisms, *Actinobacillus actinomycetemcomitans* and *Capnocytophaga*, have been identified in a large number of these patients. Interestingly the toxins produced by these organisms inhibit phagocytic cell function, which may account for the defects seen in the neutrophil and monocyte function.

Rapidly progressive periodontitis

This has been recently described in the literature. Typically the sufferers have severe and rapidly advancing lesions (Fig. 4.12). There is some disagreement as to when it first occurs, although the consensus is that it is usually seen between the ages of 25 and 35 years. The lesions are frequently generalised, with all the teeth affected to a greater or lesser degree, without any consistent pattern of destruction. The microbiology is uncertain but two organisms are often found: *Porphyromonas gingivalis* and *Actinobacillus actinomycetemcomitans*.

During the active phases of rapidly progressive periodontitis, the lesions are acutely inflamed and may proliferate

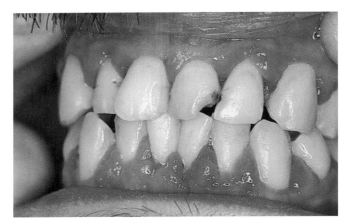

Fig. 4.12 A clinical photograph of a patient with rapidly progressive periodontitis. Note the granulomatous reaction of the gingiva to plaque.

to give rise to granulomatous gingival epulides. Some three-quarters of the patients have been shown to have functional defects of neutrophils or monocytes, and systemic manifestations including depression, weight loss and general malaise have been reported.

This type of periodontitis has been claimed to follow juvenile periodontitis in some patients and is also more commonly seen in sufferers of certain systemic diseases. There is a higher prevalence in individuals with a number of systemic disorders (Box 4.4).

Refractory periodontitis

In a small number of sites in some patients the periodontal lesion will remain active, as shown by continued signs of inflammation, pus formation or pocket deepening despite active treatment (Fig. 4.13). Although it is frequently not possible to find a cause for a site proving refractory, there may be a number of reasons for the failure of the site to heal (Box 4.5).

Inadequate oral hygiene. This may be defined as a level of supragingival dental plaque which is incompatible with marginal periodontal health. This will vary from patient to patient, but the clinical level of residual plaque should be sufficiently low as to permit the marginal gingival tissues to be free of visible inflammation. If marginal inflammation persists, then a complex subgingival flora is soon re-established and pocket activity will again occur.

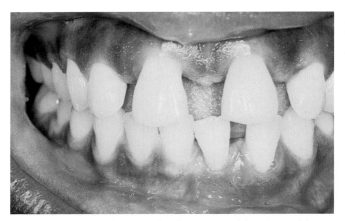

Fig. 4.11 A clinical photograph of a 16-year-old patient with juvenile periodontitis. Note the drifting of teeth despite the good oral hygiene.

Box 4.4 Systemic disorders associated with juvenile periodontitis
• Papillon–Lefèvre syndrome
• Down's syndrome
• Chediak–Higashi syndrome
• Insulin-dependent diabetes

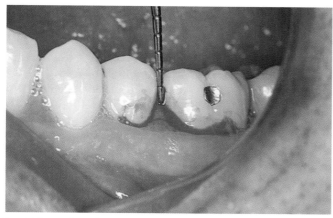

Fig. 4.13 A clinical photograph of a patient with refractory periodontitis. Note the severe inflammation despite previous root debridement.

Box 4.5 Some of the commoner reasons for refractory sites

- Inadequate oral hygiene
- Persistence of root surface deposits
- Root surface defects
- Inadequate host response
- Unidentified systemic factor
- Periodontic-endodontic lesions

Root surface deposits. These are always left after treatment, but usually the host response is able to cope with a low level of retained irritants, such as dental plaque, calculus and cementum-bound endotoxin. However, it is not always possible to debride the root surface adequately due to difficulties with access, visibility or root contour as shown in Figure 4.14. In general, anterior, single-rooted teeth are usually amenable to instrumentation, whilst posterior, multiple-rooted teeth with furcation involvement are least likely to be successfully treated.

Root surface defects. Defects such as grooves, flutes, gingival pits or enamel projections are seen in some sites with refractory inflammation (Fig. 4.15). The root surface defects prevent complete debridement and inflammation will persist.

Inadequate host response. This is seen in a small number of individuals, who usually have defects involving their polymorphonuclear leucocytes or monocytes. These defects are difficult to detect and impossible to treat. The only factor that can be changed in these unfortunate patients is to reduce the level of plaque deposits even further.

Unidentified systemic factors. Factors such as anaemia, diabetes or other similar problems occur in a very small number of patients. Although it is not appropriate to screen all patients with refractory lesions, if multiple sites are active, the tissues highly inflamed and the plaque levels low, it is worthwhile for the patient to have a haematological screening including whole blood count, film and serum chemistry.

Periodontic-endodontic lesions. Occasionally the refractory lesion may be due to primary or secondary involvement of the pulpal tissues. The source of the continued infection may be due to persistent periradicular infection and successful treatment will require both endodontic as well as periodontal therapy.

Acute necrotising ulcerative periodontitis

On occasions, the tissue destruction seen in acute necrotising ulcerative gingivitis will spread into the deeper periodontal tissues causing widespread tissue loss. When this occurs the condition can clearly no longer be termed a 'gingivitis' but justifies the term 'periodontitis'. This condition is seen very commonly when the ravages of HIV infection have reduced the host resistance to a critical level.

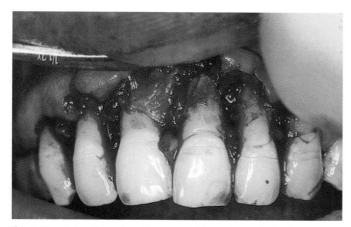

Fig. 4.14 A tooth surface that would have been difficult to instrument due to the depth of the periodontal lesions.

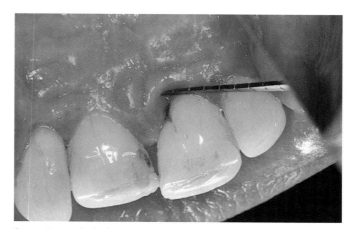

Fig. 4.15 A clinical photograph of a patient with a palatal root groove associated with severe pocketing. The groove acts as a local plaque retention factor.

HIV-associated periodontitis

Periodontitis associated with patients whose immune systems are compromised by HIV infection may show unusual features (Box 4.6). The marginal gingivitis may be intense and sometimes the overlying soft tissue will be necrotic, exposing marginal bone around the tooth. Pocketing, when present, will be deeper than expected. There is often an associated candidal infection.

Acute periodontal abscess

A periodontal abscess can occur with any type of periodontitis and is therefore not a type of periodontitis but a particular feature or symptom. A periodontal abscess forms when pus collects in the connective tissue wall of a pocket. It is important to distinguish this from a peri-radicular abscess caused by an infection emanating from the pulp, and in order to emphasise this distinction the term 'lateral periodontal abscess' is often used. The differential diagnosis may be made based on the history, clinical examination, vitality tests and appropriate radiographs.

It is unusual for a periodontal abscess to occur in the absence of severe periodontitis, although it may be initiated by acute trauma. The precipitating causes are not clearly understood and it is quite possible that they may vary from patient to patient. The main causes are shown in Box 4.7.

The abscess may present as a localised swelling with erythema of the overlying mucosa. The tooth may be tender to biting or percussion, and the patient may complain of throbbing which is relieved by pressure. The swelling is frequently, but not invariably, fluctuant. There may be systemic symptoms, such as lymphadenitis of the local lymph nodes, as well as raised temperature. This is more common when the condition is acute, but once drainage has been achieved the abscess becomes chronic with a lessening of symptoms.

Box 4.6   Manifestations of HIV periodontitis

- Inflammatory periodontal disease
- HIV-associated gingivitis
- Acute necrotising ulcerative gingivitis
- Acute necrotising ulcerative periodontitis
- Acute necrotising stomatitis
- Gingival ulceration associated with:
  - herpes simplex
  - herpes zoster
  - human cytomegalovirus
  - non-Hodgkin's lymphoma
  - Kaposi's sarcoma
  - neutropenia

Box 4.7   Commoner factors associated with an acute periodontal abscess

- Entry of organisms into the connective tissues adjacent to the periodontal pocket, which has been shown to occur in deep periodontal lesions
- The forcing of plaque, calculus and other irritant debris through the pocket lining during scaling and root debridement procedures
- Impaction of foreign bodies into the periodontal pocket. This is often quoted as a cause of the problem but the authors have never seen a periodontal abscess associated with this type of damage
- Blockage of a pocket with obstruction of drainage. Although this is a possible cause, the majority of abscesses seen are draining through the pocket on presentation
- Reduction of host resistance as seen in some conditions such as diabetes, which are associated with frequent periodontal abscesses

5 Management of inflammatory periodontal diseases

MANAGEMENT OF GINGIVITIS

Gingivitis is characterised by superficial inflammation of the gingival tissues with no loss of attachment, although swelling may cause false pocketing to be present. It is the one type of periodontal disease that has been categorically shown by experimental studies to be related to the oral hygiene of the patient. The severity of gingivitis may vary from a slight change in texture and colour of the gingival margin, to an intense erythema with a tendency to spontaneous bleeding following minor trauma. Although it is usually a chronic inflammatory process, acute episodes are common.

Early gingivitis may be completely reversed by an improvement in the standard of oral home care, provided that there are no factors such as deficient restorations or calculus that make plaque removal difficult. Later stages may pose more complex problems, such as gingival hyperplasia which may need surgical removal. The key factor in the management of all types of periodontal disease is *effective home care*.

However, it is insufficient to merely show patients how to brush their teeth and clean interdentally. They will need to be educated so they understand *why* they need to clean their teeth efficiently, and they must have the motivation to *want* to undertake thorough cleaning on a long-term basis. They also need to be instructed in the physical skills required to achieve effective plaque removal. These are the main steps for achieving control of gingivitis.

There are a number of obstacles that have to be successfully negotiated before one can achieve the restoration of gingival health in these patients:

- *The encouragement of motivation.* There are a number of ways of motivating patients, and one of the most effective is to demonstrate disease in their own mouth. The identification of periodontal pockets and bleeding, especially if there are healthy sites for comparison, will give most patients a personal interest in the measures needed to restore health.
- *Linking the disease to the cause.* Demonstrating the relationship between gingival inflammation and its cause (e.g. dental plaque) in the patient's own mouth will often motivate that person. The use of disclosing agents to colour plaque may assist in this.
- *Providing information on cleaning requirements.* Informing patients about measures that can be undertaken to remove plaque and restore health is a necessary step in their education. Realistic targets should be set for plaque control. The use of a quantitative index for the plaque level and gingival inflammation will be of great assistance in this phase of the treatment.
- *Instruction in oral hygiene.* Careful instruction in appropriate methods of oral hygiene is the last link in the

chain of home care advice and the main methods are shown in Box 5.1. In addition, it is also helpful to undertake a professional prophylaxis for patients with gingivitis. This leaves the mouth clean, starts the healing process, and has the effect of reinforcing home care. The removal of calculus and overhanging margins of restorations makes oral hygiene more effective, and the removal of stains and plaque improves motivation.

It will be necessary to follow up the patient to monitor the effect of the advice, provide feedback and reinforce the motivation. Figure 5.1 illustrates the improvement that may be obtained in these patients.

In addition to these general guidelines there are a number of specific acute types of gingivitis and the following sections describe additional measures that can be undertaken when the specific diagnosis is known.

Acute traumatic gingivitis

This condition may be caused by physical, thermal or chemical factors. Diagnosis will usually be apparent from the history, together with the appearance of the lesions. The first step in the management of patients with acute traumatic forms of gingivitis is to identify the cause. Some patients may not admit to a damaging habit and food trauma may not have been noticed, especially if the meal has been accompanied by alcohol. Once the cause has been identified, treatment is directed towards reassuring the sufferer and providing palliative measures, such as lidocaine gel, to ease the pain and antiseptic mouthwashes to decrease the duration of secondary infection. An alternative mouthwash, particularly if a thermal burn is suspected, is *benzydamine hydrochloride*, which will decrease soreness considerably. This is dispensed as a 0.15% solution and the patient should rinse with about 15 mL for 2 min every 1–3 h as required. It should not be used for more than

---

> **Box 5.1** Types and techniques of mechanical oral hygiene
>
> - *Toothbrushing*
>   - bass
>   - miniscrub
> - *Interdental cleaning*
>   - floss/tape
>   - sticks/points
>   - interdental brush
>   - superfloss
> - *Disclosing*
>   - tablets
>   - solution

7 days and may be diluted if the tissues are very sensitive. It is not suitable for children under 12 years of age.

If the condition is being aggravated by aggressive brushing then it might be advisable for the patient to stop brushing for a period and rely on the use of a chemical anti-plaque agent such as 0.2% chlorhexidine gluconate mouth rinse. This will allow keratinisation of the abraded gingiva to occur, prior to brushing being resumed. In some areas, it may be possible to cover the damage with a periodontal dressing or adhesive patch to facilitate healing and prevent further injury.

Acute non-specific gingivitis

This condition is most commonly seen as an acute exacerbation of pre-existing chronic gingivitis. There may also be local causes, such as lack of lip seal, leading to drying out of the upper incisor area; alternatively, mouth breathing, which has a similar effect palatally, may cause acute gingivitis in this area. Often, although there is no practical treatment of the precipitating cause, careful oral hygiene together with scaling and polishing will allow recovery to occur. Where the soreness of the condition makes oral

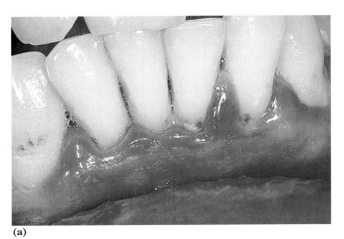

(a)

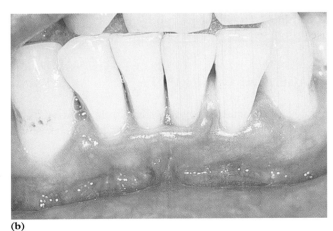

(b)

Fig. 5.1 (a) A patient with gingivitis before treatment: note the red, swollen gingiva. (b) The same patient after treatment. The gingival tissues have shrunk, reducing the swelling. The gingiva are now pink with light stippling.

hygiene difficult, the use of chemical methods of plaque control is indicated.

Acute hypersensitivity reactions

Hypersensitivity reactions to the constituents of tooth-pastes and occasionally cosmetics are sometimes seen as an 'allergic gingivitis'. An important principle in the treatment of these patients is not to expose them to further chemicals to which they may react. The urge to use a chemical anti-plaque agent should be avoided and the patient should be reassured and the toothpaste changed to allow healing to occur.

Acute necrotising ulcerative gingivitis (ANUG)

This acute gingivitis is characterised by necrotising inter-dental ulcers which spread rapidly to the other areas of the gingiva. The management of sufferers of ANUG is based on recognition of the predisposing factors. In view of the relationship between ANUG and stress, and the need for appropriate home care to prevent recurrence, a very careful explanation of the problem together with possible treatment should be provided to the patient. Advice should be given on the avoidance of smoking and the need for an adequate diet. The initial acute phase should be treated by careful debridement of the lesions with the spray from an ultrasonic scaler. Advice on home care should include the purchase of a new soft toothbrush. Although colonisation of the toothbrush bristles by the organisms involved in the condition is a theoretical possibility, the main reason for this advice is to ensure that an adequate brush is used.

Many periodontists would prescribe the drug metronidazole (Flagyl) 200 mg, taken three times a day with meals for 3 days, although for severe cases, a higher dosage used for longer would be indicated. This chemotherapeutic agent is very effective against the gram-negative organisms involved. However, there are some worries about its teratogenic potential and use in pregnancy is contraindicated. If combined with alcohol, it may cause severe nausea. Penicillin is a safe and effective alternative although it is less specific in its antimicrobial action.

It will be necessary to follow up the patient, as relapse and recurrence are common. As the condition usually occurs in patients with a pre-existing inflammatory periodontal condition, this will also require treatment once the acute phase is under control. In some patients, gingival deformities caused by the interdental ulceration will require surgical correction, by either gingivoplasty or flap surgery.

HIV-associated gingivitis

This is an acute form of gingivitis seen in AIDS sufferers. The primary treatment in these patients is directed towards coping with the HIV infection. The oral lesions should always be reported to the consulting physician as they may indicate the development of AIDS in an HIV sufferer. The oral lesions should be sampled with a smear and checked for candidal infection, as this is often present and may cause an acute form of gingivitis. Assuming that no unusual organisms are found, reinforcing the oral hygiene, together with chemical plaque control by using a 0.2% chlorhexidine gluconate mouth rinse, will help in controlling the problem.

Acute herpetic gingivostomatitis

Oral signs of acute herpetic gingivostomatitis include sore-ness of the oral mucosa, with formation of small vesicles that rapidly burst producing ulcers surrounded by a bright red halo. There is often a concomitant marginal herpetic gingivitis and also signs of systemic involvement, including malaise, fever and lymphadenitis. The most important aspect of management is to maintain fluid balance by encouraging fluid intake. Food should be soft and cold items may be soothing. This is one of the few occasions when the clinician may recommend ice-cream with no sense of guilt. Bed rest should also be advised.

The use of a 0.2% chlorhexidine gluconate mouth rinse will help to reduce the severity of secondary infection in the oral lesions. In the older patient, the use of *benzocaine* lozenges or *lidocaine* viscous paint will help to reduce discomfort during eating. *Paracetamol* or *aspirin* can also be recommended to reduce discomfort and lower temperature, and *promethazine* elixir will act as a sedative and allow sleep in the younger child.

When there are severe systemic symptoms, *aciclovir* may be taken either in tablet form or as an elixir. The cream presentation is also useful in treating the problems of herpes labialis.

MANAGEMENT OF ADULT PERIODONTITIS

Adult periodontitis is, after chronic gingivitis, the commonest of the inflammatory periodontal diseases. The management of all forms of periodontitis is very complex and time-consuming, and the main principles are as follows:

* *Assessment and diagnosis of the disease.* It is the responsibility of dental surgeons to carry out screening of patients under their care, to undertake an assessment and to arrive at an appropriate treatment plan.
* *Discussion of the findings with the patient.* This is to determine the patient's attitudes and expectations. At this stage, relief of pain, if present, may be carried out. Decisions on any teeth of hopeless prognosis, e.g. those with little supporting bone, should be made, to avoid any misunderstanding about what might be achieved with therapy. Extractions should be carried out at an early phase in the treatment plan.

- *Decision on treatment strategy.* Any decision on the type of treatment must be made in conjunction with the patient and with fully informed consent.
- *Providing advice on appropriate plaque control.* This will include advice on home care measures and the removal of plaque retention factors such as calculus. This part of treatment is often called the '*hygiene phase*' or '*cause-related*' therapy. Home care would usually involve a sub-gingival brushing technique, interdental cleaning and, for many patients, the use of disclosing agents where supragingival plaque control measures are suspect.
- *The use of chemical adjuncts.* In some patients, the use of chemical adjuncts to plaque control may be indicated and this is discussed later in the text.
- *Allowing a healing period.* During this phase of treatment, a period of time, often 6–12 weeks, is allowed for healing before the tissue response is reassessed and a decision is made on the need for further treatment (Box 5.2).

For the small group of patients who do not respond to the above regimes, it may be necessary for periodontal surgery to be undertaken.

MANAGEMENT OF AGGRESSIVE PERIODONTAL DISEASES

Prepubertal periodontitis

The overriding need of patients with prepubertal periodontitis is to undertake systemic screening to identify or eliminate systemic defects. Although in many patients the results may prove negative, the identification of a serious defect in even a small number will justify such an approach. The techniques of these investigations and their follow-up are outside the scope of this text, but should include, as a very minimum, the tests outlined in Box 5.3.

If any of the special tests proves positive then referral to a medical practitioner and further investigations would be necessary, depending upon the nature of the defect. The periodontal therapy, although secondary to the medical

---

Box 5.3 Special investigations indicated for patients with prepubertal periodontitis

- Whole blood count and film
- Differential white cell count
- Serum chemistry, including random serum glucose
- Serum folate, iron, vitamin B_{12} and total iron binding capacity
- Urine analysis, including glucose and protein using a dipstick test

---

treatment, often proves to be difficult. Some success may be obtained by the use of long courses of antibiotics, such as tetracycline, or chemotherapeutic agents such as metronidazole. The most effective therapies are thorough prophylaxis of the active sites with a low abrasive fluoride-containing paste, together with flushing of pockets with an ultrasonic scaler, making use of the cavitation and acoustic streaming effects. Oral hygiene should be kept simple and the child's parent or guardian must be involved in its supervision and monitoring.

Juvenile periodontitis

Although the treatment of these patients follows the general principles laid down for adult-type periodontitis, the rapid progression of this condition makes the monitoring much more critical. There are two areas, however, in which management does differ radically. It is now widely accepted that these patients should be treated with tetracycline to eradicate the associated organisms (Box 5.4). It is a matter of clinical judgement whether the antibiotic is given immediately the condition is diagnosed, or with mechanical root surface treatment. There is some evidence that this condition does not respond well to root debridement, and the most optimal result is obtained from a combination of early surgery and a course of systemic tetracycline.

Box 5.2 Treatment of adult periodontitis following the hygiene phase

This will depend upon the healing response and may include one or more of the following:
- When good healing has been achieved, or if there are signs that healing is occurring, the patient is monitored and treatment is provided to ensure that the tissues return to maintainable health
- If a healing response is not occurring and the home care is inadequate, the cause should be sought and further advice on oral hygiene provided
- Where the lack of healing is accompanied by an adequate level of home care, root debridement would be carried out as described elsewhere in this text

---

Box 5.4 Recommended antibiotic regimes in juvenile periodontitis

- Tetracycline or oxytetracycline – 250 mg four times a day for 3 weeks
- Minocycline – 100 mg twice a day for 1 week (both pro rata depending upon body weight)

Contraindications
- Hypersensitivity to tetracyclines
- Pregnancy or lactating
- Urinary tract disorders
- Recurrent candidal infections
- Anticoagulant therapy

Possible problems
- Care with birth control pill
- May cause nausea, vertigo or rashes
- Avoid milk products, which may hinder absorption

Rapidly progressive periodontitis

The general principles of the treatment of periodontitis apply to these patients. Recently, adjunctive treatment with tetracycline, metronidazole or a combination of metronidazole and amoxicillin has been advocated, with variable results. Box 5.5 shows possible therapeutic regimes. The use of subgingival irrigation with chlorhexidine is often helpful.

Refractory periodontitis

There are a number of actions that can be taken to stabilise refractory lesions, including checking the previous therapy and using antimicrobials. These main measures are indicated in Box 5.6.

Recheck the home care. Firstly check that the patient is using a *subgingival* brushing method, such as the bass or miniscrub techniques. It is important to note that although many methods of brushing, such as the roll technique, are quite adequate for the healthy patient, they will not cope with the presence of pocketing or gingival swelling. The use of a powered toothbrush has also been shown to improve the efficiency of plaque removal and they should be strongly recommended to these patients. Also ensure that the patient is using a disclosing agent *after* brushing to monitor residual plaque levels.

The need for good daily interdental cleansing must be stressed and insisted upon. Finally, ensure that the environment in which oral hygiene is undertaken is adequate. Good lighting, a mirror – preferably a magnifying one – and a comfortable seat are essential.

Subgingival irrigation. Some studies have shown that the introduction of a chemical antiseptic such as 0.2% chlorhexidine digluconate into the pocket will have an additional depressant effect on the subgingival flora. There are two main ways of introducing the chemical subgingivally – using a pulsed water irrigator or a syringe with a large blunt needle. The irrigation should be undertaken on a daily basis until the lesion is under control.

Repetition of root debridement. It is worthwhile repeating the root debridement on a tooth adjacent to an active site, on at least two occasions, with a period of at least 3–6 months in between. It must be remembered that it may take up to 6 months for the full effects of root debridement to be achieved. Root debridement should include the use of an ultrasonic or sonic scaler, as the flushing effect will reduce both the level of subgingival microbes and cementum-bound endotoxin. The root debridement may be combined with the use of a topical subgingival antimicrobial such as 2% minocycline, 25% metronidazole, tetracycline cord or chlorhexidine chips.

Systemic antimicrobials. The use of systemic agents such as amoxicillin, tetracycline, minocycline or metronidazole may in some cases produce dramatic improvements, provided they are combined with mechanical root surface treatment in the form of root debridement or flap surgery.

Tetracycline is the most popular antibiotic and is used in a dosage of 250 mg four times a day for 2 or 3 weeks for an average adult. Metronidazole is also a useful agent at a dosage of 200 mg three times a day for 1 or 2 weeks. Recently, a regime combining both metronidazole and amoxicillin for 2 weeks has been described, with significant improvements noted. The recommended doses are shown in Box 5.5.

Periodontal flap surgery. For those sites which persist despite previous treatment and when home care is considered adequate, the raising of a periodontal flap is necessary to permit access to the root surface for instrumentation. The commonest procedure undertaken is the replaced flap, often called the modified Widman procedure.

Professional debridement. Sometimes, when the lesions will not stabilise, it is necessary to undertake repeated professional debridement of the active sites, especially with the sonic or ultrasonic scaler. This will be sufficient in many patients to prevent extension of the lesions with the problems of further loss of attachment.

HIV-associated periodontitis

Treatment undertaken for patients with HIV involves close liaison with the physician managing the HIV infection. The most important benefit that the dentist can give to the

---

Box 5.5 Dosages of systemic antimicrobials that may be used in patients with refractory periodontitis

- Tetracycline – 250 mg four times a day for 3 weeks
- Metronidazole – 200 mg three times a day for 2 weeks
- Metronidazole plus amoxicillin
  - metronidazole 200 mg four times a day
  - amoxicillin 250 mg four times a day
  - both for 2 weeks

Box 5.6 Measures which may control refractory periodontitis

- Recheck the home care procedures, such as use of interdental cleaning
- Introduce subgingival irrigation using a pulsed irrigator
- Repeat the root debridement together with the use of a topical subgingival antimicrobial such as tetracycline, minocycline, metronidazole or chlorhexidine
- Prescribe systemic antimicrobials at the time of root debridement
- Undertake periodontal flap surgery
- Continue prolonged frequent professional debridement, using ultrasonic instrumentation

patient is to institute effective plaque control measures, which should include the regular use of chlorhexidine gluconate mouth rinse. The mouth must be monitored on a regular basis and checked carefully for signs of pathological change.

When HIV-associated periodontitis does occur, it should be treated with the usual regime of scaling, root debridement and the use of antimicrobials. If there is a candidal infection in the mouth, this needs treatment with antifungals.

The periodontitis should be managed conservatively and surgery avoided if at all possible in view of the poor healing potential of these patients. If bone denudation occurs, it should be covered with a dressing and antibiotics prescribed in conjunction with the physician responsible for the medical care.

Acute periodontal abscess

A periodontal abscess occurs when pus collects in the connective tissue wall of a pocket and is frequently seen in patients with periodontitis. The initial problem is managed by establishing drainage of this pus, so the first joint decision to be made by the operator and patient is whether this should be achieved by extracting the tooth.

If it is decided to attempt to save the tooth, initial drainage may be obtained by scaling and root debridement of the lesion. Should this not relieve the pressure then a fluctuant lesion can be incised at its most dependent point or by raising a small flap to expose the defect and allow effective debridement. Any local anaesthetic used should not be placed into the inflamed area.

The patient should be advised to use *hot salt water mouth rinses* during the healing period to encourage drainage. Once the lesion has settled, further root debridement or surgery may be required to encourage healing. This type of lesion will require careful, long-term follow-up to ensure that recurrence does not occur.

NON-SURGICAL MANAGEMENT OF THE ROOT SURFACE

A key factor in the non-surgical management of the root surface involved in an active periodontal lesion is the effective removal of root surface deposits. The acquired deposits that are found adhering to tooth surfaces include salivary pellicle, dental plaque, calculus and a variety of stains. Scaling is the procedure by which these deposits are removed from the tooth surface. Although the significance of salivary pellicle and its relationship to dental disease are unclear – it probably has a protective function – both dental plaque and calculus are associated with inflammatory periodontal disease. Scaling differs from root debridement in that the latter procedure consists of instrumentation not only to remove surface deposits, but also to smooth the root surface and remove a thin layer of cementum, thus reducing the endotoxin burden. Some authorities do not feel that effective scaling can be carried out subgingivally unless followed by root debridement. Root debridement may also be termed root cleaning or root planing. Both procedures need to be undertaken with prophylactic antibiotic cover in the patient at risk of infective endocarditis.

It is thought that root debridement reduces the amount of cementum-bound endotoxin to a biologically acceptable level and thus allows healing of the adjacent periodontal soft tissues. However, recent research has shown that endotoxin may be reduced to the level seen on healthy root surfaces by very light root cleaning, providing that the root surface in the pocket is instrumented in a thorough, systematic way. It may well be that the only difference between scaling, root cleaning and root debridement is the overall reduction in root surface contaminants and these have to be lower in some patients who have decreased resistance to the influence of dental plaque and its by-products. There are, of course, differences between the instruments used in scaling, which is often a supragingival procedure, and root debridement, which is always carried out in subgingival sites.

The three fundamentals which allow effective control of acquired tooth surface deposits are their detection, adequate removal and the prevention of recurrence.

Calculus deposits may be detected by visual and tactile methods. Visual detection can be aided by a stream of air directed at the gingival margin from the triple syringe, thus drying out supragingival calculus, which will lighten and appear chalky against the tooth surface. Subgingival calculus may appear as a dark ring often visible through the overlying gingiva, and deflecting the gingival margin with the air syringe will reveal these deposits directly (Fig. 5.2).

A variety of probes may be used to feel for calculus within the periodontal pocket and the two most useful are the World Health Organization 622 probe and the cross

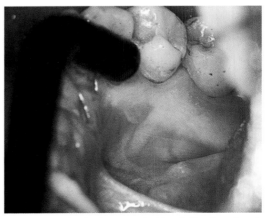

Fig. 5.2 Subgingival calculus revealed by deflecting the gingival margin with air from the triple syringe.

calculus probe (Fig. 5.3). Both of these probes are able to detect the roughness of calculus when they are run over the root surface and they will usually catch beneath the apical edge of the deposits.

Scaling instruments

All hand scaling instruments consist of three basic sections: the handle, the shank and the working tip (Fig. 5.4). Modern scaling and root debridement instruments have balanced grip handles, which give better distribution of weight and a large area of contact for the fingers. Often the handle is hollow which, besides reducing the weight, is claimed to give greater tactile discrimination. The shank is that part of the instrument connecting the working tip to the handle. The angle and length of the shank determine the access obtained by the tip to the tooth surface.

The working tip contains the cutting edge or edges which remove the acquired deposits. Scalers are classified according to the shape of the tip, and there are five basic designs: sickles, hoes, files, push (or chisel) and curettes.

Instrumentation guidelines

The successful practice of periodontics depends not only upon the ability to motivate patients in the daily use of effective oral hygiene, but also on the skilful use of instruments during scaling and root debridement (Box 5.7). For many patients these procedures may be undertaken without any form of anaesthesia. In some cases, however, especially when carrying out root debridement, some analgesia will be required. Often the use of a topical anaesthetic cream will suffice, particularly when at least 2 min is allowed to elapse between application and scaling, so that maximum anaesthesia is achieved. When topical anaesthesia is inadequate, block or infiltration anaesthesia will be required; some patients will need even this to be reinforced with inhalation relative analgesia.

The instrument should be held in the correct way, as this will determine the amount of control and thus the stability and effectiveness in use. There are three possible ways to hold a scaler:

- *Standard pen grip.* The instrument is held between the thumb and index finger and the medial part of the middle finger is used to control its movement. This grip is not commonly used (Fig. 5.5).

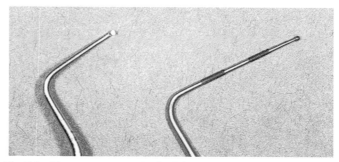

Fig. 5.3 The WHO 622 probe (right) and the cross calculus probe (left).

> **Box 5.7** Guidelines to improve the efficiency of instrumentation
>
> - Be comfortable; ensure that both you and the patient are seated comfortably
> - Position yourself for maximum visibility. If possible, work with the site in direct vision with a good, well-adjusted operating light
> - Follow an orderly sequence of instrument use and make sure they are laid out in the order of use before and after application. This will help to avoid the time wasted in searching for instruments on an untidy worktop
> - Use as few instruments as possible and know the function of each instrument
> - Maintain control of instruments during use, not only to prevent inefficient scaling but also to avoid traumatic damage caused by slipping – good finger rests are essential
> - Maintain a clear field by use of cotton wool rolls and aspiration. Both haemorrhage and saliva will require control
> - Ensure your instruments are sharp and serviceable
> - Use a slow, deliberate and methodical approach but do not confuse roughness with thoroughness
> - Always talk to the patient in a friendly and sympathetic manner not only on completion of the task but also during the procedure. This ensures that the patient adjusts to the procedure even if he or she found it difficult and time-consuming
> - Always clean up the patient before departure from the surgery. This is a courtesy appreciated by all patients
> - Use effective techniques as described in the text

- *Modified pen grasp.* This modification of the standard pen grip is used for many procedures. Instead of the side of the medial surface of the middle finger being

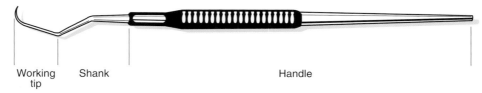

Working tip   Shank   Handle

Fig. 5.4 Component parts of a hand scaling instrument.

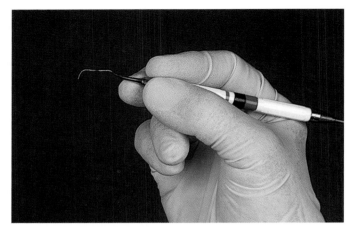

Fig. 5.5 The standard pen grip.

used, the terminal pad is utilised on the shank of the instrument, giving increased control (Fig. 5.6).

- *Palm grip.* On rare occasions during scaling, the palm grip is used to give more power, but at the price of decreased control and visibility. The handle of the instrument is held in the palm of the hand with the fingers grasping the handle and the thumb placed on the shank to control movement (Fig. 5.7).

As well as an appropriate instrument grip, it is also essential to establish a finger rest to ensure stability and lessen the possibility of slipping when applying pressure. The third or ring finger is the main source of the finger rest and the fourth or small finger is often used in addition (Fig. 5.8; see also Box 5.8).

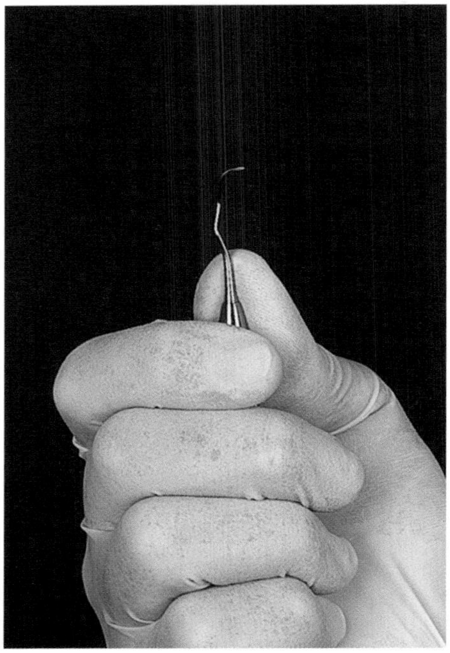

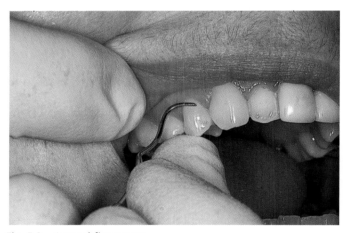

Fig. 5.7 The palm grip.

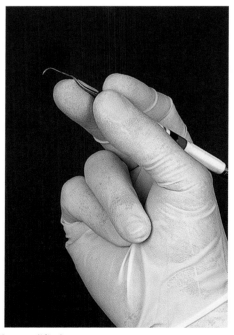

Fig. 5.6 The modified pen grasp.

Fig. 5.8 A good finger rest.

Box 5.8 Possible finger rests, in order of preference
<ul><li>On the tooth being scaled</li><li>On the adjacent teeth</li><li>On teeth in the same jaw, but some distance away</li><li>On teeth in the opposite jaw</li><li>On the external soft tissues overlying bone, e.g. on the patient's chin</li><li>In difficult cases, the fingers of the non-working hand may be rested and the finger rest placed on these</li></ul>

Most dental procedures, including scaling, are undertaken with the patient in a near horizontal position, which gives the seated operator the ability to perform most of the work using direct vision. However, working with a horizontal patient does require three important precautions to be taken:

* Eyesight protections must be provided.
* The airway must be watched carefully and protection in the form of a butterfly sponge used if necessary.
* Some method of moisture control will usually be required.

Hand instruments

The sickle scaler

This is a generic term which includes all scalers with a working tip projecting from the shank at approximately a right angle and having a sharp pointed end (Fig. 5.9). The method of use may be by pulling, such as the Jaquette no. 1, or rotation of the handle (Jaquette nos 2 and 3 and hygienist sickles). They have two cutting edges which are formed by the convergence of the top surface and the two lateral surfaces. The cross-section of the working tip is triangular in shape.

Uses. The sickle scaler is used mainly for supragingival scaling. It may also be used to scale or root plane just beneath to the gingival margin, provided the gingival pocket is fairly loose. This instrument should not be inserted too deeply into a pocket as the sharp tip will lacerate the soft tissue wall.

Method of use. The cutting edge is placed against the tooth if possible with a positive rake angle, but 90° is an acceptable compromise. It is then moved up the tooth with a pull stroke.

The periodontal hoe

This has a straight cutting edge on a short wide blade projecting at right angles from the shaft.

Uses. The hoe is the principal instrument for removing heavy deposits of subgingival calculus and for root debridement. It may also be used to remove heavy deposits of supragingival calculus. Hoes such as those in the MacFarlane set (Fig. 5.10) are suitable for scaling mesially, distally, facially and lingually, whilst modified hoes (Fig. 5.11) are useful for scaling and root debridement in furcations.

Method of use. The working tip is slid down the root surface over the calculus until the bottom edge is palpated. Pressure is applied to hold the hoe against the deposits and the shank against the crown. The instrument is then moved towards the crown to plane away the calculus.

The periodontal file

This file has a series of cutting edges set at right angles to the shank on a round, oval or rectangular base (Fig. 5.12).

Uses. The file is used for subgingival scaling and root debridement, but will not cope with heavy deposits which must be removed with a hoe scaler first.

Method of use. The instrument is slid down the root surface to the lower edge of the calculus. Pressure is applied to hold the cutting edges and the shank against the

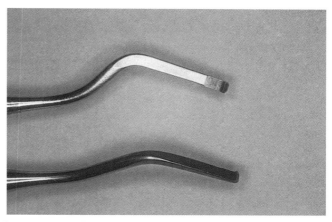

Fig. 5.10 Periodontal hoes: buccal/lingual (top) and mesial/distal (bottom).

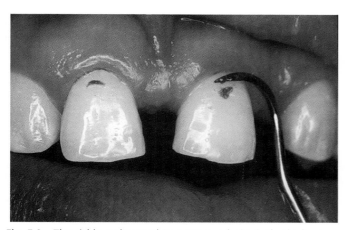

Fig. 5.9 The sickle scaler used to remove subgingival calculus in an accessible area.

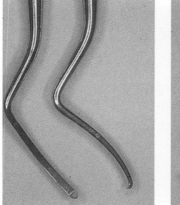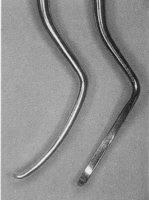

Fig. 5.11 A modified curette useful for scaling the roof of furcations.

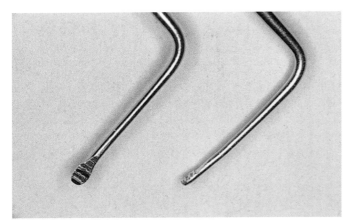

Fig. 5.12   Periodontal files.

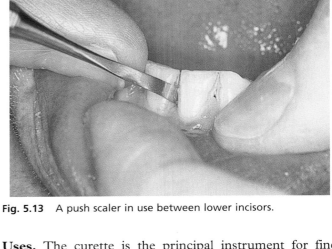

Fig. 5.13   A push scaler in use between lower incisors.

tooth, and the instrument is moved towards the crown, removing the deposits. The design of a file requires repeated strokes to be made whilst instrumenting an area.

The push scaler

The push, or chisel, scaler has a single straight bevelled cutting edge set at right angles to the shank (Fig. 5.13).

Uses. The push scaler is used to remove heavy deposits of supragingival calculus from the interdental surfaces of the anterior teeth. It should only be used when the embrasure spaces are open and sufficient space is present.

Method of use. The cutting edge is placed from the labial aspect against the tooth surface and pressure is applied to cleave away adhering calculus deposits.

The dental curette

This has a spoon-shaped working tip with a curved cutting edge. There are two principal types: the universal with two cutting edges, and the site-specific which has a cutting edge on one side only (Fig. 5.14).

Uses. The curette is the principal instrument for fine subgingival scaling, root debridement and root surface smoothing. It may also be used for curetting the soft tissue wall of the pocket, a procedure called subgingival curettage, which is no longer favoured in western Europe.

Method of use. The working tip is inserted into the base of the pocket and tilted to give a positive rake angle. It is used with a pull stroke towards the occlusal surface.

Powered scalers

Powered scalers are used in dentistry to remove plaque, calculus and stains from the teeth. The use of these automated scaling instruments makes the work of the operator much easier, and for many patients makes the scaling procedure more acceptable. They have a valuable role in the removal of gross deposits and flushing out the pocket. Ultrasonic scalers operate between 20 and 40 kilohertz (kHz) and sonic scalers in the 3–6 kHz range. Both types of instrument need a water spray, as heat is produced during use at the working tip and the cooling spray has the additional advantage of washing away dis-

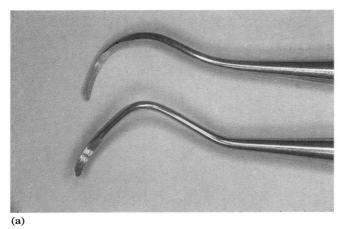

(a)

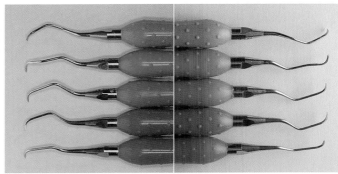

(b)

Fig. 5.14   (a) Universal dental curettes (Langer's). (b) Site-specific dental curettes (Gracey's).

lodged deposits, but also the distinct disadvantage of producing an aerosol. Box 5.9 provides a comparison between ultrasonic and sonic scalers.

Ultrasonic scaling instruments. These operate at frequencies above the level of human hearing, usually between 20 and 40 kHz. There are two different types available on the market: magnetostrictive and piezoelectronic.

Magnetostrictive types. These use a core or stack of magnetic material, usually a nickle alloy, which is acted upon by electrical windings in the handpiece producing an alternating magnetic flux. When the stack is magnetised, it contracts and as it is connected to the working tip this mechanical change is relayed to the tooth surface. The electronics of the unit changes the alternation of the magnetising current to an ultrasonic frequency, causing the tip to vibrate at a similar rate.

Piezoelectronic types. A piezoelectric material such as quartz will oscillate if an ultrasonic current is placed across it. This vibration is then transferred to the attached scaling tip.

Air or sonic scalers. Sonic scalers are operated by a pressurised air line usually connected to an air turbine. This air is passed over a reed or through an eccentric cam in the handpiece which then vibrates in the air flow. Sonic scalers operate at frequencies below that of the limit of hearing, typically in the 3–6 kHz range.

Method of action

The removal of calculus and other deposits by mechanical scaling instruments is achieved in three ways: mechanical abrading action, cavitational effects and acoustic microstreaming.

Mechanical abrading action. The action is a mixture of back-and-forth and circulatory movements and this mechanically abrades and chips away at the deposits on

---

Box 5.9 A comparison between ultrasonic and sonic scalers

Ultrasonic
- Electrically powered, tip vibration above 20 kHz
- Oscillatory pattern variable but often linear
- Cavitation occurs in water stream close to the tip
- Acoustic microstreaming occurs
- Not easily damped by loading
- Not all models are easy to sterilise

Sonic
- Air-powered, tip vibration between 3 and 6 kHz
- Oscillatory pattern usually circular or elliptical
- Cavitation not present
- Acoustic microstreaming occurs
- May be damped by excess loading
- All models are sterilisable

---

the root surface. A variety of differently shaped tips is available to achieve this result. There are differences in the oscillatory patterns of ultrasonic and sonic scalers. The ultrasonic has a higher energy output and is not easily damped by loading and is generally a linear action. The sonic scaler has a larger, usually circular and more coarse pattern of movement to compensate for the lower energy level and is more easily damped by high loading, although this may not be obvious to the operator. It is, however, easier to sterilise than the ultrasonic instrument.

Cavitational effects. These are usually seen with the ultrasonic scalers as the sonic variety do not generally have sufficient energy output at the tip to cause cavitation. All powered scalers are provided with a flow of cooling water directed at the tip to remove any heat caused by friction between the tip and the tooth surface. The water contains minute air bubbles which are expanded by the energy in the vibrating tip which causes them to have a negative internal pressure for a fraction of a second and then implode, releasing large shock waves. Such forces have been shown to remove plaque and calculus from the tooth surface. One of the side-effects of the water flow and cavitation is the generation of a large aerosol against which precautions should be taken.

Acoustic microstreaming. All powered scalers set up vigorous movements of the water around their tips and this is termed acoustic microstreaming. The large shear forces associated with this phenomenon assist in the removal of some of the tooth surface deposits and in the disruption of plaque colonies.

Both the cavitational and acoustic microstreaming effects produce an intense acoustic turbulence around the scaling tip. This has been shown to assist the root debridement process by scrubbing the root surface and disrupting associated bacteria.

Principles of use of powered scalers

Modern ultrasonic scalers are self-tuning and have a variable power control. The higher the power setting, the greater the vibration and the more likely it is for the patient to experience discomfort. In general, a low to medium setting should be used and this has the added advantage of reducing the risk of unwanted tooth surface damage. Studies have shown this to be just as effective for periodontal healing. The instrument should be positioned with the oscillating working tip almost in the long axis of the tooth with a very small rake angle. Light pressure should be applied and the tip kept constantly on the move with a light circulatory stroking action. The tip should not be held stationary in any one area for too long as this will cause excessive abrasion of the tooth in that area. Instrumentation should not be rushed and the surface should be checked from time to time for smoothness. This can be done with the tip without the power on.

Potential hazards of powered scalers

The most serious hazard from the operator's point of view is the considerable aerosol generated, especially by the ultrasonic machines. The operator should wear a good quality mask and protective spectacles, in addition to the usual gloves. The patient should be asked to rinse with an oral antiseptic such as chlorhexidine digluconate 0.2% for 1 min before the procedure, to reduce the oral flora, and high volume aspiration should be used to remove the remaining aerosol. In view of these problems, ultrasonic or sonic scalers should not be used with highly infectious patients. The tooth surface can be damaged by frictional heating if insufficient coolant is used and by abrasive scratching if the tip is incorrectly applied. Porcelain jacket crowns may be fractured by the tips and it is possible for a cement lute to be broken, so it is best to avoid contact with crown and bridgework when using powered scalers.

A potential danger exists with patients fitted with an electronic cardiac pacemaker. The ultrasonic scaler is known to emit a large electromagnetic field which may interfere with the older types of pacemaker, and it is wise to avoid its use with this category of patient. More modern pacemakers are shielded and compensated to reduce this risk but it would be unwise to test the effectiveness of this in the dental chair. The field of interference is small, of the order of 1 m, and is only likely to have an effect on the patient being treated. Sonic scalers do not operate electrically so they have no effect on pacemakers.

Older versions of ultrasonic scalers could not be effectively sterilised, as the stack containing the electrical windings could not be removed from the power cable. Recent models have removable and autoclavable stacks which reduce the risk of cross-infection.

Comparison of powered and hand instruments

The powered scaler is said to be quicker and easier for the operator and has been shown to reduce hand fatigue and strain. The water flow flushes out pockets and removes debris during scaling. Visibility may be improved by the washed field effect. It has been concluded by several researchers that the use of a powered scaler can produce a similar root finish to that achieved by a hand instrument, but this will obviously vary with the skill of the operator. A greater potential for damage exists, especially if the equipment is misused. Some patients will find instrumentation with powered scalers uncomfortable, especially if exposed cervical dentine is present. The lack of tactile sensation may also be a problem particularly if visibility is hampered by the water spray. The equipment is expensive and, like all powered items, prone to breakdown. Despite these drawbacks, it is generally agreed that their use is to be routinely recommended for most scaling and root debridement procedures.

Supragingival scaling

The removal of supragingival deposits of dental calculus is most efficiently achieved with an ultrasonic or sonic scaler. This should be applied gently to the tooth surface and moved with small overlapping or circular strokes to remove the deposits. If a powered scaler is not available, the patient cannot tolerate it, or the patient has a medical condition such as HIV infection which contraindicates the use of a powered scaler, the following hand instruments may be employed: a large excavator or cumine scaler will remove large accumulations of calculus; the push scaler can then be used between the lower incisor teeth to remove interdental deposits; a sickle or Jaquette scaler can be used on the lingual and interdental areas; and finally an appropriate hoe will remove facial and lingual calculus.

The removal of supragingival calculus is often combined with subgingival scaling.

Subgingival scaling

Ideally, supragingival scaling should be completed before subgingival scaling, as the presence of deposits on the crown of the tooth will hinder visibility and prevent the correct application of the instrument to the root.

Before activating the instrument, a series of exploratory strokes should be made to determine the location and topography of subgingival deposits. A scaling instrument or WHO probe is passed down the root surface to the base of the pocket. If any apparent obstruction is felt, the instrument is moved out from the root surface and gently extended apically to distinguish between a ledge of calculus and the junctional epithelium. As a general rule, calculus will feel hard and the junctional epithelium will be softer in consistency.

When the pocket and deposits have been mentally mapped out, scaling can commence. The best instrument to start with is the ultrasonic scaler. This will dislodge and flush out the larger deposits. Following this, a hoe scaler is used to continue the scaling, working round the site in a methodical, overlapping manner. Finally, dental curettes are used to remove fine deposits and leave a smooth root surface.

Following the scaling, the pocket should be flushed with the triple syringe or the spray from an ultrasonic scaler to remove any retained particles or microorganisms. The use of a 'through-flow' scaling tip, which delivers water into the site, is to be recommended.

Root debridement, root planing or root cleaning

Root debridement is indicated when, in the presence of good supragingival plaque control, and following the removal of all clinically detectable subgingival deposits, the activity of a periodontal pocket persists. The aims of root debridement are to remove a thin layer of endotoxin-laden cementum as well as all deposits of plaque and calculus. The root surface should be left clinically smooth. This will encourage resolution of inflammation and healing of the site.

If these aims are achieved then the root surface should be rendered biologically inert and the persistent periodontal lesion begin to resolve. For the majority of patients, local anaesthesia will be required for the teeth to be root-planed. In the maxilla this will require the use of infiltration techniques, but in the mandible, block anaesthesia together with a long buccal infiltration is necessary.

Instrumentation during root debridement is very similar to that used during subgingival scaling, but the technique is more exacting, although often there is no calculus to remove. It is again worthwhile to commence and finish with an ultrasonic scaler as there is some evidence of improved healing following its use. To permit the ultrasonic tip to reach the base of the pocket, the use of modern slimline scaling tips is essential.

The method of use of instruments also varies from scaling. The initial strokes should be made from the base of the pocket up the root surface with an overlapping technique as shown in Figure 5.15. This should be followed by a consolidating series of movements at 45° to the initial strokes. In this way the root surface is quartered by the instrument and the majority of the contaminated cementum removed. The pocket is then flushed with the water spray to remove loosened deposits. This may be achieved by using the ultrasonic scaler, provided care is taken not to further roughen the root surface following the hand smoothing. Finally the pocket is irrigated with an anti-plaque agent such as 0.2% chlorhexidine digluconate.

Contraindications to root debridement are poor patient motivation, teeth of a hopeless prognosis, severe dentinal sensitivity (which will be worsened by the procedure) and the presence of acute infection.

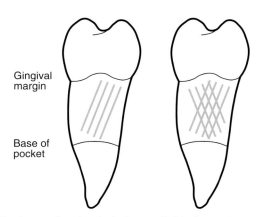

Fig. 5.15 An overlapping technique suitable for root debridement. (a) Initial overlapping strokes from base of pocket up to the enamel–cement junction; (b) secondary quartering strokes to complete surface instrumentation.

Gingival margin

Base of pocket

ANTIMICROBIAL ADJUNCTS IN PERIODONTAL THERAPY

When inflammatory periodontal diseases are present, effective removal of plaque deposits on a regular basis will usually return the inflamed tissues to health. Mechanical oral hygiene measures are sufficient to reverse early gingivitis provided that tissue swelling has not reached a level where subgingival plaque is protected from the cleaning aids, or calcified deposits hinder effective plaque removal. In these cases, additional scaling and polishing are also required.

However, it has been shown that oral hygiene does not eliminate inflammation in periodontitis where pocketing is present. Subgingival scaling, root debridement, local and systemic antimicrobials and surgery may all be required to render the root surface free from microbial deposits and permit healing. Current mechanical therapy aims at providing regular pocket debridement to eliminate most subgingival plaque and calculus, and so prevent the development of microbial complexes which may result in disease progression. A sustained reduction in the levels of pathogenic microorganisms occurs in periodontal pockets following this therapy. The results of clinical studies also support the value of regular maintenance care, and an appropriate interval for remotivation and plaque removal appears to be 3-monthly. However, oral hygiene practices may not be successful for the reasons given in Box 5.10. As a result chemical antimicrobials are often used as adjuncts in the management of inflammatory periodontal diseases.

Mouth rinses

Various chemicals have been used in the form of mouth rinses to assist in the treatment of inflammatory periodontal diseases. The influence of mouth rinses on the course of inflammatory periodontal diseases may be categorised as follows:

- They may have a bactericidal or bacteriostatic action, killing the organisms or preventing their multiplication.
- They may have anti-inflammatory actions, reducing the damage caused by the tissue response to plaque antigens.

> **Box 5.10   Reasons why mechanical oral hygiene practices may be unsuccessful**
>
> - They may be technically difficult for many patients to perform
> - They are very time-consuming to undertake effectively
> - They require a high level of motivation and habituation to be continued over a long time period
> - They are only effective at removing organisms from accessible tooth surfaces
> - They are unable to remove organisms in deep pockets

- They may alter the plaque environment by changing, for example, the acidity.

As a general rule, mouth rinses will act at either the plaque level or, to a very limited extent, at the tissue response level (Fig. 5.16). Despite these limitations, there are situations when the use of a mouth rinse is clearly indicated:

- when gingivitis does not respond to oral hygiene measures and good home care
- for patients with oral ulceration such as aphthae or herpetic lesions
- for patients suffering from oral mucosal conditions such as lichen planus and benign mucous membrane pemphigoid
- when jaws are fixed together such as following fractures or jaw surgery
- following periodontal surgery, to permit adequate healing when plaque control may be painful
- for very high-risk patients such as those who are immunocompromised, e.g. following renal, liver or heart transplants.

The general characteristics of mouth rinses are outlined in Box 5.11.

Chemicals in mouth rinses

The most effective anti-plaque mouth rinse at the present time is the bis-biguanide salt *chlorhexidine gluconate*, which has a broad antimicrobial spectrum and is active against both gram-positive and gram-negative bacteria. Another mouth rinse, in addition to chlorhexidine, which has been approved by the Council of Dental Therapeutics of the American Dental Association, is a *phenolic anti-plaque compound* with anti-inflammatory properties (Listerine). Research has shown that, although this formulation has less anti-plaque and antimicrobial activity than chlorhexidine, when used as a supplement to normal oral hygiene it has a similar effect in reducing the clinical gingivitis scores. In addition, phenolic anti-plaque compounds have been shown to have anti-inflammatory effects at subclinical concentrations.

| Box 5.11 | Characteristics of mouth rinses |

- Vary in their activity against microbial plaque
- Have differing retention times in the oral cavity (substantivity)
- Useful in the treatment of gingivitis
- Limited effect on periodontitis as they do not penetrate pockets to any significant extent
- Potential side-effects such as severe extrinsic tooth staining limit their usefulness
- Most effective when used following careful scaling and root debridement
- Retard the subsequent recolonisation of pockets following periodontal therapy and lead to a greater reduction of inflammation when used following root debridement

Amongst commercial dental companies there has been considerable interest in mouth rinses containing *cetylpyridinium chloride* (CPC). CPC in the laboratory has considerable bactericidal activity. However, the retention time or substantivity of CPC in the oral cavity is limited and therefore frequent use is required to provide any useful anti-plaque activity. These mouth rinses have a less unpleasant taste and fewer staining problems than experienced with chlorhexidine.

Another mouth rinse is 1% w/v *povidone-iodine*, a formulation which is claimed to overcome the very occasional mucosal sensitivity reactions that occur with the use of chlorhexidine. It should be noted that the prescribing information supplied by the manufacturer for this mouth rinse includes the possibility of mucosal irritation and hypersensitivity reactions, and its use is contraindicated in pregnant females and young children. Prolonged use is not recommended and it should not be used for more than 14 days.

Another chemical, *triclosan*, has proved to be very useful in toothpastes. When used as a mouth rinse combined with zinc salts or co-polymer, it has moderate substantivity and gives beneficial plaque reductions.

Chlorine dioxide-containing mouth rinses have been claimed to eliminate volatile sulphur compounds and thus reduce halitosis.

Potential problems of mouth rinses

There is a small risk when using any mouth rinse that the superficial signs of disease (e.g. redness, bleeding from the marginal gingiva) may lessen, but deeper activity in the pocket may extend, leading to insidious progression of periodontitis over a period of time. Dentists and patients should be aware of this possibility.

Two other features of mouth rinses that cause concern and which could damage the oral tissues are their alcohol (ethanol) content and the acidity levels (pH). Popular mouth rinses on sale in the UK have pH levels from 3.4 to 6.8, and alcohol levels from 0 to 27%. Ethanol in various

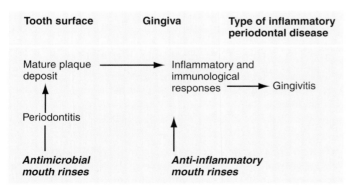

Fig. 5.16 The relationship between plaque deposits, host response and mouth rinses.

concentrations is used in many mouth rinses. Its main functions are to act both as a preservative and as a solvent, to stabilise and solubilise various flavouring and active ingredients in the mouth rinse. The pH of the rinse is usually a product of the total acid content countered by the buffering capacity of the other constituents. Recently, the adverse effects of acidic drinks on dental enamel have been documented and it is possible that acidic mouth rinses may have a similar effect.

Of concern is the fact that the concentration of alcohol in some mouth rinses equals or exceeds that in many alcoholic beverages and if used over a long term could be a contributory factor in oral cancer, but there is some disagreement over this. There is also the possibility that acute ethanol toxicity could occur following ingestion of large quantities of mouth rinse. The greater danger lies with ingestion by children, where only a small volume is needed to produce morbidity and mortality.

In response to their possible drawbacks, many manufacturers are taking steps to remove alcohol from their products and to ensure that any acidity is well buffered or that the pH is neutral.

Summary

It may be concluded that mouth rinses are beneficial for patients with gingivitis not responding to local mechanical treatment or with specific problems which prevent normal oral hygiene. For patients with periodontitis, their use is more limited, although the most effective time for using a mouth rinse is immediately following non-surgical or surgical periodontal therapy. However, as with any agent used in medical treatment, the dental practitioner should be aware of the potential disadvantages of the product, as well as the possible therapeutic gain (Box 5.12).

Box 5.12 Potential disadvantages and therapeutic gains resulting from the use of mouth rinses

Disadvantages
- Superficial reduction in inflammation, leading to loss of warning signs
- Reduction in efforts at mechanical plaque control
- Concern over alcohol content of some products
- Concern over acidity
- Problems of long-term use of chemicals
- Sensitivity to mouth rinse constituents in small numbers of subjects

Therapeutic gains
- Improved reduction in plaque levels
- Increased reduction of gingivitis
- Pleasant taste
- Plaque reduction in inaccessible areas or when conditions do not permit oral hygiene (e.g. with ulcerative conditions)
- Anti-caries effect of fluoride content

Subgingival antimicrobials

Local drug delivery has been advocated in the management of periodontitis, as an addition to mechanical subgingival debridement, in order to overcome the problem of delivering antimicrobials into periodontal pockets. In the UK, the following commercial subgingival antimicrobial systems are currently available:

- 2% minocycline gel (Dentomycin) – requires three or four applications every 2 weeks with no repetition within 6 months. It inhibits most periodontal pathogens but is rapidly cleared from pocket
- 25% metronidazole gel (Elyzol) – applied twice at 1-week intervals; this product has a slow-release base (biodegradable monoglyceride gel rich in mono-olein with sesame oil)
- 25% tetracycline hydrochloride in ethylene vinyl acetate co-polymer monofilament (Actisite) – this elastic cord is packed into the pocket and left for a 12-day period. Despite being very time-consuming to insert, Actisite has long retention and sustained release. There is, however, a subsequent need to remove the cord which is very bulky in the pocket
- 55% chlorhexidine gluconate in hydrolysed gelatine (Periochip) – this is based on a sustained-release device, which is a method of delivering the antimicrobial subgingivally over a prolonged period of time. It is very easy and quick to insert with minimum discomfort to the patient. The product is biodegradable so there is no need to remove it, and it has been shown to have effective activity over a 10-day period.

Subgingival irrigation

Another method of local drug delivery is by the use of pulsed oral irrigation systems, which are supplied with modified tips to allow professional subgingival irrigation in the surgery.

At home, local antimicrobial delivery may be achieved by irrigation using a blunt syringe or a pulsed oral irrigator. However, the syringing of periodontal pockets can be a time-consuming procedure and many patients will not possess a sufficient degree of manual dexterity to undertake effective local drug delivery. Many of the pockets may be in posterior areas and are not very accessible. Concern has also been expressed about the high pressures that can be exerted using subgingival irrigation with syringes and blunt needles. However, it has been shown that, unlike syringe irrigation, most pulsed oral irrigators produce low pressures which are tolerated by the tissues. In addition, the use of pulsed irrigation may allow lower concentrations of chemicals to be used. However, the amount of the antibacterial agent delivered to the site is the critical factor in achieving its maximum effect. For these reasons, the use of a pulsed oral irrigator has been suggested as a practical alternative to syringing.

Pulsed oral irrigation. Irrigation is achieved by the action of a small motor which activates a pump. Water is fed to the pump from a reservoir and is emitted via a handpiece into which a variety of tips can be fitted. These permit both supra- and subgingival irrigation to be undertaken. There are minor differences between the various makes, some having pressure-limiting systems to prevent excess pressure being applied whilst maintaining the pulse rate. Some machines are supplied with a range of supra- and subgingival applicators for home and surgery use.

Clinical effects. Studies have shown that pulsed oral irrigation after scaling and root debridement may further reduce plaque levels, bleeding index and pocket depths, especially when combined with an antimicrobial. With regard to the most efficacious chemical for use with such a system, chlorhexidine appears to be the agent of choice, although there is no agreement as to the most appropriate concentration. Indeed, there is considerable disagreement as to the activity of chlorhexidine in periodontal pockets. Experience in our clinics suggests that a 0.05% concentration in an oral irrigator is sufficient to improve most patients with significant periodontitis, although many other chemicals have also been shown to improve clinical parameters.

There is general agreement in the literature that pulsed oral irrigation reduces gingivitis and improves the efficiency of antimicrobial chemicals. However, when the efficacy of scaling and root debridement is compared with subgingival irrigation, the former is the most effective. Therefore, pulsed irrigation is only useful as an adjunct to standard therapy in selected patients.

In contrast, when there are problematic lesions, e.g. deep pockets, furcations, complex fixed oral appliances or refractory periodontitis not responding to standard therapy, pulsed irrigation with a suitable chemical may enable these patients to improve their periodontal healing further. It is unrealistic to expect all patients with periodontitis whose pockets exceed 3 mm – and which therefore are not accessible to the toothbrush or interdental aids – to constantly prevent colonisation with disease-associated periodontopathic organisms. Where the will and ability exist to carry out meticulous mechanical oral hygiene measures, these are at best crude and inefficient means of removing organisms from the periodontal tissues. It must therefore be concluded that pulsed oral irrigation has potential in the management of inflammatory periodontal diseases.

Safety. High irrigation pressures may propel organisms into the gingival tissues and both abscesses and bacteraemias have been reported. However, studies have shown that, provided the irrigation pressure does not exceed 480 kPA, no soft tissue injuries occur. It has been shown that a pulsed oral irrigator exerts a pressure that is tolerated by the tissues.

When using an apparatus that combines water with an electrical supply, the issue of electrical safety must also be addressed and it is preferable that a safety outlet, such as a razor socket, be used. On no account should a trailing cable be taken into the bathroom.

6 Occlusion

INTRODUCTION

Restorative dentistry is concerned with the restoration of the teeth. It is easy to consider a failing tooth as a single entity but it must always be remembered that that tooth is only one component of a functioning unit composed of:

1. the teeth and all their supporting tissues
2. the temporomandibular joints (TMJs) and their associated structures
3. the neuromusculature.

The study of occlusion involves the consideration of how these individual components interrelate and function as a whole. It should be recognised from the start that the human dentition, whilst an anatomical structure, is subject to the influences of human emotion and psychology. The interrelationship is unique to each individual. The wide variation in the ability of each individual to adapt to apparent discrepancies from the precise mechanical principles can give rise to a wide range of apparently confusing symptoms.

To understand how this system functions a thorough knowledge of the anatomy of these components and their interrelationships is required.

BASIC DEFINITIONS

The mandible is unique in that it exists as a single bone crossing the midline, with symmetrical articulating components at each end. This, in combination with the unique nature of these articulating components, leads to a complicated three dimensional geometry of movement. Secondary to the primary articulation of the TMJs is the articulation of the upper and lower teeth, and it is with this secondary articulation that the restorative dentist is involved. The relationship of the maxillary and mandibular teeth when in contact is called the *occlusal relationship* and the teeth are said to be in *occlusion*. The term occlusion defines no precise or specific tooth contact nor does it infer any particular quality of interarch contact, it defines nothing more than the existence of a state of interarch tooth contact. The teeth out of contact are said to be in *disclusion*.

Occlusal relationships may be classified not only by the quality of the relationship but also by spatial parameters. The student is referred to an orthodontic text for descriptions of the generally accepted orthodontic classifications. It should be noted, however, that the orthodontic classifications consider occlusal relation in the absence of functional movement and as such should be considered as classification of *static occlusion*.

ANATOMICAL COMPONENTS

The muscles of mastication

The muscles that give rise to mandibular movement are classified as the muscles of mastication (Table 6.1). The principal muscles of mastication comprise:

- temporalis
- masseter
- medial and lateral pterygoid muscles.

47

Table 6.1 Description of movements of muscles of mastication

Muscle	Principal Movement
Temporalis	Closes mouth
Masseter	Closes mouth Some distal movement of mandible
Medial pterygoid	Closes mouth
Lateral pterygoid	Two muscles together: Pulls mandible down and forward Separately: Moves the mandible laterally

The accessory muscles of mastication include the suprahyoid and infrahyoid muscles, most notably the digastric muscles.

The temporalis muscle originates from the temporal fossa of the temporal bone and the deep surface of the temporal fascia. The muscle fibres converge to form a tendinous attachment, passing deep to the zygomatic arch, and insert into the medial surface, apex and anterior border of the coronoid process of the mandible. Its function is to elevate the mandible and its action is to close the jaws. The posterior portion is said to exert a retracting action upon the mandible.

The masseter muscle consists of two heads, the superficial and the deep. The heads of both portions of the muscle arise from the lower border of the zygomatic arch. The superficial head inserts into the lateral surface of the ramus of the mandible; the deep head inserts into the lateral surface of the coronoid process and the superior half of the ramus. The masseter muscle's function is principally elevation and its action is to close the jaws.

The medial pterygoid muscle arises principally from the medial surface of the lateral pterygoid plate and the pyramidal process of the palatine bone adjoining the maxilla. The fibres pass laterally, posteriorly, and inferiorly, and insert into the posterior and inferior part of the medial surface of the ramus and angle of the mandible. When acting together, the medial pterygoids draw the mandible upwards. Acting alone, they draw the mandible laterally.

The lateral pterygoid muscle is a short thick muscle extending horizontally between the infratemporal fossa and the condyle of the mandible. This muscle is said to comprise two functional units, the superior and inferior heads. Both heads arise principally from the pterygoid plate of the greater wing of the sphenoid bone. The superior and medial fibres of the superior head are inserted into the anterior aspect of the articular disc. The inferior head inserts into the anterior aspect of the condyle and condylar head. Acting together these muscles pull the mandible downward and forward; separately the lateral pterygoid draws the mandible laterally. The medial and lateral pterygoid muscles are surprisingly powerful for their relative sizes and they can exert much force on the mandible during functional and parafunctional activity.

Temporomandibular joint

It is the unique anatomy of the temporomandibular joint (TMJ) that provides the range and extent of the movement of the mandible. The TMJ is a freely movable joint, a diarthrosis. It is capable of undergoing two uniquely different types of movement, a hinging movement in one plane and a gliding movement or translation (Box 6.1). It functions therefore as a hinged sliding joint and is the only joint in the human body in which the articulating bone can freely translate away from and toward its resting articular position. The capacity for these individual movements arises from its unique anatomy and therefore a thorough knowledge of the anatomy and dynamics of the human TMJ is critical to an understanding of the functional dynamics of the human dentition.

The TMJ is the principal articulation of the mandible to the cranium. Functional contact of the maxillary and mandibular teeth can be said to constitute a secondary articulation. In the ideal rest position the condylar head of the mandible, separated by the interarticular disc or meniscus, articulates with the posterior aspect of the articular tubercle of the temporal bone, the articular eminence. The joint is enclosed within a ligamentous capsule that in combination with other ligaments including the temporomandibular, sphenomandibular and stylomandibular ligaments limits the range of motion of the joint.

The TMJ is divided into two compartments by the presence of the interarticular disc (meniscus): the superior and inferior joint spaces. These joint spaces are lined by synovial membrane and contain synovial fluid that in a healthy individual lubricates the joint. The disc is biconcave in shape. The superior surface is saddle shaped, being concave anteroposteriorly and slightly convex mediolaterally to mirror the posterior surface of the articular eminence. The inferior surface is concave in both directions and is adapted to the articular surface of the condyle. The biconcave nature of the disc results in it being thinnest at its most central point. The disc is

Box 6.1 Movements within the temporomandibular joint

Upper joint space	Sliding movement (translation)
Lower joint space	Hinging movement (rotation)

attached to the medial and lateral heads of the condyle and as such the disc sits on the condyle like a cap.

BASIC MANDIBULAR MOVEMENTS

From the standpoint of mandibular movement, consideration of each muscle group in isolation can be misleading. It is important to recognise that these muscle groups must function as a coordinated and balanced whole. As such these muscles exhibit a complex dynamic interrelationship of contraction and relaxation. Not only may the mandible be elevated to close the mouth, but also lateral excursive, protrusive and retrusive movement may occur uniquely in one joint or in combination, in both joints. As a result there is usually a combination of groups of muscles functioning simultaneously to effect mandibular movement.

As stated the muscles of mastication provide the motive force for mandibular movement. Contraction of the lateral pterygoid muscles will result in both condyle-disc assemblies being pulled anteroinferiorly down the articular eminence. The movement occurs within the superior joint space and the mandible is said to translate. The hinging motion of the joint occurs within the inferior joint space, the meniscus remains static and the condyle rotates below it. In the absence of movement in the superior joint space the mandible will arc about a horizontal axis of rotation passing through the centres of rotation of each joint (terminal *hinge axis*).

Rotation of the mandible about a vertical axis through a single condyle occurs when the contralateral condyle translates anteriorly, inferiorly and medially down its associated articular eminence. The mandible is said to make a *lateral excursion* to the *working side*; the contralateral side is termed the *non-working side*. The condyle on the working side is termed the *rotating condyle* and the condyle on the non-working side is termed the *orbiting condyle* (Fig. 6.1). Applying this terminology, if the mandible moves to the left side the mandible is said to have undergone a left lateral excursion; the left condyle is said to be the rotating condyle and the right condyle is said to be the orbiting condyle; the working side is on the left and the non-working side is on the right. Some authorities alternatively term the working side the *non-balancing side* or *rotating side*. Similarly the non-working side is alternatively termed the *balancing side* or *orbiting side*.

BORDER MOVEMENTS

The extreme range of both lateral and vertical movement of the mandible is constrained by the ligamentous attachments of the TMJs and therefore the mandibular movements occur within definable boundaries. These boundaries constitute an envelope of motion. The movements of the mandible along the extreme boundaries of the envelope

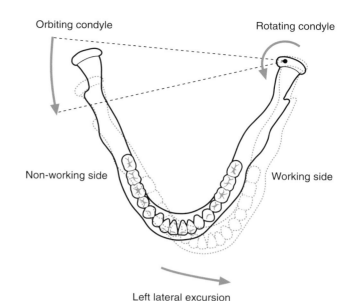

Fig. 6.1 Movement of the mandible showing the working and non-working sides. There are rotating and orbiting condyles.

of motion are termed the *border movements*. As such the anatomy of the joint and muscles gives rise to an extreme range of movements, i.e. there is a limit to how wide the mouth can open, how far forward it can move and to the left and right. The three-dimensional nature of mandibular movement, for the purposes of analysis, can be considered in the horizontal and sagittal planes.

Next we will consider the border movements of the mandible in the horizontal plane and the relationship of the TMJ function to posterior tooth morphology.

In the absence of tooth contact an arbitrary fixed point associated with the mandible, such as the contact point between the lower central incisors being on the midline of the mandible, will trace a reproducible pattern, unique to the anatomical constraints of the individual's TM joints. The outline of this tracing varies only in relation to the geometric relation of the fixed point to the joints. As suggested if the tracing is made from a point on the midline of the horizontal plane the resultant tracing, in an ideal healthy individual, will be symmetrical about the midline and is commonly termed a *gothic arch tracing*, as its outline is reminiscent of its architectural namesake (Fig. 6.2).

Likewise selected points displaced from the midline will trace similar arch-like tracings which will appear distorted and asymmetrical.

The occlusal surfaces of the adult permanent teeth are characterised by the distribution of cusps and fossae. It is sufficient to state at this level that the lower first permanent molar has five cusps, three buccal and two lingual, separated by a fossa pattern determined by the cuspal distribution. The cusp tips of the maxillary teeth may be considered to be fixed in space in relation to the occlusal surfaces of the opposing moving mandibular teeth. It can be appreciated that the imaginary tracings

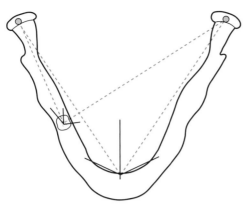

Fig. 6.2 Lateral movements of the mandible traced at the midline form a symmetrical 'gothic arch tracing'. The tracing created in the region of the lower molar coincides with the cusp–fossae lines of the occlusal morphology.

scribed by the maxillary cusp tips on the occlusal surfaces of the functioning mandibular teeth must coincide with the anatomical fossae patterns in order to avoid functional interferences. As can be observed in Figure 6.3, this tracing coincides with the anatomical distribution of the cusps and fossae of the posterior teeth.

The cusp–fossae distribution of the posterior occlusal surfaces is directly related to the functional anatomy of the TM joints.

Border movements in the sagittal plane

The TMJ confers upon the mandible the fundamental movements of rotation and translation. In considering the functional anatomy of the TM joints it has been established that in the absence of movement in the

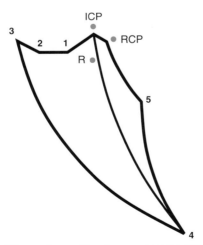

Fig. 6.3 Posselt's envelope of border movements. RCP, retruded contact position; ICP, intercuspal position; RCP → 5, rotational opening about the terminal hinge axis; 4, maximal opening; RCP → ICP, slide down deflective contact; ICP → 1 → 2 → 3, protrusive guidance; 3, maximum protrusion; 4 → ICP, path of habitual closure; R, rest position.

superior joint space, pure rotational movement of the mandible will occur about a horizontal axis passing through both condylar heads. When, in the absence of any TM joint pathology and masticatory muscle dysfunction, both condylar heads are in their most stable superior position the axis of rotation in a relaxed healthy individual with the teeth just apart is termed the *terminal hinge axis*.

The same anatomical constraints apply in the vertical dimension as has been described in the horizontal dimension, in that the extreme range of vertical movement is constrained by the ligamentous attachments of the TM joints. The border movements of the mandible in the mid-sagittal plane were first described by Posselt. In the same way that an arbitrary fixed point on the midline of the mandible will trace a horizontal outline termed a gothic arch tracing the same point, in the vertical plane will trace an outline termed *Posselt's envelope*. The point of origin of the tracing coincides with the terminal hinge axis. Initial opening is purely rotational. As the degree of opening approximates 20–25 mm, the condyle-disc assemblies begin to translate down the articular eminentiae; simultaneously, continued rotation of the condyles occurs until the mandible reaches *maximal opening*. Pure rotational movement from maximal opening to the first point of contact of the teeth establishes *maximal protrusion*. Movement back to the terminal hinge axis is influenced by the occluding surfaces of the teeth occurring principally as translation of the condyle-disc assemblies. However, some rotation of the condyles will occur to accommodate the degree of vertical overlap of the dental arches.

The border movements in both the vertical and horizontal planes can only be reliably reproduced with conscious effort or guidance from another person. *Free movements* of the mandible may describe an infinite number of patterns that resemble, but are not identical to, one another. Free movements must occur within the boundaries of the envelope of function. An individual's *habitual path* of opening and closing is a free movement, the closing end point being termed the *intercuspal position* (ICP). Intercuspal position is alternatively termed *centric occlusion*. In the intercuspal position there is maximal stable contact between the occluding surfaces of both upper and lower teeth.

RESTING ARTICULAR POSITION OF THE MANDIBLE

As stated the TMJ is the only joint in the human body in which the articulating bone can freely translate away from and toward its resting articular position. This has led to some confusion and debate as to the nature of the resting position of the joint. However, it is important from a diagnostic and therapeutic point of view to establish the nature of the resting position of the TMJ.

Intercuspal position is the occlusal relationship of the mandible to the maxilla when maximal stable intercuspation of the teeth occurs. By virtue of the anatomical fixed relationship of the condyles to the mandibular teeth the rest position of the condyles in intercuspal position is directly related to the nature and quality of the teeth. Intercuspal position is determined entirely by the position and morphology of the teeth; however, interventive dental care can, and readily does, alter the position and morphology of the teeth and as such can change or influence the resting position of the condyles.

In the absence of any dental influence the resting position of the condyles is determined by the anatomical and physiological nature of the TM joints and masticatory musculature. Under these criteria the head of the condyle appears to be accommodated in a superior position within the glenoid fossa; as a result there has existed historically a common misconception that at rest the condyle articulates superiorly. It would be reasonable to reach this conclusion if one's observations were based on assessment of tomographic radiographs of the TMJ, experience of dry specimens and the perceived wisdom of the time. Observations such as assessment of cadaver specimens, MRI images of functioning joints in healthy individuals and histological observation of the joint components provide a more rational assessment of the condylar articulation. The condylar head at rest is accommodated in a superior position within the glenoid fossa; however, the condyle articulates with the posterior aspect of the articular eminence.

When this relationship occurs the mandible is said to be in the *retruded position* (RP). This position can therefore be defined as that relation of the mandible to the cranium that occurs when the condyles are on the articular discs and located at their mid-most, most superior position on the posterior aspect of the articular eminentiae. The RP position is alternatively termed *centric relation position* (CR) and the condyles are said to be in *centric relation*.

Some authorities consider the use of the expression 'centric' potentially misleading, favouring the use of the term 'retruded'. They consider that centric relation and centric occlusion may be easily confused as a result of their similarity. They also consider that 'centric' implies centricity of the condyles in their fossae, centricity of the midline of the mandible with the midline of the face, or centricity of the cusps within the fossae of the opposing teeth, none of which may be the case. Whilst accepting the rationality of this premise, it can be argued that the use of the expression 'retruded' may give rise to at least a similar potential for misunderstanding and inappropriate technique. It cannot be emphasised enough that the RP is not the most retruded, distal or posterior position the mandible can obtain. The condyles can by means of inappropriate manipulation, especially in a less than healthy individual, be forced posteriorly.

The RP should be an unstrained and comfortable position in which the condyles are allowed to adopt their superior-anterior articulation. When the condyles are in the rest position their horizontal axis of rotation is termed the terminal hinge axis. In the absence of TMJ pathology and masticatory muscle dysfunction, the RP and associated terminal hinge axis are reproducible fixed anatomical landmarks from which accurate geometric measurements may be established. During the initial pure rotational border movement the condyles remain in the RP with the consequence that this position can occur over a limited range of mandibular opening, the resultant arc of movement being termed the *retruded arc of closure*. The mandibular position at the occlusal end point of the retruded arc of closure is termed the *retruded contact position* (RCP). Retruded contact position is alternatively termed *centric relation contact position* (CRCP).

The great majority of individuals do not exhibit perfect coincidence between RP and ICP. The relationship of the RCP to ICP is influenced by the *deflective contact*. The deflective contact may be defined as an occlusal interference the presence of which prohibits RCP–ICP coincidence. The teeth must therefore slide down or over the deflective contact to establish ICP. Posselt reported that 90% of individuals have an RCP to ICP movement of 1.25 ± 1 mm. Some authorities alternatively term the deflective contact the *premature contact*. The term premature contact should not be used in relation to the natural dentition and is more appropriate to the artificial dentition. With complete dentures, there is no natural intercuspal position, and ICP and RCP are made to coincide. The patient learns, subconsciously, to close into maximal intercuspation. When, as a result of inaccurate occlusal registration, the ICP and RCP of the complete dentures do not coincide, the patient may slide into maximal intercuspation or alternatively the dentures may move. This is known as premature contact and is clearly unsatisfactory. The artificial teeth do not have a periodontal proprioceptive system, and so the position of an artificial ICP cannot readily be detected. With a natural dentition the ICP is well recognised by the neuromuscular mechanism and the mandible closes habitually into ICP in the majority of involuntary closing movements. It may not be so in the dental chair when the mandible is brought under voluntary rather than involuntary control. In these circumstances, even if the first contact appears to be a premature contact, this should not be assumed to be the normal pattern of closure, but only the result of the patient concentrating on a movement that is usually entirely automatic. For these reasons the term premature contact should be avoided in relation to the dentate patient.

OCCLUSAL INTERFERENCES AND OCCLUSAL HARMONY

The deflective contact has been presented as an example of an occlusal interference. An occlusal interference may be defined as any occlusal contact that gives rise to disharmony in the free gliding movements of the mandible whilst it maintains occlusion with the maxilla. In considering the horizontal border movements of the mandible, it was established that in an ideal occlusal relationship the cusps of the functioning lower first permanent molar can pass the occluding cusps of the opposing maxillary molar harmoniously only if the fossae pattern of the lower molar is in harmony with the functional anatomy of the TM joints. If the cusp–fossae pattern is altered, for example by tooth migration, over-eruption or inappropriate restoration, the functioning cusps will collide, the resultant contact being described as an occlusal interference.

It has been previously stated that the majority of individuals exhibit some degree of occlusal interference to which they adapt satisfactorily with no significant problems. Indeed normal occlusion can be described as a malocclusion in which the requirements of function and aesthetics are satisfied but the individual has adapted satisfactorily to minor occlusal interferences. Occlusal interferences are only considered significant if they are associated with a degenerative or pathological condition, such as tooth fracture, mobility or excessive wear. It is generally accepted that an individual's ability to adapt to the presence of occlusal interferences is strongly influenced by their emotional and psychological state.

An occlusal contact on the non-working side that causes either disclusion of the teeth on the working side or displacement or pathology of the non-working side tooth is termed a non-working interference. An occlusal contact on the working side that disrupts the smooth harmonious movement of the functioning tooth contacts is termed a working interference.

CONCEPT OF MUTUAL PROTECTION

A theory of occlusal harmony in relation to the border movements of the mandible has been considered. However, an individual's normal range of function occurs within the envelope of motion in the form of free movements. To provide for harmony of the infinite number of free movements, the posterior teeth would have to be effectively cuspless. Indeed some individuals present with extreme tooth wear, the consequence of which is that the cusps of the posterior teeth have been obliterated. In view of these observations, to allow for the harmonious functioning of cusps some other feature of the occlusal relationship must confer some element of protection.

The TM joints, musculature and teeth can from the standpoint of mechanics be considered as a lever system (Fig. 6.4). The joints constitute the fulcrum, the musculature the applied force and the teeth the load. The masticatory muscles as a whole insert onto the ramus of the mandible and its associated structures and the teeth lie anterior to the musculature. As the fulcrum is the joint this distribution of force and load constitutes a class III lever.

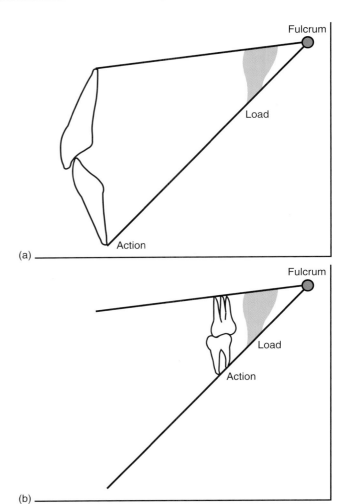

Fig. 6.4 A class III lever as related to the temporomandibular joints, musculature and teeth. Posterior teeth positioned closer to the applied load (musculature) are subjected to greater axial force than corresponding anterior teeth.

The mechanical advantage of such a distribution is inversely proportional to the distance of the load to the force. The anterior teeth will be subject to fewer loads per unit force than the posterior teeth. The posterior teeth therefore must be able to withstand substantial vertical load. Anterior teeth are subjected to fewer loads both vertically and laterally relative to the posterior teeth. The inclined overlapping occluding surfaces of the anterior teeth do not readily withstand vertical load but are ideally suited to distributing lateral load. The long single roots of the anterior teeth further aids in withstanding lateral loads whereas the multiple rooted nature of the posterior teeth aids in withstanding vertical load. The nature of the anterior teeth confers upon them the ability to protect the posterior teeth from the potentially damaging effects of lateral interferences by providing a discluding influence. This relationship between anterior and posterior teeth is termed *mutual protection*. The posterior teeth provide posterior stops to closure of the mandible and the anterior teeth provide a disclusive influence, which causes the posterior teeth to disclude on lateral excursions of the mandible thereby protecting them from lateral contact. Consideration of the mechanics suggests that the most appropriate tooth to provide the anterior disclusive influence would be the most anteriorly placed teeth in the arches, the incisors, this being termed *incisal guidance*. The canine teeth are commonly the most substantial of the anterior teeth and as such particularly well suited to withstand the associated lateral load. Their position lateral in the anterior arch is well suited to provide the anterior disclusive influence. The guiding influence provided by the canine teeth is termed *canine guidance* (Fig. 6.5).

If the guiding influence is not specific to the incisors or the canines but distributed between them the term *shared* or *group anterior guidance* may be applied. The capacity for the teeth to withstand load is dependent on such factors as their periodontal status and root integrity. A simple rule of thumb in establishing the therapeutic quality of the anterior guidance is to place it on the healthiest anterior teeth capable of withstanding lateral load. In some cases the quality and distribution of the anterior teeth requires that the discluding influence be shared with posterior tooth cusps. The teeth are then said to be in *group function* (Fig. 6.6).

It is most important in establishing group function that the lateral load is distributed evenly and simultaneously over all the teeth involved. Failure to do so will only potentially introduce lateral interferences.

COMPLETE REMOVABLE PROSTHETIC CONSIDERATIONS

As has been alluded to in consideration of the term premature contact, complete removable dentures give rise to a range of unique occlusal criteria. The lack of periodontal support leads to both a modified and diminished proprioceptive awareness and reduced stability. In the case of complete dentures there is no natural ICP and ICP and RCP are made to coincide. Adequately extended dentures,

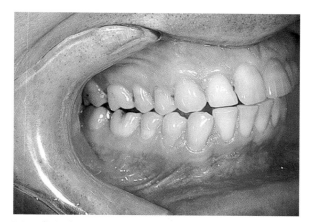
Fig. 6.6 Clinical example of group function.

constructed to ICP–RCP coincidence, will provide good stops to vertical closure. However, if the tooth alignment is constructed to the criteria of mutual protection the resultant anterior guidance will tend to compromise the stability and retention of the denture bases. With a view to improving the stability, the occlusal relation of complete dentures is constructed to the criteria of *bilateral occlusal balance* (Fig. 6.7).

The prerequisites of *occlusal balance* are ICP–RCP coincidence; on the working side the buccal inclines of the maxillary palatal cusps are set in even group function with the lingual inclines of the mandibular buccal cusps. Simultaneous with the working side contacts, on the non-working side the palatal inclines of the maxillary buccal cusps are set in even group function with the buccal inclines of the mandibular buccal cusps. In the protrusive excursion the incisal edges of the maxillary six anteriors are set in even group function with the incisal edges of the mandibular eight anterior teeth. All the posterior teeth have balancing functional contact simultaneously with the anterior teeth.

The angle of the protrusive anterior guidance is normally less than the angle of the protrusive path made by the condyles passing down the articular eminentiae. In order to establish protrusive bilateral balanced occlusion the angles of the cusp inclines of the more anterior posterior teeth must be set shallow relative to the most posterior teeth, and the inclines of the cusps must get steeper as they are set more posteriorly. Commercial denture teeth are constructed to a prescribed single cusp angle. In order to establish a graduated cusp incline the denture teeth must be set on an anteroposterior curve termed the *compensating curve of Spee*.

OCCLUSAL FUNCTION AS AN AETIOLOGICAL FACTOR IN DENTAL PAIN

Individuals do not normally make prolonged occlusal contacts during normal functional activity. During eating,

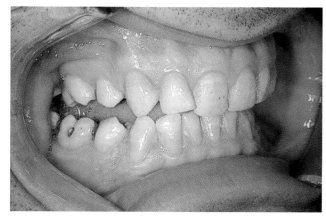
Fig. 6.5 Clinical example of canine guidance.

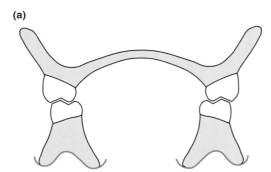

Occlusal balance in complete dentures – the teeth are meeting together bilaterally at rest

(b)

Working side   Balancing side

Direction of movement of mandible

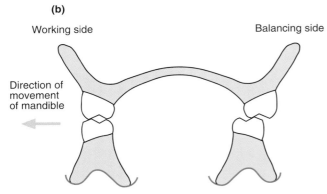

Occlusal balance in complete dentures – the teeth are meeting together bilaterally during movement of the mandible without any cuspal interference

Fig. 6.7 (a) Occlusal balance in complete dentures: the teeth are meeting together bilaterally at rest. (b) Occlusal balance in complete dentures: the teeth are meeting together bilaterally during movement of the mandible without any cuspal interference.

speech and at rest the teeth only make contact for comparatively short periods, applying relatively moderate force. Abnormally forceful prolonged occlusal function is termed *parafunction* and is commonly an expression of masticatory muscle hyperactivity. The prolonged forceful nature of parafunctional activity gives rise to a considerable increase in the load applied to the occluding teeth. Such increased loading may give rise to a range of signs and symptoms including cracking of the teeth which may be excessive enough as to give rise to pulpal inflammation with resultant symptoms of pain. In extreme cases catastrophic failure of a tooth may occur, presenting as cuspal fracture or more severe root fracture. Parafunctional activity is commonly associated with abnormally high rates of tooth wear, especially in individuals with an unusually raised acidic dietary component such as fruit juices or carbonated drinks. Such tooth wear may present with symptoms of pain and sensitivity.

Any clinical procedure that seeks to modify intentionally or that unintentionally changes the occluding surfaces of the teeth may potentially influence the intercuspal position. Humans possess a unique capacity for cognitive thought and memory and as such are subject to the influence of hindsight. Fortunately the majority of individuals are able to adapt to minor changes in their occlusal relationships with no specific or long-term disadvantages. This capacity, however, should not be considered as an excuse for poor clinical practice; clinical procedures should have as their goal a stable harmonious occlusal interrelationship which avoids the introduction of potentially harmful contacts and interferences. The cerebral higher centres influence an individual's neuromuscular feedback and proprioceptive capacity. Therefore, the individual's capacity for adaption to change may be heavily influenced by their mood and psychological state. Relatively minor changes to the occlusal morphology, such as the provision of a new crown, which the patient rationally perceives as being a specific physical change, may expose an incapacity for that particular individual to adapt within normal limits to such change. Signs and symptoms, the primary aetiology of which the patient perceives to be changes in occlusal form or relationship, should more correctly be considered secondary to the patient's primary underlying altered psychological state. A classic example of this is the group of conditions collectively termed temporomandibular disorder (TMD). Historically, it has been held that the presence of a deflective contact and or occlusal interferences may give rise to masticatory muscle hyperactivity leading to the pain and symptoms of TMD. In reality there is very little well-constructed, reproducible research data to support this hypothesis. Indeed the reverse argument is more tenable. Changes in the patient's mood or psychological state, as a result of stress and specific life events, alter the capacity to tolerate or adapt to occlusal discrepancies. Through the capacity for cognitive thought and hindsight the patient rationalises these discrepancies as the primary cause of the pain rather than secondary to the primary aetiological factor, the altered psychological state or mood. Modification of the interarch relationship to provide for a stable harmonious occlusal relationship conforming to the criteria of an optimal occlusion will eradicate the secondary occlusal factor and in many individuals can lead to reduction in TMD symptoms. Such occlusal modification is achieved by means of the provision of an appropriate prosthesis rather than by the destructive and potentially irreversible adjustment of individual tooth contacts and cusp inclines. The prosthesis should take the form of a rigid, removable appliance designed to give full coverage of the occluding surfaces of one or other dental arch.

This will give rise to even opposing tooth contact coincident with RCP, axial loading of the posterior teeth with mutual protection provided by the inclusion of an anterior guiding incline that establishes posterior tooth disclusion on protrusive and lateral excursions (Fig. 6.8).

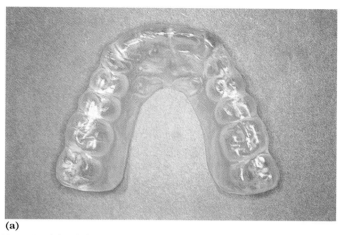

(a)

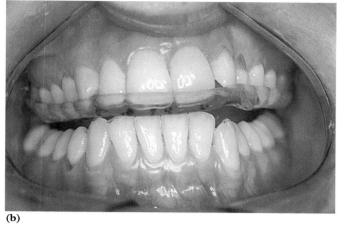

(b)

Fig. 6.8 (a) Full coverage occlusal appliance constructed for maxillary arch. (b) A clinical view of appliance in place providing right lateral guidance.

RESTORATIVE CONSIDERATIONS

Certain clinical procedures, such as the provision of complete dentures, full mouth reconstruction involving the provision of multiple indirect restorations or comprehensive orthodontic treatment, have as their primary objective the establishment of a therapeutically prescribed intercuspal position. Such prescribed treatment modalities may be said to provide *reorganisational care*. As has been previously established, in the absence of pre-existing tooth contacts the only reproducible interarch relationship is the retruded position or centric relation position. To this end reorganisational care has as its objective the provision of harmonious occlusal contacts where the intercuspal position and retruded contact position (centric relation contact position) are coincident and therefore a deflective contact is absent. The occlusal relationships should conform to the criteria of optimal occlusion. Such treatment objectives should not be viewed as the end result of all restorative procedures, only those where insufficient occlusal contacts exist to provide a stable comfortable pre-existing ICP. Where a stable pre-existing ICP occurs, restorative procedures should be undertaken such as not to alter the ICP and should be completed to a standard that does not introduce occlusal disharmonies. Such care is said to be *conformative* as the restorations provided conform to the pre-existing ICP. The treatment objectives of conformative care include maintenance of the existing ICP and avoiding the introduction of non-working contacts and deflective contacts on the restored tooth.

When a mouth is to be restored with multiple restorations that include both the anterior and posterior teeth, it should be remembered that the anterior teeth provide the anterior controlling influence of the occlusion, i.e. the anterior disclusive influence. The anterior teeth should be constructed first in order that the posterior tooth morphology may be constructed so as to be in harmony with both TMJ function and the anterior guidance.

Where multiple anterior teeth require restoration and the pre-existing anterior guidance is to be reproduced, a customized anterior table may be fabricated to provide a three-dimensional record of the anterior guidance and function.

ARTICULATORS

The movements of the mandible may be mimicked by an artificial jaw known as an articulator. They range from a simple hinge (Fig. 6.9) to a fully adjustable articulator.

The simple hinge will only provide movement in a vertical direction and therefore there is no provision for side-to-side movement. It has some use in providing a relationship between two casts but it should be avoided at all times due to its severe limitations in reproducing jaw movements.

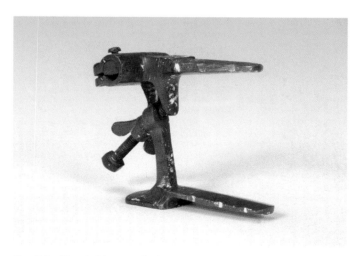

Fig. 6.9 Simple hinge articulator.

55

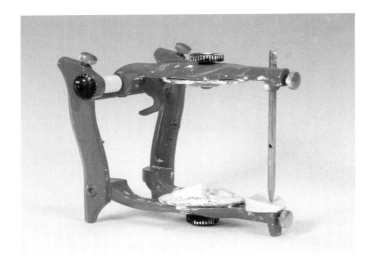

Fig. 6.10   The average movement articulator.

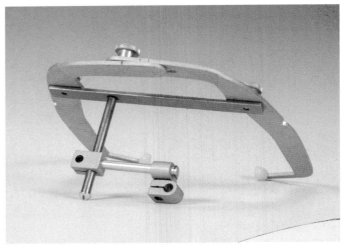

Fig. 6.12   The face bow is used to relate the condylar axis to the occlusal plane and provides further accuracy in replicating the movements of the patient's mandible.

The average movement articulator (Fig. 6.10) introduces some lateral movement to the assembly. The condylar guidance angle is set at 30° to the horizontal. This is taken from an average value of the general population and attempts to reproduce the movement of the mandible moving downwards in the glenoid fossa. There is an incisal pin which is set to contact a guidance table. The table has an average guidance of 10° which once again is a representative value taken from the general population.

An adjustable articulator such as the Whipmix articulator (Fig. 6.11) allows for the side shifting of the artificial condyles to take place. There is also the ability to adjust the guidance angles of both the condyles and the incisal table to take account of individual movements. Articulators allow a face bow transfer to be attached at the time of positioning the upper cast.

The face bow is used to relate the terminal hinge axis to the occlusal plane and provides further accuracy in replicating the movements of the patient's mandible (Fig. 6.12). Articulators may be classed as being either arcon or non-arcon. Arcon stands for *articulator condyle* and the term relates to whether the condyles are fixed to the lower arm such as with the Whipmix (arcon) or to the upper arm (non-arcon).

Finally there are fully adjustable articulators available which may be made to closely reflect the individual patient's jaw movements and are beyond the scope of this text. The use of articulators covers a broad spectrum of movements from the simple hinge which only allows for an opening movement in the vertical plane to the fully adjustable articulator which attempts to fully reproduce all the possible movements of the natural temporomandibular joint. The use of the articulator will be discussed further in Chapter 12.

SUMMARY

Occlusion is an important consideration in the restorative care of a patient. An understanding of the movements of the mandible and how restorative dentistry may influence them should be considered in any treatment plan. Most patients, happily, can accommodate small changes in their occlusal relationship but large disruption of the occlusal scheme is more likely to give rise to symptoms which may shorten the life of any restorative care undertaken.

A small but significant group of patients will find minor modifications to their occlusal scheme to be highly destructive and/or disharmonious and lead to symptoms that are out of proportion to the size of the discrepancy. Such alterations should be avoided at all costs.

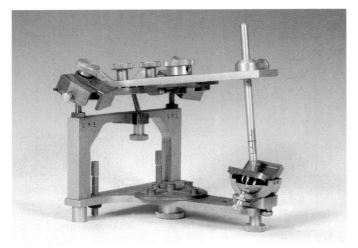

Fig. 6.11   Whipmix articulator.

7

Caries and other reasons for restoring teeth

INTRODUCTION

There are a multitude of reasons for making the clinical decision to 'restore' a tooth and patients have increasing expectations that not only the function, but also the aesthetics of a tooth will be restored or even enhanced. Dental hard tissues can suffer from a number of insults that result in loss of structure either in a gross fashion, for example in the case of trauma, or more chronically, for example as a result of erosion. A decision to restore a tooth may be made in the absence of significant loss of material, for example in the case of intrinsic or extrinsic staining, or perhaps to alter the shape of a tooth to improve a contact point or access for cleaning.

While considering treatment plans, clinicians should always bear in mind that an option for no active treatment, but instead to monitor a tooth, should always be considered. As our understanding of, for example, the dynamics of the caries process increases, we should also consider how we can prevent diseases progressing and even how we can improve the chances of regression. Treatment plans can involve the stabilisation of the dentition by identifying and removing potential causes of tooth damage and are helped by a close relationship between clinician and patient, with patients being encouraged to take ownership of their own health outcomes.

It should also be remembered that the majority of restorations placed are replacements of those that are perceived to have failed. The decision to place a restoration should not be taken lightly, as it will, invariably, commit the patient to a series of increasingly complex replacements throughout the lifetime of the tooth (Fig. 7.1). Equally, clinicians should assess the replacement need of a restoration carefully and consider the possibility of monitoring or repair.

DENTAL CARIES

Despite common misunderstandings among both lay and professional persons, caries is not a disease of the past and remains the commonest cause of tooth damage and loss. Over 40% of 5-year-olds still have caries and this has a long-term impact on their oral health throughout life. Significant advances in our understanding of the caries process have enabled us to describe a dynamic system; between the biofilm (composed of pellicle, plaque and saliva) and the host tooth surface there is an almost constant interchange of ions and this is increased following eating or drinking. In most cases any demineralisation that occurs can quickly be replenished from stocks of calcium, phosphate and magnesium within the saliva. Only when this delicate balance of demineralisation and remineralisation is disrupted does the accumulation of mineral loss lead to the development of a carious lesion. Such an imbalance occurs when the causative factors outweigh the protective factors over an extended period. (Fig. 7.2). Development of the lesion is by no means certain, and there are several points at which the process may either stop (arrest) or even regress (recover).

Aetiology

The factors leading to a caries lesion are now well understood. The biofilm on the tooth surface consists of bacteria that will produce acids (typically lactic acid) as a metabolic by-product. These bacteria are named acidogenic bacteria;

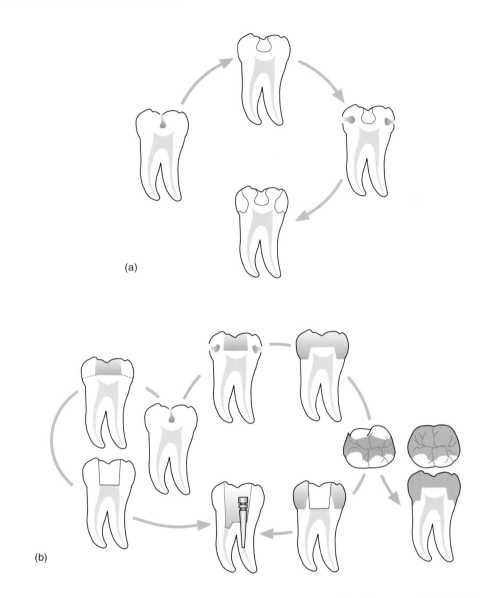

(a)

(b)

Fig. 7.1 The restorative cycle. (Adapted from Dietschi & Spreafico 1997, with permission of Quintessence Publishing.)

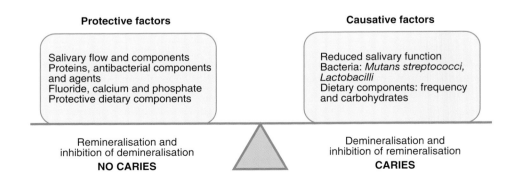

Protective factors

Salivary flow and components
Proteins, antibacterial components
and agents
Fluoride, calcium and phosphate
Protective dietary components

Causative factors

Reduced salivary function
Bacteria: *Mutans streptococci,
Lactobacilli*
Dietary components: frequency
and carbohydrates

Remineralisation and
inhibition of demineralisation
NO CARIES

Demineralisation and
inhibition of remineralisation
CARIES

Fig. 7.2 The caries balance. (Adapted from Featherstone J D (1998). Prevention and reversal of dental caries: role of low level fluoride. *Community Dentistry and Oral Epidemiology*;27(1):31–40. Munksgaard International Publishing. With kind permission of Blackwell Publishing.)

i.e. they produce acid following the metabolism of fermentable carbohydrates. Typical examples of fermentable carbohydrates include glucose, sucrose, fructose and uncooked starch. The acids produced diffuse through the plaque and into the porous subsurface enamel (or exposed dentine). As they travel through this system they dissociate, producing hydrogen ions that can readily dissolve the mineral component of the teeth freeing calcium and phosphate into solution. Hence the process of demineralisation occurs. If this mineral loss is not halted or reversed the demineralisation will spread rapidly through dentine and may threaten the vitality of the pulp.

The two most important groups of acidogenic bacteria are the mutans streptococci and the lactobacilli. Each of these groups contains several species, all of which are cariogenic. Examples include *Streptococus mutans* and *S. sobrinus*. These two groups of bacteria can be described as the primary causative agents of dental caries. The production of acid following consumption of food can be rapid, reaching the so-called 'critical pH' (around pH 5 for enamel) within minutes. Recovery of a normal, neutral plaque may, however, take up to an hour. This is well illustrated by the Stephan curves of plaque pH (Fig. 7.3). The buffering role of saliva is crucial in the recovery of the Stephan curve and this is well demonstrated by the disastrous effects that significant xerostomia causes to the dentition (see Box 7.1 for medications that may reduce salivary flow).

Caries terminology and progression

Caries is a chronic, normally slowly progressing disease that is rarely self-limiting, with the end point of the disease being tooth destruction and loss. The caries process can occur on enamel, dentine and cementum, and lesions are often described using the anatomical structure affected; for example root caries referring to caries limited to, or initiated on, exposed dentine surfaces. Other terms for lesions include primary caries, that which occurs on previously sound, unrestored surfaces, and secondary caries, that which is associated with or immediately adjacent to a dental restoration. It can be useful to provide an indication of lesion activity, especially as this can impact on management, and so terms such as 'arrested lesion' can be seen in patient notes (Box 7.2).

The carious process commences as a small subclinical subsurface demineralisation which appears white, the so-called 'white-spot' lesion. In its earliest phase this will only appear when the tooth is dried, emphasising the need for careful clinical examination. The surface at this stage is especially prone to damage from probing and, with an increased surface porosity, to the take-up of stain. The degree of demineralisation at this stage is unlikely to cause a loss of mineral density detectable on a radiograph, although some of the novel techniques of caries detection may be able to visualise these lesions (see next section). Most importantly, white-spot lesions have the potential to be remineralised, and this can be augmented by the use of remineralising treatments. During the remineralisation and demineralisation cycle, the dissolution of the

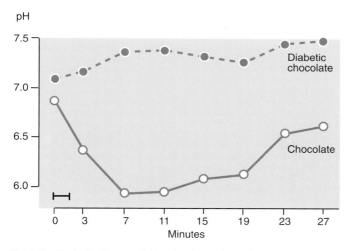

Fig. 7.3 Typical pH curve following ingestion of two types of chocolate.

Box 7.1   Medications which may reduce salivary flow

- Antidepressants, tranquillisers and hypnotics
- Antihistamines and anti-nausea drugs
- Anticholinergics and muscle relaxants
- Antihypertensives and diuretics
- Appetite suppressants

Box 7.2   Caries terminology

Anatomical
- Enamel caries
- Root caries
- Occlusal caries
- Smooth surface caries
- Interproximal caries

Condition of site
- Primary caries
- Secondary caries/recurrent caries
- Residual caries

Activity
- Active lesion
- Arrested or inactive lesion
- Remineralised lesion
- Chronic lesion

Others
- Rampant caries
  - Bottle (nursing caries)
  - Early childhood caries
  - Radiation caries
  - Drug-induced caries
- Hidden caries
- Incipient lesions

hydroxyapatite, in the presence of fluoride, permits the incorporation of further calcium and phosphate to create a surface coating of fluorapatite which has a reduced solubility (critical pH) and hence it confers some caries protection to the lesion surface (Figure 7.4).

The extent of the subsurface lesion may progress and involve the underlying dentine, become radiographically visible and yet still retain a visually intact surface. Such lesions may still be amenable to remineralising therapy; and, depending on both tooth and patient factors, a decision to monitor may be justified. If demineralisation continues, the undermining of the surface will eventually lead to cavitation, creating a protected environment in which acidogenic bacteria can thrive. The further complication of a difficult to clean site renders further remineralisation a remote possibility. Further spread into dentine results in bacterial colonisation of the hard tissue with resulting dentine softening and continued undermining of enamel. In rare cases, extensively cavitated lesions may remineralise, their bases becoming black and hardened as a result of improved access and cleaning. However, rapidly progressing caries quickly overtakes the protective mechanisms of the pulp and vitality is hence threatened.

Caries of root surfaces is essentially the same physiological process although the differences in presentation and natural history are important. The differing biochemical and optical properties of dentine preclude the development of a white spot and hence the initial mineral loss may be difficult to detect clinically. Unlike enamel when lesions are well hydrated there is often little loss of profile or structure. The softened dentine is particularly susceptible to further physical or chemical damage, but is also amenable to remineralisation and long-standing dentine lesions that are hard, black and shiny are not uncommon. In an ageing population that are retaining their teeth for longer, root caries is likely to be a major challenge in terms of detection, diagnosis and management.

The stage of the lesion is one variable in the clinical decision-making process to treat a tooth; either by preventative or surgical means. However, the caries diagnostic process is a complex one involving a variety of assessments that should be carefully weighed by the clinician before a treatment strategy is developed.

Caries detection and diagnosis

An important distinction should be made between caries detection and diagnosis. Detection is the process of identifying an area of demineralisation, and this can be undertaken either visually, or by one of several novel devices. However, the process of diagnosis is undertaken by a trained clinician, who collates information from a variety of sources before deciding upon a diagnosis and appropriate treatment plan. In caries diagnosis, there should be the identification of a lesion (presence of demineralisation), the severity of the lesion (depth) and whether or not it is progressing (active) or if it is arrested; therefore intrinsic within caries diagnosis is an assessment of activity. Such an inclusion is essential as it will inform, to a great degree, the treatment plan that will follow the diagnosis. For example, it would be inappropriate to restore an arrested lesion that was of no aesthetic concern to the patient.

To identify a caries lesion, the tooth surface must be clean and dry. In fact the individual drying of teeth with

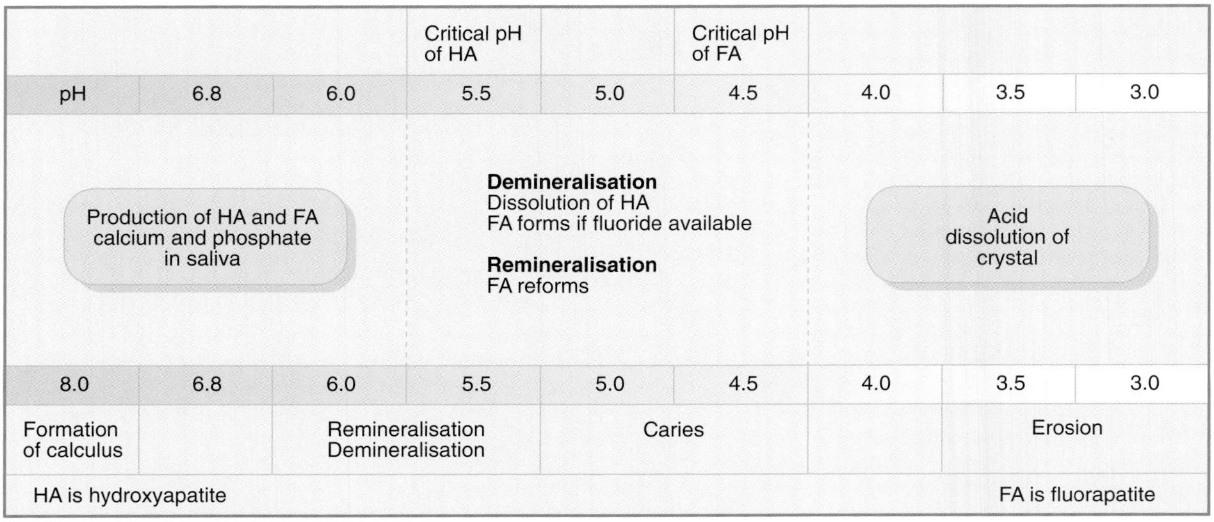

			Critical pH of HA		Critical pH of FA			
pH	6.8	6.0	5.5	5.0	4.5	4.0	3.5	3.0
	Production of HA and FA calcium and phosphate in saliva		**Demineralisation** Dissolution of HA FA forms if fluoride available **Remineralisation** FA reforms				Acid dissolution of crystal	
8.0	6.8	6.0	5.5	5.0	4.5	4.0	3.5	3.0
Formation of calculus		Remineralisation Demineralisation		Caries			Erosion	
HA is hydroxyapatite							FA is fluorapatite	

Fig. 7.4 Demineralisation and remineralisation cycle for enamel caries. (Adapted from. Mount G J & Hume W R (1998) *Preservation and Restoration of Tooth Structure* with permission of Mosby.)

compressed air is an essential step in the classification of lesions; and may be an indicator of their potential to remineralise. On smooth surfaces, the classic 'white spot' is seen although long-standing lesions may become darker as they take up extrinsic stain (Fig. 7.5). The use of a sharp probe is not recommended as this can damage early lesions causing cavitation and make remineralisation more problematic. Some dentists believe that moving a probe from lesion to lesion will facilitate the spread of microorganisms. Bite wing radiographs are an essential aid in the diagnosis of approximal caries, although the radiographs will underestimate the extent of the histological lesion by as much as a third. Bite wing radiographs are of little use in the detection of early occlusal caries (when it can be seen, it is invariably well into dentine), which remains a difficult diagnostic challenge, even for the most experienced clinicians. Bite wings should always be taken using a film holder to ensure that the beam is at right angles to the film and the contact areas of the teeth. (Fig. 7.6).

There are a number of techniques that can augment visual examinations, for example fibreoptic transillumination (FOTI). In this technique a high intensity light is shone down a narrow aperture probe on to the surface of the tooth. Due to backscattering caused by demineralised enamel, carious lesions restricted to enamel appear dark, with those extending into dentine appearing orange (Fig. 7.7). FOTI provides an increased sensitivity to visual examinations and enables clinicians to discriminate more easily between those lesions restricted to enamel and those extending into dentine. An advanced version of the system incorporates a small camera enabling the images to be viewed on a computer screen and retained for longitudinal monitoring; this system is known as digital image FOTI, or DiFOTI (Fig. 7.8). A further technique of use in a visual examination is the use of orthodontic elastics to separate adjacent teeth allowing, after 5–7 days of placement, to visualise directly the proximal surface of the tooth.

Other techniques for caries diagnosis include laser fluorescence (DiagnoDent, KaVo), light fluorescence (QLF, Inspektor), electronic caries monitor (ECM, Lode) as well as some more developmental systems such as ultrasound or thermal imaging. The DiagnoDent device (Fig. 7.9) is a small, compact unit that uses the fluorescence of bacteria, or their metabolic products, to detect if a lesion is present. Two tips are supplied with the system, one for smooth surfaces and the other for fissures, and this is simply placed on the area of interest. Within a second a digital readout presents a number from 0 to 99. A number of researchers have suggested interpretative indices so that clinicians can relate these values to a clinically relevant description, i.e. >30, caries into dentine. The system is simple to use but research suggests that it is adversely affected by stain, and the angulation of the tip is critical to obtaining meaningful results. The QLF system uses an intraoral camera to capture fluorescent images of tooth surfaces. The system enhances the contrast between sound

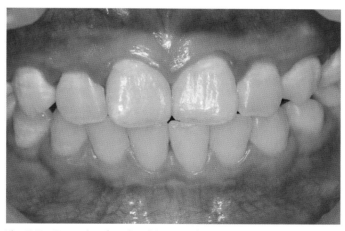

Fig. 7.5 Example of early white-spot lesions on the labial surfaces of maxillary incisors. Such lesions are amenable to remineralisation.

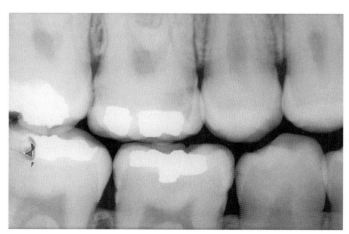

Fig. 7.6 Example of a bite wing radiograph. Note caries between the mandibular first molar and second premolar.

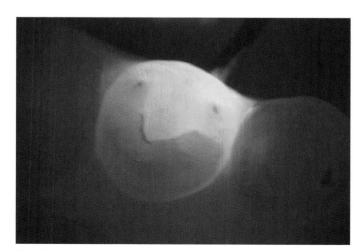

Fig. 7.7 Example of fibreoptic transillumination highlighting dentine caries in a premolar.

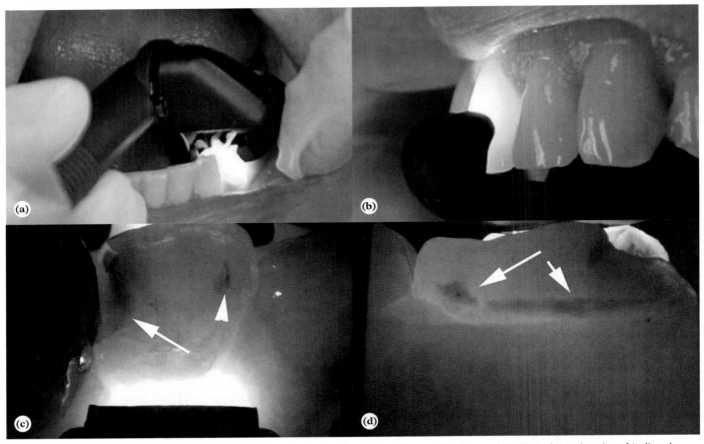

Fig. 7.8 Example of digital fibreoptic transillumination (courtesy of Professor George Stookey and Dr M Ando, University of Indiano). (a) Imaging of occlusal and interproximal surfaces. (b) Imaging of smooth surfaces. (c) Demonstrating image of occlusal and interproximal lesions. (d) Example of a smooth surface lesion.

and demineralised enamel by at least ten times, and hence it is easier to visualise early caries (Fig. 7.10). Software accompanying the system permits dentists to quantify the degree of mineral loss and then monitor the lesion over time to determine if a given tooth is responding to preventative care, or if restorative intervention is required.

The electronic caries monitor measures the resistance of the tooth to a mild electrical stimulus and is related to the porosity of the lesion (Fig. 7.11). Used in combination with a 5-second compressed air jet, the system relates the time taken to stabilise, with larger, wetter lesions taking longer to stabilise then smaller, dryer ones. The ECM tip is very small, and suffers from issues of reliability when successive measurements, so important in measuring caries activity, are taken over time. All of these systems should be considered as additional tools in the armamentarium of the clinician and enhance, but do not replace, effective diagnosis by a clinician.

Once the presence of demineralisation has been established, the next stage of the process is to determine the likely severity of the lesion, most often interpreted as the depth of the lesion. Caries progresses in a generally predictable way, but the visual indications can be confusing, for example 'hidden caries' where visually intact occlusal surfaces are revealed, following radiography, to have extensive dentine lesions. However, careful clinical examination of clean, dry teeth, combined with careful, selective and properly indicated radiographic views, should enable the clinician to gauge the likely severity of most lesions.

The final stage in the diagnostic sequence is establishing whether or not the lesion is active. It can be argued that the only way that this can be truly established is by monitoring the lesion over time and detecting changes. Before the advent of the QLF and DiagnoDent systems this was impossible in all practical clinical situations, as one simply cannot recall accurately the status of the lesion from one visit to the next. However, both of these systems enable *early* lesions to be followed and their activity determined. It is interesting to note that the QLF system can detect the products of bacterial metabolism, and these are shown in red on fluorescent images. It has been proposed that lesions that exhibit this red fluorescence are at an increased risk of progression as they contain metabolically active bacteria. Should clinical trial evidence support this, it could be one method by which activity could be measured in a single visit (Fig. 7.12).

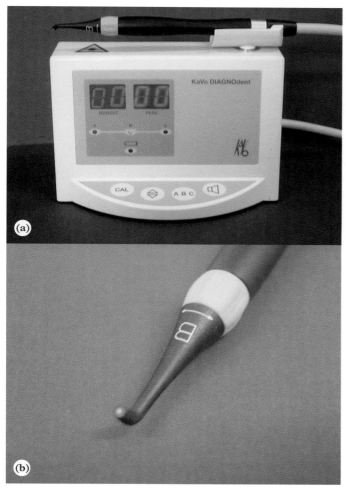

Fig. 7.9 The DiagnoDent device (**a**) The system box, indicating current and maximum readings. (**b**) The tip employed in the assessment of pit and fissure caries. (Courtesy of KaVo.)

appear darker, and may be black, are frequently shiny and hard to gentle examination by a blunt probe or excavator.

Caries risk assessment

Once all of the components of a caries diagnosis are complete; a calculation of the patient's caries risk should be conducted. Patients have a range of risk and modifying factors and these should be identified and managed as part of any treatment plan. A system has been developed with 16 major risk factors for caries, divided into 11 primary and 5 modifying factors. These are shown in Table 7.1. Each of these factors has a direct or indirect influence on the biofilm, and many work in combination. For example, high frequency intake of fermentable carbohydrates produces an acidic biofilm which further favours the development of acidogenic bacteria which in turn further lowers the pH. Caries activity is best assessed by examination of the patient's dentition, given that clinical evidence may be considered the most useful indicator of caries risk. The patient who gives a history of repeated restorations, who has multiple new lesions on clinical or radiographic examination, or who has a large number of crowns at a comparatively young age is an obvious high caries risk. Other methods of caries assessment include salivary flow tests and saliva buffering capacity. Since there is some evidence that individuals with low levels of streptococci may have low risk of caries, and that high levels of lactobacilli may indicate high caries activity, kits have been

It is, however, possible to assess the likely activity of a lesion using visual methods, again, on impeccably clean and dry teeth. On smooth surfaces active lesions tend to be adjacent to the gingival margin, or other plaque stagnation areas (such as a poor restorative margin), and are dull in appearance. Running a *blunt* probe over such lesions results in a sensation of roughness. Inactive lesions are often distant from the gingival margin (i.e. achieved during tooth eruption) and have a surface lustre or shine. Examination with a blunt probe reveals a smooth, glass-like surface. Some of these lesions will have discoloured, being dark black or brown due to the incorporation of extrinsic stain. Obviously these examinations are complicated in the case of pit and fissure caries and those on the interproximal surfaces of teeth.

Root surface caries presents initially as well-defined discoloured lesions in areas of plaque accumulation, often close to a recessed gingival margin. Active root surface lesions are soft or leathery in consistency and may exhibit a loss of surface contour or cavitation. Arrested lesions

Table 7.1   Risk factors for the development of caries.

Primary risk factors	
Saliva	1. Ability of minor salivary glands to produce saliva
	2. Consistency of unstimulated (resting) saliva
	3. pH of unstimulated saliva
	4. Stimulated salivary flow rate
	5. Buffering capacity of stimulated saliva
Diet	6. Number of sugar exposures per day
	7. Number of acid exposures per day
Fluoride	8. Past and current exposure
Oral biofilm	9. Differential staining
	10. Composition
	11. Activity
Modifying factors	
	12. Past and current dental status
	13. Past and current medical status
	14. Compliance with oral hygiene and dietary advice
	15. Lifestyle
	16. Socioeconomic status

Modified from Ngo H & Gaffrey S (2005) Risk assessment in the diagnosis and management of caries. In: Mount G J & Hume W R (eds) *Preservation and Restoration of Tooth Structure*. Sandgate, Queensland: Knowledge Books and Software, pp. 61–82.

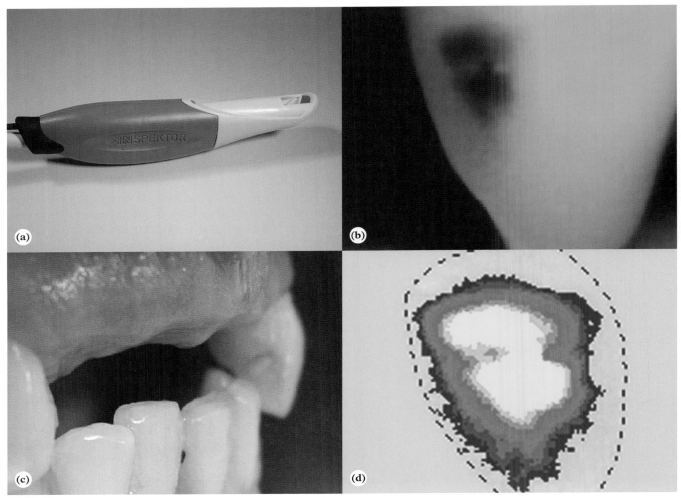

Fig. 7.10 The QLF device. **(a)** The QLF handpiece, with disposable mirror tip. **(b)** Example of a lesion under normal conditions on the mesial surface of the maxillary left canine. **(c)** View of the same tooth under QLF conditions, with tenfold increase in lesion enhancement. **(d)** Analysis of this lesion, a coloured map of the degree of demineralisation illustrating that the centre of the lesion is the most severely effected. This lesion would be amenable to remineralisation therapy. (Courtesy of Inspektor.)

manufactured to measure *Streptococcus mutans* and *Lactobacillus* counts many of which are suitable for use in general practice. Given the function of saliva in clearing the mouth of food and debris, as well as its buffering capacity, a reduction in salivary flow, due to either disease or medications, is likely to predispose to caries (Box 7.1).

Following the diagnostic processes and the assessment of risk, it should be possible to make a decision on the need (or otherwise) to *treat* a caries lesion. The decision *not* to actively treat should not be interpreted as *no treatment* but suggests that the patient is given oral hygiene instruction and perhaps dietary advice. In these circumstances the whole mouth is considered, rather than an individual lesion. If active treatment is to take place a decision on whether or not this will include surgical intervention should be reached. If the degree of the caries has been properly assessed then a non-surgical remineralisation treatment may be indicated. If surgical removal of infected dentine is required this is normally associated with

a decision on the most appropriate restorative material to be used following cavity preparation. Further details on the preventative and surgical approach to caries management can be found in Chapter 8.

TOOTH FRACTURE

Tooth fractures are a significant dental problem and are reported to be the third most common cause of tooth loss, after caries and periodontal disease. The majority of tooth fractures are associated with a restoration and are therefore not the cause of a restoration per se; rather, they are the cause of an enlarged restoration. In a significant number of cases, tooth fracture occurs subgingivally or involves a vertical root fracture and may render the tooth unrestorable. Fractures may be complete or incomplete:

- Complete fracture–visible separation at the interface of the segments along the line of the fracture

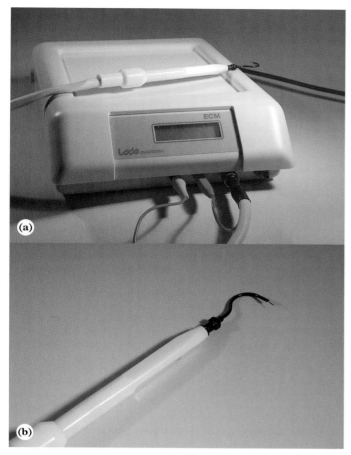

Fig. 7.11 The electronic caries monitor (ECM). **(a)** The ECM device with digital readout. **(b)** The ECM tip–compressed air is released during the measurement process. (Courtesy of Lode.)

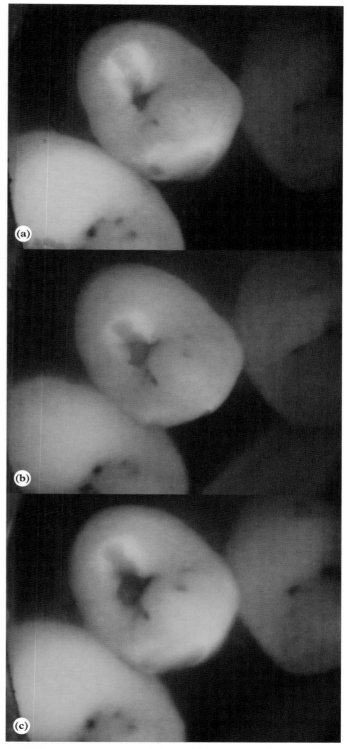

Fig. 7.12 Red fluorescence (RF) on QLF images may be related to lesion activity. **(a)** This occlusal lesion demonstrates RF at a baseline examination. **(b)** Six months later the lesion has progressed. **(c)** Twelve months later further progression can be seen.

- Incomplete fracture–demonstrable fracture but with no visible separation of the segments.

Diagnosis of the complete fracture is usually straightforward, but the diagnosis of an incomplete fracture may be problematic. Diagnostic signs for the incomplete fracture, or cracked tooth, include pulpitis-like symptoms in a vital tooth, tenderness of one cusp (the fractured one) to percussion, with the patient experiencing pain on biting (Fig. 7.13). Tooth fracture is normally associated with increased force on a tooth. This may be caused by direct trauma from an external body (*exogenous* trauma) or by impact forces originating from the dentition (endogenous trauma). In case of trauma this is commonly combined with other oral-facial injuries. Early recognition and management of traumatic fractures can greatly improve tooth survival and functionality. Approximately 82% of traumatised teeth are maxillary, with the distribution on the central incisors (64%), lateral incisors (15%) and canines (3%). Exogenous trauma may result from falls and collisions, physical abuse (which, in children, the dentist has a duty to report), assaults, accidents and sporting injuries; trauma from oropharyngeal intubation has recently been added to this list. When examining complete fractures the Ellis classification system can be used:

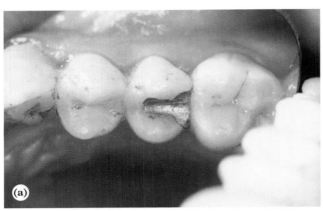

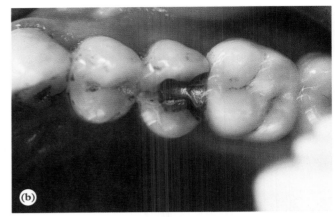

Fig. 7.13 Patient reported tenderness of one cusp on biting. The diagnosis was not obvious until the fractured cusp was found to be separated from the remaining tooth (b).

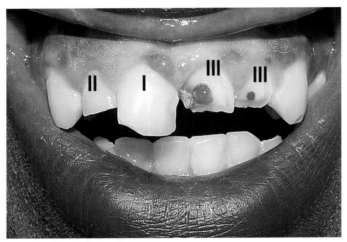

Fig. 7.14 Clinical example of trauma with all three grades of Ellis fracture presented.

- Ellis I – fractures only involving enamel, and are usually minor chipping with roughened edges.
- Ellis II – fractures involving enamel and dentine. Patients may complain of pain to touch and sensitivity, especially younger adults.
- Ellis III – fractures involving enamel, dentine and pulp. Patients complain of significant pain to touch, air and temperature.

See Figure 7.14 for a clinical example of each of these. The Ellis classification is a helpful system as it generally indicates a likely treatment plan; for example, an Ellis III will almost certainly require endodontic treatment if this has not previously been undertaken. Non-traumatic crown-fractures have typically been described when large forces result from biting unexpectedly on a hard object, with the force being concentrated on a small area of one or two teeth, and there are several occlusal factors that can contribute to this (Box 7.3).

Cavity preparation increases the risk of tooth fracture substantially; the risk is further increased by the following:

- a greater number of surfaces involved
- a deep pulpal floor
- an isthmus width greater than one-third of the inter-cuspal distance.

Restorations with no cuspal protection also increase the risk, as does endodontic access and preparation and the placement of dentine pins. Restorations with cuspal coverage tend to prevent future fracture – a sound restorative principle which often involves only minimal additional preparation/loss of tooth substance to accomplish in a large cavity. Failure to provide such coverage, especially in endodontically treated teeth, will significantly increase the risk of tooth threatening fractures (Fig. 7.15).

An additional restorative concept is that of the restoration which fractures in such a manner that the remaining tooth structure is easily restored, i.e. the restoration 'protects' tooth structure and acts as a 'fail-safe', rather than fracturing synergistically with the tooth in such a way that the tooth is rendered unrestorable.

It is important to remember that root fractures can occur either in isolation or in combination with a crown

Box 7.3   Occlusal relationships considered to predispose to tooth fracture
<ul><li>Anterior open bite and posterior cross-bite or edge-to-edge relationship</li><li>Altered cusp–fossa relationship of Angle's class II and III malocclusions</li><li>Poor posterior disclusion</li><li>Tight interlocking occlusion</li><li>Parafunctional activity</li><li>Strong masseter muscles</li><li>Drug-related clenching</li><li>Non-working side interferences</li><li>Excessive working side contacts</li></ul>

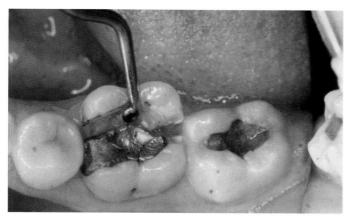

Fig. 7.15 Tooth fracture in an endodontically treated tooth with heavy occlusal loading demonstrating the need for cuspal coverage.

fracture and are generally classified as complete/incomplete and horizontal or vertical. For example, Figure 7.16 demonstrates a complete horizontal fracture. Such fractures are complex to treat and may result in the ultimate loss of the tooth, although this may be delayed by many years with appropriate treatment.

TOOTH SUBSTANCE LOSS

Apart from dental caries and fractures, the main mechanisms for loss of tooth substance are attrition, abrasion and erosion. In this text, the term *tooth substance loss* (TSL) will be used to describe the loss of enamel and dentine from each of these processes.

As individuals in the developed world continue to live longer and retain more of their teeth into old age, it is likely that the prevalence of TSL will increase. TSL has a number of aetiological factors and the interrelationship of these factors is often difficult to determine. However, it is rare to see all teeth in a particular mouth affected by TSL to the same degree; indeed, TSL may affect the anterior teeth only, and often only the teeth of one arch. Reports from colleagues in the UK seem to suggest an increasing incidence of TSL in both the elderly and the young, and this is likely to give rise to a parallel increase in the need for restorative care.

The mechanisms of TSL often act concurrently. As a general rule, in patients with severe, progressive TSL, the clinician should look for a multifactorial aetiology.

Attrition

This type of TSL occurs due to tooth-to-tooth contact in the absence of food or other material and is often seen on the incisal edge of teeth. Some minor TSL may also occur interproximally. There may be varying degrees of attrition, such as physiological, intensified and pathological,

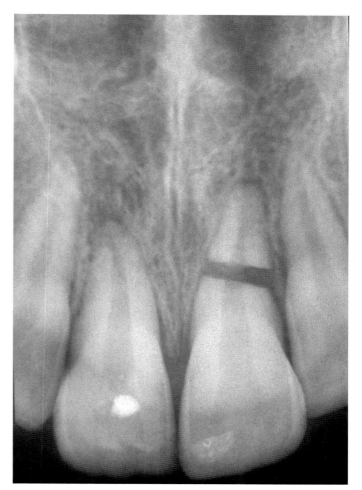

Fig. 7.16 Example of a horizontal root fracture.

the latter being used to describe extreme TSL. Physiological TSL occurs throughout life, and in most individuals will be of no clinical consequence. Pronounced attrition-related wear may be associated with parafunctional activity, with teeth showing distinct faceting, and with the facets in one arch matching those in the opposing arch in positions of contact (Fig. 7.17). Additionally, iatrogenic wear may result from contact between tooth substance and an abrasive, hard surface such as a poorly polished ceramic restoration. Bruxism is a common cause of attrition, and in those with canine guided occlusions, it is these teeth which will most often demonstrate the classic pattern of cuspal flattening. Indeed attrition can result in a shift from canine guidance to a group function occlusal system.

Abrasion

Abrasion can be described as the 'wearing of tooth substance that results from the friction of exogenous material forced over the surface by incisive, masticatory, and grasping forces'. Abrasions can be distinguished from

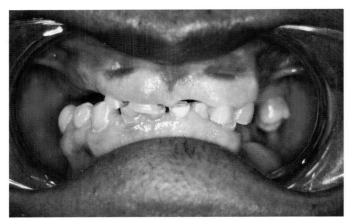

Fig. 7.17 Example of severe attrition demonstrating effects on both upper and lower arches.

an attrition facet as they tend to result in rounded or blunt tooth cusps and occlusal surfaces may well be pitted. Age is an important factor in abrasion, with newly erupted teeth demonstrating less abrasion than those that have been in function for some time. In Western populations with soft, processed diets, the main cause of abrasion can be attributed to over-vigorous oral hygiene measures such as toothbrushing and flossing. This can be enhanced by the use of abrasive dentifrices, and is seen especially in areas of gingival recession when the softer, more easily abraded, dentine is exposed. Other examples of abrasion include loss of tooth substance due to repeated chewing of a pipe stem, using a toothpick or biting thread. Certain professions such as electricians, hairdressers and seamstresses will often exhibit occupation related abrasion as a result of, for example, stripping wires or holding pins between the teeth (Fig. 7.18).

Erosion

Erosion may be described as the loss of dental hard tissues due to acid dissolution not involving bacterial activity. The source of the acids can be described as either intrinsic (gastric regurgitation), occupational (workers in chemical plants, wine tasters) or dietary (acidic foods or drinks) (Box 7.4). The clinical presentation of erosion will typically depend on its aetiology. Intrinsic acid principally affects the palatal surfaces of the upper teeth, with the incisors being particularly at risk. Dietary acid principally affects buccal, occlusal and incisal surfaces. Surfaces affected by erosion will present as smooth, rounded areas of TSL, with loss of the normal tooth surface detail. Restorations in amalgam may appear 'proud' of the remaining tooth surface in patients with severe erosive TSL, such as those with bulimia (Fig. 7.19). As erosion begins, there is an initial loss of surface definition, with the enamel edges becoming rounded and characterless. The enamel surfaces become concave, smooth and glossy although, especially with palatal erosion, a marginal area of sound, non-affected

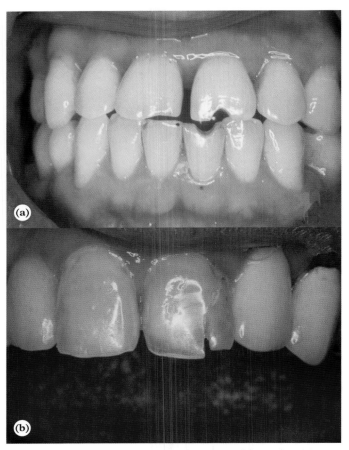

Fig. 7.18 Occupational examples of abrasion. **(a)** An electrician who uses his teeth to strip electrical wires. **(b)** A seamstress who held pins in her maxillary left central incisor.

enamel may remain, and these teeth often look as if they have been prepared for indirect veneers. Once the enamel has been breached and dentine is exposed, the process accelerates rapidly. Sensitivity is often a feature of active erosion lesions into dentine. In the presence of a reduced salivary flow the effect of both intrinsic and extrinsic acid will be accentuated. The buffering effect of saliva is the best protection against erosion, in combination with behavioural

---

Box 7.4   Causes of dental erosion

Intrinsic factors
- Regurgitation of acid food
- Gastric reflux disease (GORD)
- Chronic vomiting (e.g. eating disorders, alcoholism)

Extrinsic factors
- Acid foods, such as citrus fruits
- Acid drinks, such as carbonated drinks, sports drinks, juices and wine
- Medications, such as asthma inhalers
- Occupational exposure, such as workers in the chemical industry or professional wine tasters

---

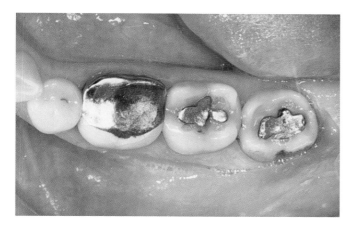

Fig. 7.19 Restorations in amalgam may appear 'proud' of the remaining tooth surface in patients with severe erosive tooth substance loss, such as those with bulimia.

and diet changes as required. Individuals should be advised against toothbrushing following an episode of vomiting or acidic food intake, and should instead be recommended an alcohol-free, fluoride mouth rinse.

Measuring tooth surface loss

Recording TSL is a difficult procedure and a number of indices have been used. One of the more commonly accepted is the Smith and Knight index as discussed earlier (p. 19, Table 3.3). A simple method of recording the amount of TSL that has occurred is the use of a silicone index. Impressions are taken of the teeth and the resulting casts are given to the patient for safe-keeping. At subsequent future appointments (i.e. 6 months later), silicone putty impressions are taken of the teeth, sectioned and relocated on the original casts. Any TSL can be identified by discrepancies between the impression and the silicone index

(Fig. 7.20). Several more advanced methods exist, such as the use of laser scanners to determine loss based on serial impressions, although these are outwith the scope of clinical practice and are largely restricted to use in research.

ABFRACTION

Non-carious cervical lesions (NCCLs) are wedge-shaped areas of loss of tooth structure limited to the cervical area of the tooth (Fig. 7.21). Their cause is the source of some debate. Traditionally, the pathogenesis of class V NCCLs has been associated with abrasion or erosion. Their prevalence is increasing, particularly in older patients, and gender differences have also been reported. It may therefore be the case that other factors are involved in the pathogenesis of NCCLs. It has been suggested that tensile stresses resulting from occlusal overload may be involved, the so-called 'occlusal' theory. Bending stresses may cause disruption of the surface enamel in the cervical area, resulting in increased susceptibility to dissolution and abrasion at the affected sites and in the development of lesions (Fig. 7.22).

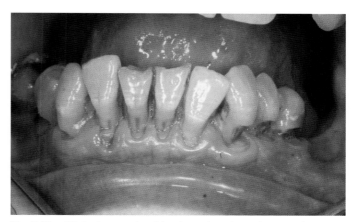

Fig. 7.21 Clinical example of both wedge-shaped non-carious cervical lesions and abrasion.

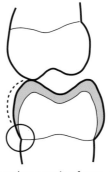

Fig. 7.22 The occlusal pathogenesis of non-carious cervical lesions. Chipping of the cervical enamel occurs when the tooth flexes, exposing an area which may then be affected by other forms of tooth substance loss.

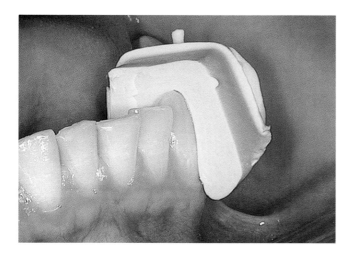

Fig. 7.20 Use of a silicone index to record tooth wear.

These NCCLs have also been termed 'abfractions', which is an engineering term derived from the Latin for 'to break away' and relating to stress corrosion. Increasingly, tooth flexure is becoming accepted as a mechanism for the loss of dental hard tissue, although this is the least studied of the processes thought to cause TSL.

TOOTH DISCOLORATION

Tooth colour is dependent on the intrinsic pigmentation of the tooth, which is naturally/genetically controlled. The majority of natural tooth colour is determined by the dentine (yellow to brown), the enamel being relatively transparent contributing blue, green and pink tints. Historically tooth discoloration has been divided into intrinsic or extrinsic, with a further category of internalised stain or discoloration recently being suggested. It is essential when considering treatment of a discoloured tooth to determine the aetiology of the stain. Failure to do so may result in an overly aggressive treatment (e.g., porcelain veneers for extrinsic staining) or a treatment unlikely to succeed (e.g. tooth bleaching for severe tetracycline staining).

Intrinsic discoloration

Intrinsic tooth discoloration is a result of a structural change in either the thickness or composition of the dental hard tissues. Examples of causes are provided in Box 7.5. The most common examples are the brown discoloration, known as mottling, caused by excessive intake of fluoride (Fig. 7.23), and the yellow/grey discoloration resulting from administration of tetracyclines (Fig. 7.24).

Fortunately, staining due to tetracycline is not as prevalent as in the past, due to medical awareness in the prescrip-

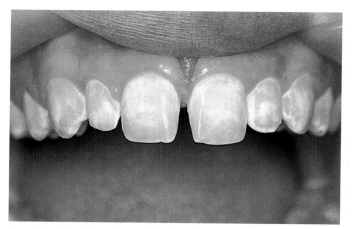

Fig. 7.23 Mottling of enamel caused by excessive intake of fluoride.

Box 7.5 Causes of tooth discoloration

Intrinsic factors
- Alkaptonuria
- Congenital erythropoietic porphyria
- Amelogenesis imperfecta
- Dentinogenesis imperfecta
- Tetracycline staining
- Fluorosis
- Enamel hypoplasia
- Pulpal haemorrhagic products
- Root resorption
- Ageing

Extrinsic factors
- Metallic
- Non-metallic

Internalised discolorations
- Developmental defects
- Acquired defects:
    Tooth wear and gingival recession
    Dental caries
    Restorative materials

---

tion of this drug to susceptible age groups, and while excessive intake of fluoride rarely causes mottling in the developed world, there is still a risk of over-ingestion of fluoride to the extent that enamel opacities are becoming more prevalent. As a result, children under the age of 6 years who are at low risk of developing dental caries should use a toothpaste containing no more than 600 ppm of fluoride; children at higher risk of caries should use a standard (1000 ppm) or higher (1450 ppm) fluoride toothpaste, and accept that there may be a small risk of developing enamel opacities. In the UK fluorosis is likely to be mild, presenting as white striations, or 'ice caps' on the incisal edge. Fluorosis should be distinguished from demarcated enamel opacities which are usually the result of trauma to the developing permanent dentition. Such lesions are deeper than the somewhat superficial fluorotic hypomineralisation and, if treatment is required, this is usually more aggressive than that for fluorosis.

Intrinsic tooth discoloration cannot be polished away without the use of special abrasive techniques. In cases where the discoloration is severe and of concern to the patient, restorative intervention may be warranted. The least invasive techniques are hydrochloric acid microabrasion, macroabrasion and veneering with resin composite or ceramic. There has been reported success using tooth bleaching techniques (using hydrogen peroxide in custom trays) to reduce the aesthetic impact of fluorosis. In these cases the whiteness of the tooth is increased, creating a more homogeneous appearance. Some success with this technique has also been described for cases of *mild* tetracycline staining.

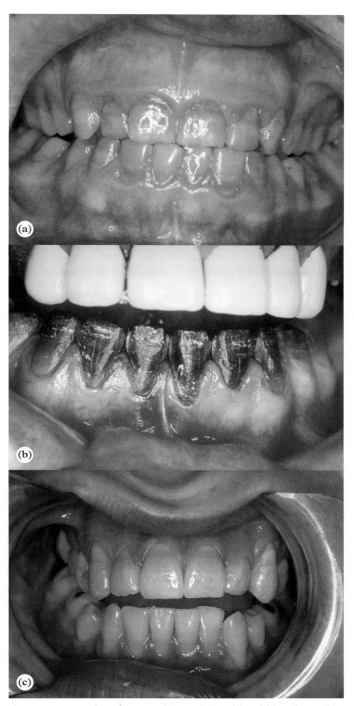

Fig. 7.24 Examples of tetracycline staining. (a) Mild banding with the stain restricted to mainly cervical areas. This degree of stain may be amenable to tooth bleaching treatment, either alone, or to facilitate the placement of more translucent (and hence aesthetically acceptable) ceramic veneers. (b) Severe tetracycline staining from long-term use. The upper teeth have been restored with veneers but due to their opacity they are aesthetically poor. Such cases are difficult to treat. (c) Case exhibiting the greyness of this form of staining. This mild form may respond well to long-term home use bleaching.

Extrinsic discoloration

Extrinsic staining may result from two main mechanisms: those compounds that become incorporated into the pellicle and produce a stain based on their innate colour and those that result in a discoloration by chemical interactions at the tooth surface. Direct staining comes from, for example, tobacco or dyes from foodstuffs. Additionally, the oral microflora may contain chromogenic (pigment-producing) microorganisms which may cause black, brown, green or yellow/orange stains. Indirect staining is associated with cationic anti-septics and metal salts. Typically the causative agent is without colour, or of a different colour to the resultant stain. An example of this is chlorhexidine. There is some evidence that suggests that the salivary composition of individuals can make them more or less susceptible to stain. Extrinsic staining may be polished away using conventional prophylaxis. In certain cases, a more thorough technique, such as microabrasion, is indicated.

Restorative materials may also discolour intrinsically as a result of chemical changes occurring following initial set, but this is an undesirable factor which has largely been overcome in modern materials. Restorative materials should ideally have a surface morphology which resists the accumulation of extrinsic stains. The development of stain around the margins of restorations is usually indicative of poor marginal adaptation, especially when using tooth-coloured restorative materials and these should be polished, repaired or replaced as indicated.

Internalised discoloration

Teeth may possess either developmental or acquired defects that result in an increased porosity and thus propensity to stain. Developmental defects are those described under 'intrinsic' staining, but post-eruptively these defects can acquire further stain. Conditions that cause any form of enamel hypoplasia are especially prone and exposed dentine is especially vulnerable to the uptake of dietary chromogens. Acquired defects result from the use, misuse and abuse of teeth over their lifetime and include such things as caries and gingival recession both of which are associated with an increased uptake of stain. The treatment of this type of discoloration must be determined after a careful consideration of the aetiology. For example, inactive, highly stained caries on an occlusal surface would be treated quite differently to stained dentine following gingival recession.

REPLACEMENT OF RESTORATIONS

The reasons for replacing restorations are often subjective. Replacement has sometimes been carried out because of confusion between secondary caries and marginal leakage, the former being diagnosed erroneously. In fact, the correlation between secondary caries and marginal leakage is low, and in cases where there is doubt, the astute clinician will smooth and polish a rough margin and then observe, rather than replacing the restoration. Replacement should be avoided because of the potential for further insult to pulpal tissues and because tooth substance is invariably lost when a restoration is removed. Conservative cavity preparation designs should be encouraged, not only for restorations which adhere to tooth substance but also for amalgam and other non-adhesive materials. This is of particular relevance in approximal restorations, given the potential for a mesial-occlusal-distal restoration to weaken tooth substance and predispose to cuspal fracture, especially in premolar teeth.

Marginal staining may be considered a reason for replacement of tooth-coloured restorations, but the clinician should be aware that the principal motivation in this case is aesthetics, rather than a high risk of secondary caries. As for marginal gaps, the correlation between marginal staining of composite restorations and secondary caries is not well defined. Poor aesthetics may be a reason for replacement of a restoration, but this is something for the patient to consider rather than the clinician.

SUMMARY

Any damage or aesthetic change to a tooth may require a form of restoration to be placed, although other treatment alternatives such as preventative care may be indicated. The correct diagnosis and identification of the aetiology of tooth damage are the clinician's responsibility. As with all diagnoses, careful application of special tests, such as radiographs, should be employed only when necessary and likely to result in an increase in diagnostic yield. Written notes on diagnostic decisions should be copious and, remembering that many dental hard tissue conditions are chronic, the clinician may choose, in the absence of pain, and in the presence of a diagnostic dilemma, to make careful notes of the presentation and review any lesion until a definitive answer is achieved. The decision to restore should not be taken lightly as one is committing a tooth to a lengthy and perhaps ultimately destructive restorative cycle and the tenets of minimally invasive practice should be adhered to when possible. Only when a firm clinical diagnosis is made can the treatment planning for the restoration of the tooth take place.

8 Restoration of teeth (simple restorations) and preventative dentistry

patient and therefore an accurate history is an essential first step in preventative practice. Key questions on diet and oral hygiene are essential and these should be tailored to the patient's age. For example, in younger individuals it is likely that high-volume, high-frequency fermentable carbohydrate intake may be responsible for caries, while in the elderly a failure to control plaque combined with reduced salivary flow may result in demineralisation. Once the causative factors have been identified, it is possible to develop a preventative treatment plan that reflects the aetiology and natural history of the disease.

Role of oral hygiene and caries prevention

Oral hygiene alone has been shown to have little effect in reducing caries development. The value of toothbrushing is mainly related to the delivery of fluoride via a fluoridated dentifrice. Plaque removal is secondary and has an obvious benefit in periodontal disease. There are a number of toothbrushing techniques that have been described in the literature, and these mainly relate to achieving adequate plaque removal around gingival margins. The main aim must be to instigate a regular, habitual twice daily brushing with fluoride dentifrice. It is recommended that individuals brush their teeth in the morning and before bedtime. Given the increasing consumption of acidic fruit juices at breakfast time, it may be advisable to brush before breakfast and then after the evening meal.

An assessment of toothbrushing efficiency can easily be carried out by using disclosing tablets and these are as

PREVENTATIVE DENTISTRY

Introduction

As described in Chapter 7, caries is a multifactorial disease and hence attempts at prevention must be based on a multifactorial approach. Demineralisation of dental tissues can be influenced by a number of factors (Box 8.1). The importance of any one of these factors will vary between

---

Box 8.1   Factors associated with demineralisation of tooth structure

- High-volume, high-frequency intake of fermentable carbohydrates
- Reduced salivary flow
- Inadequate plaque control
- Unfavourable microflora
- Unfavourable anatomy, plaque retention sites

useful on adults as children, many of whom are surprised at the amount of plaque remaining on the teeth. Similarly, adults and teenagers will report brushing for two minutes (the recommended time) yet when a stop-clock is used they are often amazed to see that less than a minute has elapsed. Some individuals will have particular difficulties in toothbrushing, for example those with muscular or arthritic problems, and in these groups the use of wide-handled or electronic brushes may be recommended.

Certain individuals will require more extensive oral hygiene procedures, and these may need to be augmented by additional medicaments. Individuals with reduced salivary flow, high sugar medication users, those with fixed orthodontic appliances and removable partial denture wearers will all benefit from the use of floss or other inter-dental cleaning aids, therapeutic mouth rinses (especially those containing fluoride) and more regular brushing with high (2800, 5000 ppm) fluoride dentifrices.

Role of fluoride in preventative dentistry

As was described in Chapter 7, caries is a dynamic process, and, in the presence of fluoride, fluorapatite can be formed following dissolution of hydroxyapatite. This is of benefit to the tooth surface as fluorapatite is more resilient to acid attack with a critical pH of 4.5 rather than 5.5 for hydroxyapatite. Fluoride also directly inhibits the demineralisation process and promotes remineralisation, and, if present in high enough concentrations, will prove toxic to cariogenic bacteria, inhibiting their metabolic pathways. Other evidence suggests that fluoride will inhibit further plaque formation and reduce the 'wettability' of the tooth structure (Box 8.2). Fluoride is not only helpful at inhibiting early lesions, but can cause the arrest of larger lesions (Fig. 8.1) and in adults, this is frequently in root caries.

There are numerous vehicles for fluoride delivery and the choice of mechanism should be based on a careful assessment of the patient, including a thorough examination of current sources of fluoride, including dentifrice use, drinking water and any self-administered supplements. By far the most prevalent method of delivering fluoride to the oral hard tissues is via the use of a dentifrice. 1000 ppm fluoride pastes have been shown to reduce caries levels by as much as 30% even in the absence of any form of dietary control. Fluorides in toothpastes differ across manufac-

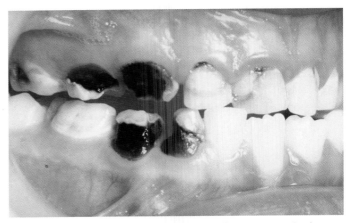

Fig. 8.1 Example of a primary dentition where gross caries has been arrested by the provision of preventative measures including fluoride and increased oral hygiene. Note that where restorations have been placed (UR1, UR2), active caries can be seen.

turers, and there is no evidence suggesting that one is more effective than another. Examples include sodium fluoride (NaF) and mono-fluorophosphate (MFP). Levels of fluoride also vary, with some pastes being targeted at young children, with 250–500 ppm, adult pastes with 1000–1500 ppm and pastes designed for those at high risk of caries, both adults and children, with levels between 2500 and 5000 ppm (Fig. 8.2).

Other methods of delivering fluoride include solutions, tablets, gels and varnishes as well as over-the-counter products such as chewing gums and mouth rinses. Concentrated gels are normally applied in trays and are generally prescription only. Fluoride concentration of these gels may be up to 12 300 for APF (acidulated phosphate

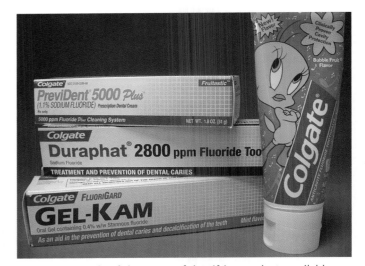

Fig. 8.2 Example of the range of dentifrice products available, including those for children, children at high-risk and also high-risk adults. Products with high fluoride should be prescribed with care. (Courtesy of Colgate.)

Box 8.2	Mechanisms of fluoride action

- Produces fluorapatite – a more acid-resilient mineral
- Inhibits bacterial metabolism at high concentrations
- Inhibits demineralisation and promotes remineralisation
- Inhibits plaque formation

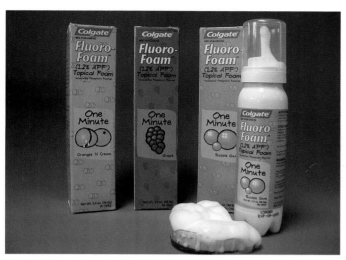

Fig. 8.3 Example of topical fluoride application. These products are fluoride foams that can be used in stock trays. Their pleasant taste makes them especially suitable for children. (Courtesy of Colgate.)

fluoride). In high-risk individuals such applications may be used at up to 6-week intervals. Such products are often made into pleasant tasting mousses for younger children, (Figs 8.3, 8.4). Varnishes have the benefit of longer retention times in the oral cavity and can be site specific, i.e. targeting those tooth surfaces with lesions amenable to remineralisation therapy. Varnishes may contain up to 2600 ppm fluoride and are generally viscous coloured resins. When planning fluoride therapy one should remember that the probable toxic dose for adults is 5 mg/kg body weight per day. It is also important to remind adults who are provided with high-fluoride dentifrices for home use that these should be kept away from small children.

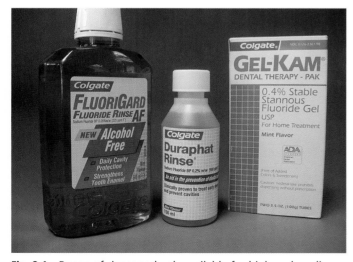

Fig. 8.4 Range of rinses and gels available for high-and medium-risk patients such as those with reduced salivary flow, or removable partial denture wearers. (Courtesy of Colgate.)

Role of diet in preventative dentistry

The role of diet as a causative factor in caries cannot be underestimated. The presence of persistent acidogenic challenges caused by 'grazing' foods inhibits the buffering capacity of saliva and ensures that the oral pH is always at a critical level. This shifts the dynamic of the caries balance resulting in net demineralisation and the initiation and progression of caries. Change in diet will require a highly motivated and cooperative patient who must be prepared to complete a diet questionnaire and diary as well as be willing to undergo changes. Younger patients will frequently imbibe large amounts of sugary drinks and their consumption of sweets may also be significant and almost constant throughout the day. In adults, the addition of sugar to hot drinks is often a highly contributory factor. As with all causative factors in caries, diet should not be assessed in isolation, but rather in combination with other factors, such as salivary flow which may well modify the quantities of fermentable carbohydrates that can be considered a risk for demineralisation.

Role of fissure sealants in preventative dentistry

The use of targeted, well-placed fissure sealants has a wealth of supportive research evidence. They have been shown to be a highly effective measure against the development of carious pits and fissures in young children and for all age groups at high risk of caries. Some authors advocate their use for erupting third molars as these are often difficult to clean. Fissure sealants can play an important role in the management of patients with special needs, particularly if they are unable to control the causative factors themselves. There is mounting evidence that fissure sealants that are placed on early demineralisation will arrest such lesions, although case selection is crucial. Indeed, it is in applications such as these that the new caries diagnostic tools may be helpful. Fissure sealants based on glass-ionomer, with fluoride release, may remineralise existing incipient lesions, but those based on unfilled composite resins will prevent further demineralisation but will not promote remineralisation.

Summary

There is a spectrum of treatment need for any given lesion; this is not solely based on the severity of the demineralisation, but on the assessment of a number of factors including diet, oral hygiene, ability to attend, attitude to change etc. The clinician must work through a complex set of decisions before embarking on a potentially destructive restoration, or on a plan of preventative work that may fail, leading to an increased treatment need. Such decisions are influenced by experience and careful history-taking as well as communication with the patient.

RESTORING TEETH

Until recently, cavity design for the restoration of teeth affected by caries followed the recommendations of G.V. Black which were proposed at the end of the 19th century. Today, with the increasing use of adhesive materials, cavity preparations no longer require the potentially tooth-destructive retentive features that were necessary for non-adhesive materials.

Contemporary restorations may therefore be divided into two groups, depending on the restorative material and placement technique utilised: non-adhesive and adhesive (Box 8.3).

This classification is not absolute, given that some materials may be placed in cavities either with or without adhesive techniques. For example, while amalgam restorations have, until recently, been placed without the use of adhesive techniques, the bonding of amalgam to tooth substance is now becoming more common. Furthermore, while ceramic restorations have frequently been luted with traditional non-adhesive luting materials, it is now recognised that their performance is enhanced if these are bonded directly to teeth using enamel and dentine bonding systems. As a result, resin cements are increasingly being used, especially in ceramic restorations. The advantage of cavity designs for adhesive materials is primarily the saving of tooth substance that accrues from not having to prepare retentive features in the cavity, such as occlusal keys and undercuts. This will ultimately lead to a reduced risk of subsequent tooth fracture. Furthermore, this reduced preparation leads to fewer dentinal tubules being opened and less likelihood of pulpal damage, although the degree of pulp damage, per se, is also dependent on other factors such as the placement of a material that bonds to the dentine and does not permit microleakage.

AMALGAM

An amalgam is defined as an alloy of mercury. Dental amalgam is a mixture of mercury, tin, silver, copper and other elements. It has been used in dentistry since 1826.

Box 8.3   Materials used in tooth restoration

Adhesive
Composite (using intermediate bonding layer)
Glass ionomer and derivatives
Ceramic (using bonding techniques)

Non-adhesive
Amalgam
Gold
Ceramic (using 'traditional' luting materials)

Box 8.4   Advantages of high-copper amalgams

- Less easily deformed
- Stronger in compression
- Reduced potential for corrosion
- Less marginal deterioration than traditional amalgams

Dental amalgams are classified according to their composition or particle shape.

The main categories of amalgam are low-copper alloys, which were commonly used until the 1970s, and high-copper alloys, which have been available since the 1970s (Table 8.1). High-copper amalgam (Box 8.4) contains smaller concentrations of Sn–Hg compound (gamma-2 phase). This compound is relatively softer than the rest of the amalgam, resulting in a set material which may deform or flow under occlusal stress, an undesirable property known as creep. The gamma-2 phase is also responsible for an increased susceptibility of the low-copper alloys to corrosion.

Amalgams may also be classified according to the shape of the alloy particles, this being spherical, lathe-cut or admixed. Spherical alloys are prepared by an atomisation process in which the molten alloy is sprayed into an inert atmosphere, with the spherical particles forming on solidification. Lathe-cut alloys are irregularly shaped, with sharp edges, having been cut on a lathe. Admixed alloys are a combination of lathe-cut and spherical alloys. The alloy

---

Table 8.1   Composition of low- and high-copper amalgam alloys

	Low-copper amalgam alloys	High-copper amalgam alloys
Silver	70%	40–60%
Tin	25–27%	25%
Copper	3–5%	30%
Palladium and other elements	Small amounts to improve strength and corrosion resistance	
Resultant mixture	45–50% mercury by weight	Smaller concentration of Sn–Hg compound (gamma-2 phase)

particle shape does not affect the physical properties of the set amalgam, but it does affect the handling characteristics, with spherical alloys requiring less force for adequate condensing than lathe-cut alloys. In addition, the suggested instruments for condensing spherical alloys should be of a larger diameter than those used for lathe-cut alloys.

Cavity preparations for amalgam

Non-bonded amalgam restorations depend entirely upon mechanical features built into the cavity preparation to achieve their retention. The principles of cavity design for such restorations are derived from those presented by G.V. Black towards the end of the 19th century.

In brief, the principles of cavity preparation following removal of caries are as follows:

- *Resistance to displacement in an occlusal direction.* Originally this was achieved by production of an undercut cavity, but it is now generally accepted that a cavity with parallel, or minimally divergent, walls will suffice.
- *Resistance to displacement in an approximal direction.* For class II cavities, this is achieved by the production of occlusal 'locks' (Fig. 8.5), or, less frequently, by grooves in the approximal 'box' (Fig. 8.6).

It is the loss of occlusal tooth substance in forming the occlusal key which predisposes most to the fracture of posterior teeth, especially premolar teeth. This is more of a risk if the cavity is a mesial-occlusal distal preparation. Retentive cavity features which obviate the need for occlusal keys should be encouraged. It is no longer considered necessary to extend a cavity into self-cleansing areas in a buccolingual direction. However, it is essential that an approximal cavity is prepared through the contact area in a gingival direction, given the potential for caries at the contact area (Fig. 8.7). This will also help with matrix band placement.

Achievement of resistance form

This is intended to produce a cavity which will adequately resist occlusal forces, i.e. the cavity floor should ideally be at a right angle to the direction of the occlusal forces. Furthermore, the cavity should allow for the placement of a sufficient depth of restorative material compatible with its physical properties. With amalgam and composite materials, this is generally considered to be approximately 2 mm.

Enamel margins should be finished so that there is no unsupported, overhanging enamel. Failure to achieve this will result in fracture of the margin if loaded, with the production of a defect at the cavity margin.

ADHESIVE RESTORATIONS

'Adhesive' cavity design principles may be applied when using materials such as resin composite, which may be bonded to tooth substance, and glass ionomer which itself forms a bond to enamel and dentine (Table 8.2).

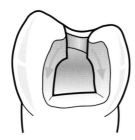

Fig. 8.5 The occlusal 'lock' or 'key' was an integral feature of nonadhesive cavity designs.

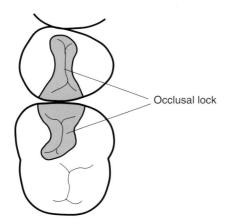

Fig. 8.6 Grooves in the approximal 'box' may provide the retention required for a non-adhesive restoration.

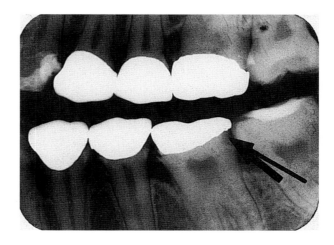

Fig. 8.7 If a cavity is not prepared through the contact area, there is a potential for caries to recur beneath the restoration, with the diagnosis of such caries being difficult other than by radiographs. Approximal cavities should therefore be prepared through the contact area in a gingival direction.

Occlusal lock

Table 8.2   Principles of cavity preparation

Traditional	For adhesive materials
Outline/convenience form	Access form
Caries removal	Caries removal
Resistance and retention form	Bonding form
Cavity toilet	Cavity cleansing

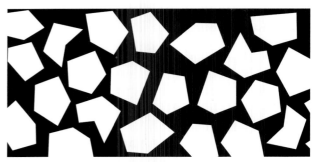

Fig. 8.9   Macrofilled composites contain fillers of between 5 and 10 µm.

Resin composite

Composites of polymers and ceramics, known as resin composites, are now widely used in restorative dentistry (Box 8.5). Early materials contained methyl methacrylate, but in the mid-1960s, dimethacrylate polymers, such as Bis-GMA (Fig. 8.8), were developed and used in dental restorative materials. Since that time, considerable development has taken place, especially in the filler technology. Contemporary composite materials are ceramic-filled dimethacrylates. These materials are widely used and are now finding a growing application in posterior teeth, as patients increasingly request tooth-coloured restorations, and as a general alternative to amalgam as concern grows among patients about the use of mercury-containing materials.

Box 8.5   The components of a contemporary composite material

Principal monomers
Bis-GMA
Urethane dimethacrylate

Diluent monomers
Ethylene glycol dimethacrylate
Triethylene glycol dimethacrylate (TEGDMA)

Inorganic fillers
Small/large particle fillers (1–7 µm)
Microfilled fillers (circa 0.04 µm)
Nanofillers

Silane coupling agents
Initiator/activator components
Chemical – benzoyl peroxide
Light cure – α-diketone (camphorquinone and an amine)

Basic principles

Many composites are based on an aromatic dimethacrylate system, such as the monomer Bis-GMA, which is the reaction product of bisphenol-A and glycidyl methacrylate. This is a highly viscous monomer which polymerises to form a rigid cross-linked polymer. Because of the viscosity Bis-GMA, it is necessary to add diluent monomers to the composite restorative so that its handling is appropriate for intraoral use. A smaller number of composites contain urethane dimethacrylate as their principal monomer.

Diluent monomers are typically low-molecular-weight monomers which reduce the viscosity of the material. In general, low-viscosity resins have greater polymerisation shrinkage than high-molecular-weight resins. These low-molecular-weight resins contribute substantially to the overall polymerisation shrinkage of the composite material. A number of manufacturers have recently developed and introduced alternative resin systems to the 'traditional' systems described above.

Early composites, termed macrofilled composites (Fig. 8.9), contained fillers of between 5 and 10 µm, but these materials produced restorations which were difficult to polish and of poor wear resistance. Microfilled composites (Fig. 8.10), which contained colloidal silica filler particles of about 0.04 µm, were developed in the mid- to-late 1970s and are still available. Restorations in these materials were easily polished. Current materials may contain fillers of lithium aluminosilicates, crystalline quartz, or barium aluminoborate silica glasses. The filler in materials designed for use in posterior teeth should be radio-opaque. Many composites contain a combination of a barium glass and another filler – these are termed hybrid composites (Fig. 8.11). Their mean filler particle size is typically in the range 1–2 µm.

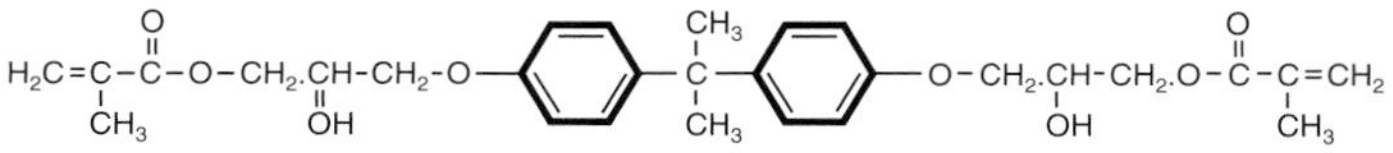

H₂C=C–C–O–CH₂.CH–CH₂–O–⬡–C–⬡–O–CH₂.CH–CH₂.O–C–C=CH₂

Fig. 8.8   A dimethacrylate polymer, Bis-GMA, which is the reaction product of bisphenol-A and glycidyl methacrylate.

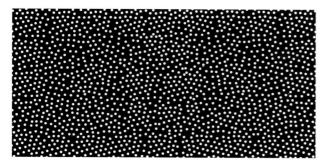

Fig. 8.10 Microfilled composites contain colloidal silica filler particles of approximately 0.04 µm.

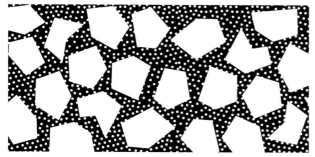

Fig. 8.11 Hybrid composites typically contain filler particles in the range of 1–7 µm with colloidal silica fillers and macrofillers.

Most recently, research has been carried out on the use of nanofillers, which have particle sizes below the wavelengths of visible light. Since these nanofillers do not scatter or absorb visible light, they may provide a method for incorporating radio-opacity into a material without interfering with its aesthetics. They may also allow high filler loading levels to be obtained, with a consequent reduction in polymerisation shrinkage.

Silane coupling agents (vinyl silane compounds) are incorporated into composite materials in order to bond the filler particles to the resin. The polymerisation of resin composite materials may be achieved by chemical means, using benzoyl peroxide as the initiator. Tertiary amine activators are also present. However, visible light cure (VLC) composites which contain an α-diketone such as camphorquinone and an amine are much more frequently used. On application of visible light of wavelength 460–485 nm, free radicals are generated, initiating polymerisation. Because of the advantage of 'command' set, VLC materials are now widely used. Light sources of adequate intensity will polymerise most light-cured materials to a depth of 3 mm.

Causes of undercuring of composites are as follows:

* the light source is not sufficiently close to the material surface
* the light source is of insufficient intensity

* light is attenuated by a restoration or tooth substance
* darker material shades, which absorb more light.

Overcuring is not harmful, so longer curing times should be used rather than shorter.

Physical properties

Contemporary resin composite materials possess adequate physical properties for all classes of restoration. Wear resistance is substantially improved in comparison with older materials. These materials do not form a bond to tooth substance, and an intermediate bonding system is therefore required. Resin composite materials are generally supplied in a wide range of shades. Their aesthetic properties are good.

Stress in composite

The forces generated by polymerisation shrinkage may be sufficient to damage the bond to dentine, or cause stresses to develop within the restoration. If the stress exceeds the adhesive or cohesive strength of the substrates involved, separation will occur. Stresses are greatest in cavities with a high ratio of bonded to unbonded surface area (Fig. 8.12). This ratio is termed the configuration factor. The occlusal cavity has the highest area of bonded surface when compared with its unbonded surface (the occlusal surface) and is therefore the cavity in which, potentially, the greatest stresses can develop (Fig. 8.12).

Methods to reduce the formation of stresses include:

* the use of a material which has a low modulus of elasticity (e.g. microfill composites)
* the use of a flowable composite (see below) of lower modulus to fill part of the cavity
* slowing the polymerisation of the material by:
  - using a light source which gradually reaches maximum intensity over a period of 30 seconds (ramped curing)

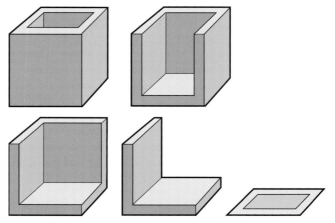

Fig. 8.12 Diagrammatic representation of the various cavity designs. The design at the top left has the lowest ratio of unbonded to bonded surface area.

- curing the restoration through tooth substance
- bringing the light to the restoration gradually
- use of bulk fillers such as ceramic inserts to reduce the volume of material that shrinks
- incremental packing, with each increment touching only one wall of the cavity.

Uses of composite materials

Composite materials possess suitable physical characteristics for their use in all Black's classes of cavity. Problems of poor wear resistance for class I and II restorations have been addressed in contemporary materials and the principal difficulties are in placement technique and the achievement of a firm contact point in class II restorations. Clinical assessments of posterior composite restorations have indicated 'high clinical performance' in a meta-analysis and 'adequate clinical service for 10 years'. This would appear to indicate that the performance of the materials used in these studies is better than the early materials which exhibited poor wear resistance and marginal discoloration. In addition, recent reviews of the literature have indicated that resin composite restorations in posterior teeth perform at least as well as amalgam restorations.

Resin composite may also be used for indirect restorations – the composite inlay technique. Indications are for larger cavities in which difficulties may be anticipated in achieving the correct anatomical form. However, these difficulties have been reduced by the introduction of matrix systems which have been designed specifically for resin composite restorations.

The glass ionomer family (Box 8.6)

Glass ionomer cements contain a fluoroaluminosilicate (FAS) glass which reacts with a water-soluble polyalkenoic acid to form a cement. Fluoride is an important component of the glass. It lowers the fusion temperature during the manufacture of the glass and potentially contributes to the therapeutic value of the cement. In materials designed as bases, radio-opaque glasses are used in which calcium may be replaced by barium or strontium. In its original form, poly(acrylic acid) was used, but many current materials use a copolymer of acrylic acid with itaconic or maleic acid. In general, this will be referred to as a poly(alkenoic acid). Tartaric acid is added to produce materials with a clinically acceptable setting time.

In contemporary materials, the polymer is often supplied as a dry powder blended with the glass and this is mixed with water. Some materials are supplied in encapsulated form. On mixing the glass with the poly(alkenoic acid), an acid–base reaction occurs. The outer layers of the glass particles are decomposed, releasing Ca^{2+} and Al^{3+} ions (Fig. 8.13). These ions cross-link the polyalkenoate chains, causing hardening of the material. As the material may take 24 hours to mature, it is recommended that

Box 8.6 Types of glass ionomer
• Conventional glass ionomer • Metal-reinforced glass ionomer (cermet) • Resin-modified glass ionomer • Resin-modified glass ionomer luting materials • Reinforced glass ionomer materials for use in the atraumatic restorative treatment (ART) technique

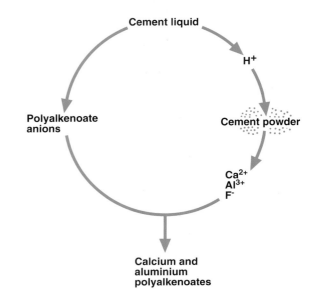

Fig. 8.13 The setting reaction of glass ionomer materials. The outer layers of the glass particles decompose, releasing Ca^{2+} and Al^{3+} ions.

the freshly set cement is protected from exposure to moisture by unfilled resin. The set cement contains a core of unreacted glass particles bound together by the matrix of reaction products. The set material contains water and is therefore susceptible to drying in mouths where there is reduced salivary flow, or if held under rubber dam for long periods.

Properties (Box 8.7)

Glass ionomer materials release fluoride and adhere to tooth substance. They are biocompatibile unless placed within 1 mm of the pulp, in which case a sub-base of calcium hydroxide should be placed. Cariostatic properties may result from the release of fluoride by these cements, although these properties have been questioned. The amount of fluoride released is high soon after placement but reduces to a constant, lower, level within 1 week with most materials (Fig. 8.14). The fluoride has been shown to be incorporated into surrounding enamel, but the amount of fluoride in solution around the restoration may not be sufficient for long-term cariostasis.

Box 8.7   Properties of glass ionomer cements

- Adhere to enamel, dentine and base metal casting alloys
- High compressive strength
- Brittle with low tensile strength (therefore not to be used in load-bearing areas)
- Aesthetic properties
  - traditional cements have high opacity
  - resin-modified cements have satisfactory aesthetics

Box 8.8   Advantages of compomers

- Generally simple to use and easy to handle
- Stronger, more aesthetic and less soluble than glass ionomer materials
- Wear resistance is less than resin composite
- Fluoride release is substantially less than glass ionomer materials

---

Uses of glass ionomer materials

Glass ionomer cements may be used for abrasion and erosion cavities, restoration of deciduous teeth, restoration of class III and class V carious lesions, and tunnel restorations, and may also be combined with resin composite in the laminate or 'sandwich' technique. Their high opacity also makes glass ionomer materials suitable for repairing defective margins around crowns. In view of their less than adequate tensile strength, conventional glass ionomer materials are contraindicated in load-bearing situations in permanent teeth and in core build-ups. Glass ionomer materials may also be used as bases under amalgam or gold restorations. More recently introduced high-viscosity materials (p. 82) have improved physical properties when compared to conventional glass ionomers.

Compomers

Compomer materials (polyacid-modified composite resins) were introduced in the early 1990s. The original manu-facturer's concept was to produce a material with the handling and aesthetics of composite (Box 8.8), but with the fluoride-releasing properties seen in glass ionomers. In this respect, while resin-modified glass ionomers (p. 82) are true glass ionomers with some additional resin charac-teristics, compomers are composite resins with some glass ionomer characteristics. The similarities between compomers and glass ionomers are principally that they contain similar acid-decomposable FAS glasses and release fluoride, although in compomers this is less than one-tenth of the fluoride released by glass ionomer materials. The acid–base reaction typical of glass ionomer materials does not occur in compomers, at least not to an extent that will lead to setting of the material in the dark. Compomers are therefore light-cured materials.

In compomer materials, polyacrylic acid molecules are incorporated in the resin monomer which forms the matrix. Compomers are presented as anhydrous one-component materials, and it is considered that, when the material hydrates after being placed in the mouth, a glass ionomer-type setting reaction takes place, leading to the

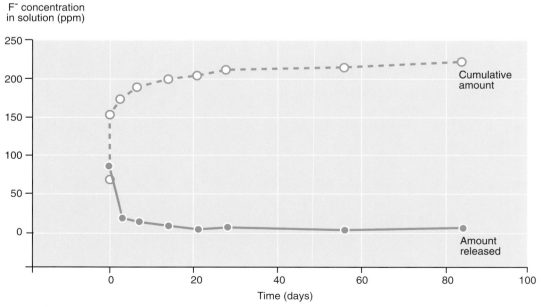

Fig. 8.14   The amount of fluoride released from glass ionomer materials is high soon after placement but reduces to a constant, lower, level within 1 week.

small amount of fluoride release which is seen. Early compomer materials used a self-etching primer for tooth conditioning and bonding, but more recent materials have incorporated a phosphoric acid etching stage prior to placement. It has been demonstrated that microleakage is reduced when enamel margins are etched prior to restoration placement.

A wide variety of compomer materials are currently available. Their resin matrices vary. One early material contained an elastomeric resin which added flexibility to the bonding mechanism. Another material contains an acid monomer, termed TCB resin (a bi-ester of 2-HEMA and butane tetracarboxylic acid). This contains two acidic polycarboxylate groups and two polymerisable methacrylate groups which enable polymerisation by light and an acid–base reaction when water is present. Water is taken up to a maximum of 3% by weight in a period of months following placement. This diffuses through the restoration and an acid–base reaction takes place between the strontium fluorosilicate glass and the polycarboxylate groups of the monomer. This acid–base reaction leads to further cross-linking of the matrix and release of a small amount of fluoride.

Compomers are not adhesive to enamel and dentine, so an intermediate bonding system must be employed. Bonding via the systems supplied with compomer materials produces a hybrid layer similar to that produced by dentine bonding systems, but there may be some adhesion from an ionic bond to the inorganic part of the tooth. Bond strength measurements produce values which are not as high as with dentine bonding systems to resin-based composite, but retention of restorations in non-retentive cavities does not appear to be a problem. The mechanical properties of compomers are generally inferior to resin-based composite materials but superior to glass ionomer materials. Filler loading of a typical compomer is approximately 70% by weight, and polymerisation shrinkage is 3–4%. A wide variety of shades is available with many systems and, as a result, compomer materials may produce restorations with good aesthetics. Clinical trial data on the use of compomer materials in class III and V cavities in permanent teeth, and in the restoration of primary teeth are positive.

Cermets

In CERamoMETal cements, an ion-leachable glass and fine silver powder are heated to over 1000°C to form an amorphous mass which is ground to make a powder that is then mixed with a poly(alkenoic acid) to form a set cement. These materials have similar adhesion to dentine and enamel as do conventional glass ionomers and slightly improved physical properties. However, the fluoride release is lower. Their applications include core build-ups and as filling materials for deciduous teeth. However, the value of cermet materials has diminished somewhat since the

introduction of more heavily filled viscous glass ionomer materials.

Resin-modified glass ionomer cements

Resin-modified glass ionomers (RMGIs) contain a FAS glass and poly(alkenoic acid), but also incorporate a monomer such as 2-hydroxyethyl methacrylate (HEMA) or Bis-GMA. These products set by two mechanisms:

- by the curing of the monomer – light cure or chemical cure, or both
- by the conventional glass ionomer acid–base reaction.

These materials will therefore set without light curing, as a result of the acid–base reaction (Fig. 8.15).

RGMIs are true glass ionomer materials and are of similar biocompatibility to conventional glass ionomers, with higher rates of fluoride release and better physical properties, especially with regard to tensile strength. Wear resistance is similar to that of conventional glass ionomers, while the aesthetic properties are better. Applications for RMGIs include core build-ups, restoration of class V cavities, linings and bases.

High-viscosity glass ionomer materials

High-viscosity glass ionomer cements were developed in the early 1990s following the introduction of the atraumatic restorative treatment (ART) technique – a minimal instrumentation technique designed for less industrialised communities (p. 86). These materials, if mixed to the correct consistency, have high viscosity and may therefore be condensed into a cavity in a manner similar to amalgam. The increased viscosity is a result of finer particle size and the addition of poly(acrylic acid) to the powder of some materials. These materials possess improved physical

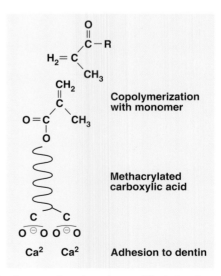

Fig. 8.15 Setting reactions in resin-modified glass ionomer materials.

properties, in particular tensile strength, abrasion resistance and wear resistance, compared with conventional glass ionomer materials. Adhesion to enamel and dentine, and fluoride release are similar to conventional glass ionomers. The improvement in physical properties has expanded the range of applications to include conventional glass ionomer applications, core build-ups, small load-bearing cavities in permanent posterior teeth where the load is not excessive, and ART.

CAVITY PREPARATION PRINCIPLES FOR ADHESIVE RESTORATIONS

Cavity preparations for adhesive materials differ principally from those for non-adhesive materials in that they are not required to achieve resistance to displacement in occlusal and approximal directions, and there is a potentially substantial reduction in the loss of non-carious tooth substance during the preparation (Fig. 8.16). However, the achievement of a cavity which possesses some innate resistance and retention form would appear to be desirable (provided that this does not require the removal of excessive tooth substance), as this will 'protect' the bond between tooth and restoration from excessive loading. In this respect, it may be argued that a bond which is protected from torquing, tensile and shear forces may be likely to survive for longer periods of time than one which is subjected to such forces.

OCCLUSAL CAVITY DESIGNS: THE PREVENTIVE RESIN RESTORATION

In the class I situation, once the finished cavity is made caries-free, consideration should be given to the application of sealant to the remaining fissure system. This is the

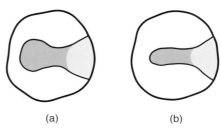

Fig. 8.16 Tooth substance is conserved by the use of 'adhesive' principles (shaded areas). **(a)** Typical Black's design class I cavity. **(b)** The occlusal key may be reduced in size for adhesive restorations or may not be required, with a commensurate saving in tooth substance (red shaded area).

concept of the preventive resin restoration (Fig. 8.17a–c) in which the caries is removed and a resin composite is bonded to the cavity using a dentine bonding system.

During the bonding procedure, the etchant is also applied to the remaining fissure system, to which unfilled resin is applied at the same time as the placement of the composite restoration. High rates of success have been reported. Glass ionomer materials have also been suggested for use in preparations of this type.

APPROXIMAL CAVITY DESIGNS FOR DIRECT-PLACEMENT RESIN COMPOSITE RESTORATIONS

In the case of approximal caries, the need to extend the approximal cavity is only in a gingival direction through the contact point in order to facilitate the placement of a matrix. There is no need for buccolingual extension for prevention. The subsequent management differs from the traditional non-adhesive approach in that there is no need to provide resistance from displacement in an occlusal or

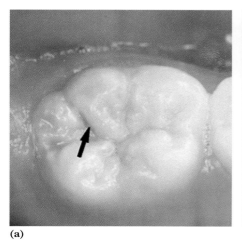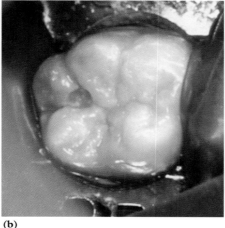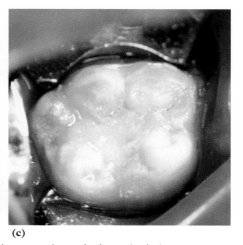

(a)   (b)   (c)

Fig. 8.17 A preventive resin restoration. **(a)** Caries is diagnosed. **(b)** Minimal cavity preparation removing only the caries lesion. **(c)** The cavity is restored with resin composite and the remaining fissure system is sealed. (Reproduced by courtesy of George Warman Publications, Guildford, UK, publishers of Dental Update.)

approximal direction. Furthermore, the adhesive material will offer some support to unsupported enamel and dentine margins. However, the limiting factor in contemporary cavity design may be the need to cut sufficient access in order to remove caries (Fig. 8.18). In this respect, the use of magnifying loupes may be considered essential for the accurate viewing of minimal cavity preparations. Indeed, the use of magnification may be considered essential in most areas of restorative dentistry.

PLACEMENT OF CLASS II COMPOSITE RESTORATIONS

The clinical sequence involved in the placement of a class II composite restoration is outlined in Table 8.3.

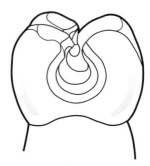

Fig. 8.18 Cavity design may be limited only by the need to cut sufficient access to permit identification and removal of caries, and allow placement of a matrix.

Table 8.3 Placement of class II composite restoration

Operation	Rationale
Select shade	A slight mismatch is desirable in posterior teeth so that cavity margins can be visualised and enamel damage reduced during finishing procedures
Check occlusal relationship	This is done to visualise the ideal final contour of the occlusal surface, and it avoids the need for time-consuming removal of excess material
Remove caries; smooth rough or gross overhanging margins	
Extend through contact point in a gingival direction	Allows placement of matrix
Obtain isolation, preferably by rubber dam	The performance of composite materials is compromised when contaminated by saliva or blood
Place matrix and wedge	A firmly fitting matrix is essential to the correct contour of the restoration
Place base if indicated	Bases are only indicated in cavities in close proximity to the pulp
Apply components of dentine bonding system	Follow manufacturer's instructions implicitly
Apply layer of flowable composite to the base of the interproximal box and the occlusal floor and cure for a period in excess of the manufacturer's instruction	A layer of flowable composite will reduce microleakage at the gingival margin. Curing in excess of the manufacturer's suggested radiation time will ensure proper curing as the layer is furthest from the curing light
Apply increments of composite which only touch one wall of the cavity at a time and light cure	Increments placed in this manner may minimise stresses within the final restoration
Use a non-stick, non-slumping composite which can be packed against the matrix	Achieving a tight contact is essential, but difficult to achieve
Build occlusal contours with incremental build-up. Use sectional matrix and 'bi-time' ring	Overbuilding requires removal of excess and costs time
Remove rubber dam	
Check occlusion in centric relation and lateral excursions, adjust as necessary and finish using composite finishing burs	
Apply unfilled resin 'glaze' and light cure	Re-curing the surface will ensure maximum conversion and optimal physical properties of the outermost layer of composite. The unfilled resin will fill any microscopic defects

Box 8.9   Causes of thermal sensitivity following restoration replacement

- Direct thermal shock to the pulp as a result of temperature changes transferred through the (metal) restoration
- Pulpal hydrodynamics due to a space between restoration and tooth permitting the slow outward movement of dentinal fluid
- Bacterial invasion of any space between tooth and restoration may result in invasion and inflammation of the pulp

Box 8.10   Mounts classification

This takes account of the site, size and complexity of the caries lesion:
- *Site 1 lesions* are similar to pit and fissure class I lesions
- *Site 2 lesions* are those at contact areas:
  - size 1 (minimal)
  - size 2 (moderate)
  - size 3 (enlarged)
  - size 4 (extensive)
- *Site 3 lesions* are those originating close to the gingival margin and continuing around the full circumference of a tooth

The use of bases under resin composite restorations

Bases or liners were traditionally placed below metal restorations as a means of providing additional thermal insulation, and under resin-based restorations because the restorative material was considered to be irritant to pulpal tissue. However, no artificial material which may be placed in a cavity provides greater protection than dentine. The causes of thermal sensitivity following restoration placement are listed in Box 8.9.

In deep cavities, the number and size of the exposed dentinal tubules increase, and there may be a corresponding increase in the volume of fluid flow, a possible explanation for the fact that deeper restorations may be more sensitive than restorations in shallow cavities. The application of a dentine bonding agent to 'seal' dentine prior to placement of a restoration will occlude the tubules, prevent fluid flow and reduce postoperative sensitivity.

It is generally considered that placement of a layer of flowable composite over the occlusal floor and the interproximal box will reduce the potential for microleakage at the gingival margin, probably because of the 'stress-absorbing' properties of the materials and the ease with which they may be applied. However, failure to place a matrix that is tightly adapted at the gingival margin will result in a damaging excess of material flowing into the gingival crevice.

CONTEMPORARY CAVITY DESIGNS FOR GLASS IONOMER RESTORATIONS

Contemporary cavity classifications

For proximal lesions, Mount and Hume (1997) considered that some modification from conventional cavity design was necessary, and further developed this idea, suggesting a new classification for cavities which may be particularly appropriate for 'new' caries situations such as are seen in gerodontics, e.g. circumferential cavities at gingival level and proximal lesions which are not appropriate for conventional class II preparations (Box 8.10). It can therefore be envisaged that these would also include those lesions referred to as Black's class V lesions, including cavities occurring on the mesial or distal tooth surfaces following gingival recession (Fig. 8.19).

Site 2, size 1 (2.1) lesions would therefore be appropriate for restoration by a tunnel, slot or other minimal cavity preparation designed to maintain the maximum amount of tooth structure. Glass ionomer would be an appropriate material for such cavities. This revised classification of caries lesions is more appropriate to modern, adhesive restorative materials such as glass ionomer than that suggested by G.V. Black almost a century ago.

Tunnel restorations

In this application, glass ionomer material is syringed into a proximal preparation prior to the restoration of the occlusal access cavity with a resin-based material (Fig. 8.20). This procedure will leave the marginal ridge intact.

There is a divergence of opinions on the effectiveness of tunnel restorations, with some workers reporting no cases of marginal ridge fracture or recurrent caries in 'dozens' of restorations. The consensus view from laboratory experiments is that the strength of the marginal ridge of teeth

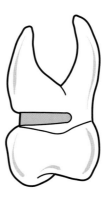

Fig. 8.19 A circumferential class V cavity, designated 'site 3' in the Mount classification.

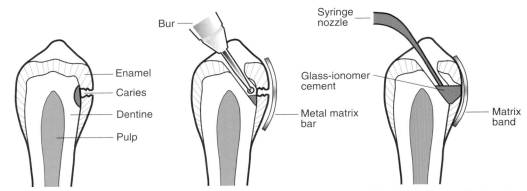

Fig. 8.20 The tunnel preparation. (Adapted with permission from Davidson CL, Mjor A, eds (1999) Advances in glass-ionomer cements. Berlin: Quintessence Publishing Company.)

restored with tunnel cermet restorations is as great as that of unrestored sound teeth. Other workers concluded that 25% of the glass ionomer and 10% of the cermet tunnel restorations failed, while none of the small amalgam class II restorations placed as controls required replacement. Furthermore, it has been demonstrated that caries is not removed in a proportion of cases.

Anecdotal evidence suggests that this approach is technique-sensitive and the use of magnification techniques is essential when carrying out tunnel restorations. Caries detection solutions may also be helpful in ensuring complete removal of the lesion. Intraoral video cameras may be helpful in viewing of the preparation.

An alternative approach to the operative management of the small proximal lesion of caries may be the 'lateral' tunnel or slot preparation (Fig. 8.21), using either a bur or ultrasonic means of preparation. In this technique, the proximal lesion is accessed from the lingual or buccal surface, with the preservation of substantial amounts of

tooth tissue, including the marginal ridge. Optical aids and fibreoptic illumination are required to view the lesion and its preparation satisfactorily. This technique may find particular application for patients who have suffered gingival recession, which permits easy access to the lesion of caries. As with the tunnel concept, a radio-opaque glass ionomer is most appropriate, so that the proximal area may be checked radiographically for recurrent caries.

Atraumatic restorative treatment (ART) technique

The ART technique was first developed in the mid-1980s, along with interested manufacturers of materials. The concept is based upon hand excavation of caries and the use of an adhesive restorative material and/or sealant. Currently, a reinforced glass ionomer is employed. ART may be considered appropriate for persons living in underdeveloped countries and other groups such as refugees. However, ART is only one component of treatment, which should also include promotion of other dental health messages such as good oral hygiene and avoidance of cariogenic foods and drinks.

The ART concept has its basis in minimal cavity preparation and prevention. It may therefore be applied in the restorative treatment of many child patients, rather than confining the concept to less industrialised countries. It is also a treatment option for handicapped patients and those in domiciliary care.

The ART technique has been shown to be effective, with results of studies on the longevity of restorations placed under field conditions using ART with glass ionomer restorations indicating reasonable success rates. ART has been well received by the majority of patients.

The principal stages in the ART technique are as follows:

- isolation of the tooth with cotton rolls
- cleaning the tooth with wet cotton wool
- making access to the caries with a hatchet or similar instrument

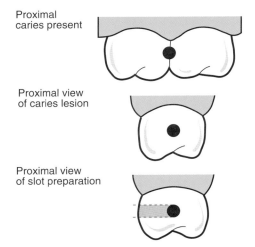

Proximal caries present

Proximal view of caries lesion

Proximal view of slot preparation

Fig. 8.21 The 'lateral' tunnel or 'slot' preparation. (Adapted with permission from Davidson CL, Mjor A, eds (1999) Advances in glass-ionomer cements. Berlin: Quintessence Publishing Company.)

- removal of caries with an excavator
- providing pulpal protection where necessary
- placement of the restoration
- checking the occlusion
- removal of any excess material before it has hardened
- coating the glass ionomer restoration with varnish or petroleum jelly.

ART is most appropriate to minimal cavities in permanent teeth and to the majority of cavities in deciduous teeth, provided that access is possible without the use of conventional rotary instruments.

ADHESIVE RESTORATIVE TECHNIQUES WITH BONDED AMALGAM

It has been demonstrated that it is possible to bond amalgam restorations to the cavity wall and/or base by the use of adhesive resins. The bond strengths which are obtained are, in general, not as high as those achieved between tooth substance and enamel/dentine bonding systems, and further work is required to evaluate the performance of the amalgam/resin bond under conditions of occlusal loading. However, the restoration/tooth interface is not stressed in the way that a resin-based composite restoration margin may be stressed by polymerisation contraction, and amalgam does not contract on setting. The clinical technique involves the use of an autopolymerised dentine bonding system placed in accordance with the manufacturer's instructions, followed by condensation of the amalgam into the cavity before the autocuring bonding system is polymerised.

Box 8.11   Advantages and disadvantages of the amalgam bonding procedure

Advantages
- Reduced need for preparation of retentive features in the cavity
- Reduced need to use pins
- Reduced marginal leakage and postoperative sensitivity
- Potential reinforcement of tooth structure

Disadvantages
- Increased time for the placement of the restoration
- Increased in cost
- Lack of data on long-term clinical effectiveness

The advantages and disadvantages of the amalgam bonding procedure are outlined in Box 8.11.

SUMMARY

There has been a progression in restorative dentistry from mechanical to adhesive retention, and along with the advent of new filling materials, this had led to considerable advances in the techniques involved in the restoration of teeth. The use of adhesive restorations should result in a reduction in the amount of tooth substance lost in providing retention for non-adhesive restorations. This, in turn, will mean a reduced incidence of cusp fracture because of weakened tooth substance, and reduced potential for pulpal irritation.

Management of pulpal and periradicular disease

INTRODUCTION

The field of endodontology has undergone rapid growth over recent years. In particular, there has been a revolution in the technology available for use in treatment. These developments, however, have not changed the fundamental reason for treatment, i.e. pulpal and periradicular disease, which is principally bacterial in origin. The aim of treatment is therefore to eliminate these bacteria from within the root canal system and seal the root canal and tooth to prevent re-entry.

PULPAL AND PERIRADICULAR PATHOLOGY

Pulpal or periradicular inflammation results from irritation or injury usually from the following sources:

- bacterial
- mechanical
- chemical.

Bacteria, usually from dental caries, are the main sources of injury to the pulpal and periradicular tissues and enter either directly or through dentine tubules. The link between bacteria and pulpal and periradicular disease is well established, as in the absence of bacteria periradicular pathology does not develop. Some modes of entry for bacteria are listed in Box 9.1.

Box 9.1   Modes of entry for bacteria into the root canal system

- Caries
- Periodontal disease (dentine tubules, furcal canals, lateral canals)
- Erosion, attrition and abrasion (dentinal tubules)
- Trauma with or without pulpal exposure
- Developmental anomalies
- Anachoresis (the passage of microorganisms into the root canal system from the bloodstream)

Examples of mechanical irritation include trauma, operative procedures, excessive orthodontic forces, sub-gingival scaling and over-instrumentation with root canal instruments. Chemical irritation may be caused by bacterial toxins or some restorative materials/conditioning agents, while periradicular irritation may occur as a result of irrigating solutions, phenolic-based intracanal medicaments or extrusion of root canal filling materials.

PULP DISEASE

Irritation from any of the sources mentioned above causes some degree of inflammation. The response of the pulp depends on the severity of the insult and the resultant inflammation could be either transient (reversible) or irreversible, eventually proceeding to pulp necrosis.

There is an inconsistent relationship between clinical symptoms and histological findings in pulpal disease. Diagnoses are therefore usually based on patient symptoms and clinical findings. Pulpal disease may result in changes to both the soft and hard tissues.

Soft tissue changes

Reversible pulpitis is a transient condition which may be precipitated by caries, erosion, attrition, abrasion, operative procedures, scaling or mild trauma. The symptoms are usually as follows:

- pain does not linger after the stimulus is removed
- pain is difficult to localise (as the pulp does not contain proprioceptive fibres)
- normal periradicular radiographic appearance
- teeth are not tender to percussion (unless occlusal trauma is present).

Treatment involves covering up exposed dentine, removing the stimulus or dressing the tooth as appropriate. Reversible pulpitis may progress to an irreversible situation.

Irreversible pulpitis usually occurs as a result of more severe insults of the type listed above. Typically it may develop as a progression from a reversible state. The symptoms are as follows:

- pain may develop spontaneously or from stimuli
- in the latter stages, heat may be more significant
- response lasts from minutes to hours
- when the periodontal ligament becomes involved, the pain will be localised
- a widened periodontal ligament may be seen radiographically in the later stages.

Treatment of irreversible pulpitis involves either root canal therapy or extraction of the tooth.

Hyperplastic pulpitis

This is a form of irreversible pulpitis otherwise known as a pulp polyp. It occurs as a result of proliferation of chronically inflamed young pulp tissue. Treatment involves root canal therapy or extraction.

Pulp necrosis

Pulp necrosis occurs as the end result of irreversible pulpitis and treatment involves root canal therapy or extraction.

Hard tissue changes
Pulp calcification

Physiological secondary dentine is formed after tooth eruption and the completion of root development. It is deposited on the floor and ceiling of the pulp chamber rather than on the walls and, with time, can result in occlusion of the pulp chamber. Tertiary dentine is laid down in response to environmental stimuli as reactionary or reparative dentine. Reactionary dentine is a response to a mild noxious stimuli, whereas reparative dentine is deposited directly beneath the path of injured dentinal tubules as a response to strong noxious stimuli. Treatment is dependent upon the pulpal symptoms.

Internal resorption

Occasionally, pulpal inflammation may cause changes that result in dentinoclastic activity. Such changes result in resorption of dentine, and clinically a pink spot may be seen in the later stages if the lesion is coronal. Radiographic examination reveals a punched-out outline that is seen to be continuous with the rest of the pulp cavity. Root canal therapy will result in arrest of the resorptive process, but where destruction is very advanced extraction may be required.

CLASSIFICATION OF PERIAPICAL DISEASE

Acute apical periodontitis

Causes of acute apical periodontitis include occlusal trauma, egress of bacteria from infected pulps, toxins from necrotic pulps, chemicals, irrigants or over-instrumentation in root canal therapy. Clinically the tooth is tender to biting, and widening of the periodontal space may be seen on a radiograph. Treatment depends on the pulpal diagnosis, and may thus range from occlusal adjustment to root canal therapy or extraction.

Chronic apical periodontitis

Chronic apical periodontitis occurs as a result of pulp necrosis. Affected teeth do not respond to pulp sensitivity tests. Tenderness to biting, if present, is usually mild, but some tenderness may be noted on palpation over the root apex. Radiographic appearance is varied, ranging from minimal widening of the periodontal ligament space to a large area of destruction of periapical tissues. Treatment involves root canal therapy or extraction.

Condensing osteitis

Condensing osteitis is a variant of chronic apical periodontitis and represents a diffuse increase in trabecular bone in response to irritation. Radiographically, a concentric radio-opaque area is seen around the offending root. Treatment is only required if symptoms/pulpal diagnosis indicate a need.

Acute apical abscess

An acute apical abscess is a severe inflammatory response to microorganisms or their irritants that have leached out into the periradicular tissues. Symptoms vary from moderate discomfort or swelling to systemic involvement such as raised temperature and malaise. The teeth involved are usually tender to both palpation and percussion. Radiographic changes are variable depending on the amount of periradicular destruction already present, but there is usually a well-defined radiolucent area, as in many situations an acute apical abscess is an acute exacerbation of a chronic situation. A well-recognised event is that of a phoenix abscess, which refers to an acute exacerbation of a chronic situation during treatment. Initial treatment of an acute apical abscess involves removal of the cause as soon as possible. Drainage should be established either by opening the tooth or by incision into a dependent swelling. An antibiotic may need to be prescribed depending on the patient's condition. Once the acute symptoms have subsided, root canal therapy or extraction may be performed.

Chronic apical abscess

In chronic cases the abscess has formed a communication through which it discharges. Such communications may be through an intraoral sinus or, less commonly, extraorally. Alternatively the discharge may be along the periodontal ligament, such cases mimicking a periodontal pocket. Usually these communications or tracts heal spontaneously following root canal therapy or extraction.

RADIOGRAPHIC LESIONS OF NON-ENDODONTIC ORIGIN

Although lesions noted on radiographs are usually of endodontic origin, this is not always the case. Other causes may be normal anatomical structures and benign or malignant lesions (see Box 9.2; this list is not exhaustive and readers should refer to an appropriate text on oral pathology).

Box 9.2 Radiographic lesions of non-endodontic origin

Normal anatomical structures
- Maxillary sinus
- Mental foramen
- Nasopalatine foramen

Benign lesions
- Cementoma
- Fibrous dysplasia
- Ossifying fibroma
- Primordial cysts
- Lateral periodontal cyst
- Dentigerous cyst
- Traumatic bone cyst
- Central giant cell granuloma
- Central haemangioma
- Ameloblastoma

Malignant lesions
- Squamous cell carcinoma
- Osteosarcoma
- Chondrosarcoma
- Multiple myeloma

Certain normal anatomical structures may mimic radiolucencies. In these situations the associated teeth will respond normally to pulp sensitivity tests and a radiograph taken from a different angle will reveal that the lesion is not closely related to the root. Benign lesions may mimic endodontic pathology, but in such situations the lamina dura will be intact around the teeth and final diagnosis will rely on appropriate biopsy. Malignant lesions are usually associated with rapid hard tissue destruction.

MANAGEMENT OF PULPAL AND PERIRADICULAR DISEASE

Endodontic treatment must be considered as part of an overall plan of care in such a way that it represents the patient's best interests and wishes. The past dental history will provide much information about attitude towards treatment. Good endodontic management takes time, requiring a commitment from both clinician and patient, and should be performed in a healthy oral environment.

Sequencing of treatment involves the:

1. management of pulpal or periodontal pain as a priority
2. extraction of unsaveable teeth
3. stabilisation of large carious lesions
4. institution of a preventive regimen, including periodontal therapy.

Irreversible pulpal damage occurs as a result of bacteria entering the pulp space. Treatment should be performed in an aseptic manner with the aim of preventing entry of further bacteria (e.g. rubber dam and coronal seal) and eliminating those already present. The adoption of the following antiseptic principles is therefore of paramount importance:

- chemomechanical debridement of the pulp cavity
- removal of infected dentine
- use of antimicrobial agents.

CHEMOMECHANICAL DEBRIDEMENT

Cleaning of root canals is carried out using a combination of irrigating solutions (chemo) and hand and automated instruments (mechanical); the use of rubber dam is mandatory (Fig. 9.1, Box 9.3).

Hand instruments

Hand instruments include barbed broaches, and Hedstrom and K type files (Fig. 9.2). Barbed broaches are placed loosely within the canal and turned through 90° to engage their barbs. They are used for removing vital pulp tissue or soft foreign objects such as cotton wool or paper points from root canals. Hedstrom files have a sharp cutting edge (positive rake) and are used in a linear manner, not in rotation. Hedstroms are not as popular as K type files for instrumentation, but they are useful for flaring canals and in retreatment.

K file designs are the type most commonly used in manual root canal instrumentation. The standard taper of hand

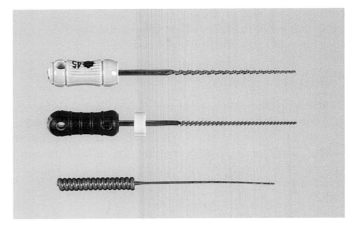

Fig. 9.2 Various types of root canal hand instruments (from top): Hedstrom, K type and barbed broach.

instruments is 0.02 mm/mm and they have a variety of tip sizes ranging from 0.06 to 1.40 mm. The increase in tip size is not uniform, with relatively bigger jumps in the smaller sizes, for example, the change from size 10 to 15 represents a jump of 50%, whilst that from size 55 to 60 represents a jump of 9% (Fig. 9.3). This 50% increase can lead to difficulty in negotiating narrow canals and has led to manufacturers constructing files of intermediate sizes, e.g. 0.12 mm.

The two most commonly used motions with K type files are watchwinding and balanced forces. Watchwinding refers to the gentle side-to-side rotation of the file (30° each way). This motion is useful for all stages of canal preparation, especially initial negotiation and finishing the apical third. Balanced forces (in many ways a development from watchwinding) involves rotating the instrument 60° clockwise to set the flutes and then rotating it 120° anti-clockwise whilst maintaining apical pressure sufficient to resist coronal movement of the file. Balanced forces is an efficient cutting motion and has been shown to maintain a central canal position even around moderate curvatures whilst allowing a larger size to be prepared apically as compared with other hand instrumentation techniques.

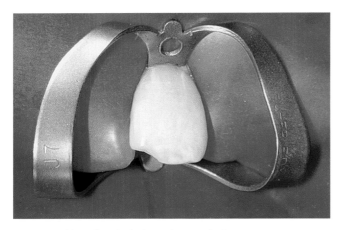

Fig. 9.1 Rubber dam isolation of upper incisor.

Box 9.3	Advantages offered by rubber dam

- Improved visibility
- Soft tissue protection
- Confinement of excess irrigant
- Prevention of saliva contamination
- Reduced liability in the medicolegal sense

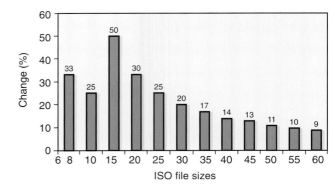

Fig. 9.3 Graphical representation of percentage increase in file tip diameter.

Other methods of movement include reaming and filing. Reaming infers rotating the root canal instrument clockwise; this motion draws the instrument into the canal and cuts dentine. Filing infers a linear motion of the instrument in a push–pull manner. Filing may be performed around the perimeter of a root canal, especially if it is oval or dumb-bell-shaped; such instrument manipulation is termed circumferential filing.

Nickel titanium (NiTi) alloy files

Root canal instruments have traditionally been manufactured out of stainless steel. Nickel titanium, noted for its hyperelasticity and shape memory, has radically changed endodontic file design and instrumentation techniques. Two features of nickel titanium have proved particularly beneficial to endodontics. Firstly, the increased flexibility has allowed files of a taper greater than the standard 0.02 mm/mm used for stainless steel instruments. Such variably tapered files range from 0.02 to 0.12 mm/mm. A 0.06 taper file, for example, is three times more tapered than a conventional 0.02 mm/mm file. Secondly, the superior resistance of nickel titanium to torsional failure compared with stainless steel has allowed the production of files that can be used in 360° rotation.

Greater taper (GT) files are an example of increased taper hand files. They are available in a tip size of 20 and have four different rates of taper: 0.06, 0.08, 0.10 and 0.12 (Fig. 9.4). The files all have a maximum flute diameter of 1 mm to restrict enlargement coronally. The flutes of the files are machined in a reverse direction and a balanced force movement is recommended for their use, but in reverse, in view of the flute direction. The handle on these

files is increased in size in order to make this reverse balanced force manipulation easier. The increased taper of these files reduces the need for stepping back of 0.02 taper instruments to taper the canal preparation.

A recent development is the introduction of hand ProTaper files (Fig. 9.5). This assortment of instruments includes three Shaper and three Finisher files and they are described in more detail in the rotary nickel titanium section (p. 94). They are used by hand in either a continuous rotations or watchwinding motion. The sequence of use for the hand ProTaper is as for the rotary ProTaper and is described in Box 9.6.

Automated instrumentation

There is considerable interest in trying to make the mechanical aspects of canal preparation easier and quicker. The most obvious example of this is the use of rotary stainless steel Gates-Glidden burs to create space coronally. File activation by means of a handpiece to speed up the creation of shape deeper in the canal system is also popular. Historically these have used a reciprocating action or oscillatory motion (ultrasonic or sonic), but the introduction of nickel titanium has allowed rotary instrumentation to be used over the full canal length in many situations.

Reciprocating handpieces

Developments in endodontic handpieces include a refinement of the reciprocating motion to one of 60°, as opposed to 90°, which provides a watchwinding type motion. A variety of file designs with a latch grip attachment are available for such handpieces; however, the M4 handpiece allows root canal files (Fig. 9.6) with conventional handles to be placed in it. Most instruments for use with the reciprocating type handpiece are manufactured from stainless steel and should be used with a light touch to prevent

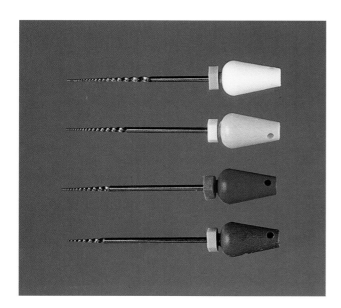

Fig. 9.4 Greater taper hand files.

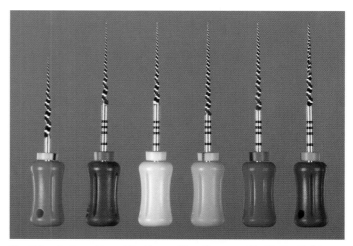

Fig. 9.5 Series of hand ProTaper files. Shapers: S1, S2, Sx; Finishers: F1, F2, F3.

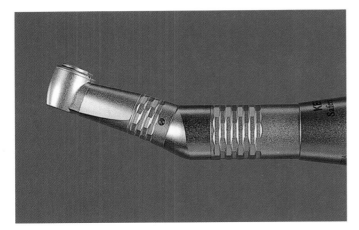

Fig. 9.6 M4 reciprocating handpiece.

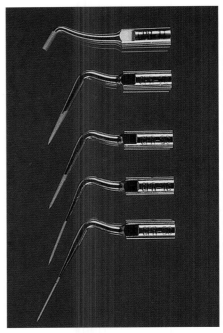

Fig. 9.8 Range of ultrasonic inserts for use with Spartan ultrasonic unit.

gouging of canal walls or instrument fracture. The watch-winding motion provided by such handpieces is particularly useful for negotiating and enlarging fine calcified canals using small files with a light touch.

Ultrasonic and sonic units

Particular advantages of the vibratory systems (Fig. 9.7) include the use of concurrent irrigation and the associated microstreaming which produces excellent canal debridement. The shaping ability of these instruments has proved to be disappointing and attention has turned to the use of rotary handpieces. The use of a size 15 file in an ultrasonic handpiece with irrigation, however, remains an excellent way of irrigating root canals. Ultrasound does retain a prominent position in endodontics, in particular for vibration of posts/crowns prior to removal, identifying canal orifices, removing fractured instruments and in apical surgery (Fig. 9.8).

Rotary nickel titanium (NiTi) instrumentation

Nickel titanium has allowed the production of files that can be rotated continuously in a handpiece through 360°. The advantages of the present generation of rotary nickel titanium instruments include increased debris removal in view of the continuous rotation, reduced canal transportation and smoother, faster canal preparation with less operator fatigue. Rotary instruments manufactured from nickel titanium can be classified into two groups: first, those that resemble conventional files but have varying tapers (e.g. Orifice shapers, ProFiles, rotary GTs; see Fig. 9.9, Table 9.1); and second, the Lightspeed (Fig. 9.10),

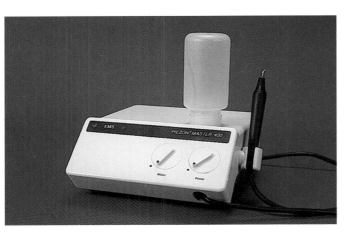

Fig. 9.7 The Piezon ultrasonic unit.

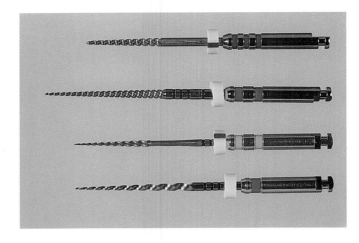

Fig. 9.9 A range of rotary nickel titanium (NiTi) files (from top): Orifice shapers, ProFile, Rotary GT and ProTaper.

Table 9.1   A representative selection of rotary nickel titanium (NiTi) instruments

Instrument	Tip size	Taper
ProFile, K3	Variable, 15–40+	Fixed 0.04 or 0.06
Standard GT files	20, 30, 40	Fixed 0.06, 0.08, 0.10
Accessory GT files	Variable 35, 50, 70	Fixed 0.12
Orifice shapers	Variable 20/0.05, 30/0.06, 40/0.06	Fixed 50/0.07, 60/0.08, 80/0.08
ProTaper finishing files	Variable 20/0.07, 25/0.08, 30/0.09	Progressive
Lightspeed	Variable	No taper

which has a thin shaft and cutting bud at the end similar to a Gates-Glidden bur. ProTaper files offer variable tip sizes but have multiple tapers along their length.

Irrigation

Irrigating solutions are usually delivered using a syringe with a 27 or 28 gauge needle, as this allows deeper penetration into the canal. Care should be taken to ensure that the needle does not bind and that irrigating solution does not pass into the periapical tissues. The role of the irrigant is to remove debris and provide lubrication for instruments. Specifically, an irrigant such as sodium hypochlorite will dissolve organic remnants and, most importantly, also has an antibacterial action. This may be used in a range of concentrations, from 0.5 to 5.25% (2.5% is popular). Sodium hypochlorite is caustic and can cause damage if extruded out of the tooth. Typically this will result in pain, swelling and profuse bleeding. If a hypochlorite accident occurs then the patient should be reassured and the tooth monitored for about 30 minutes. If the exudate continues to be profuse, then leaving the tooth on open drainage for 24 hours should be considered. In severe cases, an antibiotic and analgesic may need to be prescribed.

It is important that the irrigant is changed frequently. Ideally, irrigation should be performed between each file, at least every two to three files being the minimum. Instrumentation of the root canal wall results in the production of a smear layer. If removal of the smear layer is desired then an EDTA-containing irrigation solution should be used. There is no clinical consensus as to whether or not smear layer removal should be practised.

An effective way of delivering irrigating solutions is through an ultrasonic handpiece. Ultrasonic agitation (acoustic microstreaming; Fig. 9.11) has been shown to be effective in removing debris from canals. Sodium

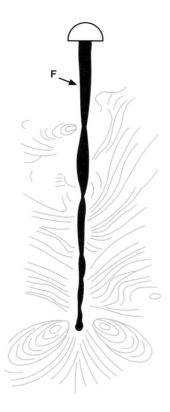

Fig. 9.11   Acoustic microstreaming associated with ultrasonic irrigation.

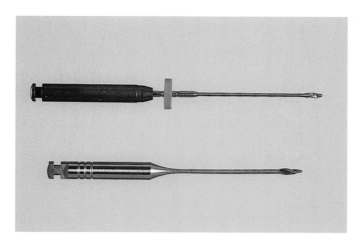

Fig. 9.10   Lightspeed nickel titanium (NiTi) instrument (top) and stainless steel Gates-Glidden bur (bottom).

hypochlorite is, however, corrosive and may rapidly cause deterioration of metallic components in handpieces.

Summary

The aim of root canal preparation is to debride the pulp space, rendering it as bacteria-free as possible, producing a shape amenable to obturation. This is complicated by root canal system anatomy, which is complex and makes complete cleaning impossible. Gross debridement of the root canal is performed using hand and automated instruments. These instruments remove infected dentine but also, most importantly, create space within the canal which allows the irrigating solutions to work effectively as it is not possible to clean root canals using instruments alone.

ROOT CANAL PREPARATION

Current thinking on canal preparation emphasises the development of shape in a crown-down manner, removing infected dentine as it is encountered, starting with the access cavity. Further cleaning of the canal is done using root canal irrigants (in particular, sodium hypochlorite because of its antimicrobial and tissue-dissolving properties). Root canal preparation involves gaining access to, cleaning and shaping the root canal system. It has both biological and mechanical objectives:

- Biological objectives – eliminate the pulp, bacteria and related irritants from the root canal system
- Mechanical objectives:
  produce a continuously tapering preparation
  - maintain the original anatomy
  - maintain the foramen position
  - keep the apical foramen as small as practical.

The sequence of canal preparation is as follows:

1. Access
2. Canal identification
3. Straight-line radicular access and preparation of coronal two-thirds
4. Length determination
5. Apical third preparation.

Access

Access to the root canal system involves both coronal access to the pulp chamber and radicular access to the root canals. The coronal access should:

- provide an unimpeded path to the root canal system
- eliminate the pulp chamber roof in its entirety
- be large enough to allow light in and enable examination of the pulp chamber floor for root canal orifices or fractures
- have divergent walls to support a temporary dressing between visits
- provide a straight-line path to each canal orifice.

The ideal access cavity will achieve the key objectives but will preserve as much sound coronal and radicular tissue as possible. Occasionally, however, it may be necessary to enlarge and deflect the access to enhance the preparation of roots that are especially curved in their coronal thirds. In these situations, access preparation is dynamic, developing as instrumentation progresses.

Assessment

Access to the root canal system is aided by examination of the following:

- coronal anatomy
- tooth position and angulation
- external root morphology
- preoperative radiograph (or preferably more than one taken at different angles), which affords information on:
  - the size of the pulp chamber +/– calcifications
  - the distance of the chamber from the occlusal surface; overlay the access bur to determine the maximum safe depth
  - the angle of exit of root canals from the floor of the pulp chamber; this provides an indication of the amount of coronal third root canal modification required to obtain straight-line radicular access
  - the number of roots, degree of root curvature and canal patency.

Endodontic access openings

Incisor and canine teeth. The access cavities for maxillary central and lateral incisors are similar and generally triangular in shape (Fig. 9.12a). Access cavities for maxillary and mandibular canines are almost identical and more ovoid in shape (Fig 9.12b). Access for mandibular central

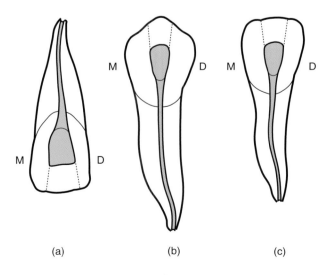

(a)   (b)   (c)

Fig. 9.12 Access cavity outline for upper incisor (**a**), canine (**b**) and lower incisor (**c**) teeth.

and lateral incisors are triangular in shape and a second canal may be present in 40% of cases. In general, extend the access in anterior teeth towards the incisal edge and under the cingulum (Fig 9.12c).

Premolar teeth. The maxillary first premolar in most cases contains two canals and the access cavity is extended more buccolingually than in single-rooted premolars (Fig. 9.13a). Five per cent may have a third root/canal placed buccally. In such situations, the access will be triangular in outline with the base towards the buccal.

The maxillary second premolar and both the mandibular first and second premolars usually have one centrally located root canal. However, if the canal appears to be situated under either the buccal or lingual cusp, look carefully for a second canal under the opposite cusp. The opening is a narrow oval in shape. The maxillary second premolar access is centred over the central groove. Access for mandibular premolars is buccal to the central groove (Fig. 9.13b).

Maxillary molars. The maxillary molar access is generally triangular in shape with the base to the buccal and the apex to the lingual. Usually one palatal and two buccal canals are identified; however, two canals may be present in the mesiobuccal root in 70% of cases (Fig. 9.14a).

Mandibular molars. The mandibular molar access is more trapezoidal in shape, with its base to the mesial and apex to the distal. Mandibular molars usually have two roots, with two canals in the mesial root and one in the distal. There is a possibility of a second canal in the distal root (33%) (Fig. 9.14b).

Access technique

On occasions, it may be deemed appropriate to initiate access prior to placement of rubber dam, as this allows better appreciation of external root contour and tooth position. Rubber dam should be placed as soon as the pulp chamber is identified for the reasons highlighted in Box 9.3. Broken-down teeth should be restored with

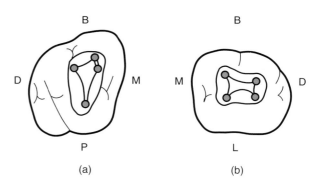

Fig. 9.14 Access cavity outline for upper (**a**) and lower (**b**) molar teeth.

amalgams, copper bands or temporary crowns when it is not possible to isolate them with rubber dam. It may be preferable to perform crown lengthening. Additionally, reduction of the occlusal table makes weakened cusps less vulnerable to fracture, simplifies canal identification and instrumentation as well as providing a level point of reference.

Prior to access cavity preparation, remove:

- as much restoration as necessary prior to entering the chamber, in order to reduce the likelihood of filling material entering the canal system
- all temporary materials when feasible
- crowns when feasible (full coverage crowns are frequently not oriented to the original tooth anatomy)
- all caries prior to entering the pulp chamber.

The access cavity is outlined provisionally on the tooth and progress is directed pulpally, being constantly mindful of the depth of bur penetration into the tooth. A round-ended bur is preferred, as flat-ended burs may gouge the access cavity walls. It is wise to compare depth of penetration of the bur with the apparent pulp chamber depth on the preoperative radiograph. If there is vital pulp tissue (haemorrhage), remove the coronal pulp with an excavator and/or radicular pulp with broaches and irrigate with sodium hypochlorite as good visibility is important. Once the pulp chamber has been identified, it is de-roofed using a slow-speed round bur (long-neck bur if necessary) directed coronally. The walls can then be smoothed and flared using a tapered bur in the air turbine.

Canal identification

Knowledge of dental anatomy and undulations in the floor of the pulp chamber in multi-rooted teeth are used as a guide. Magnification and coaxial lighting are particularly useful in helping to identify small root canal openings and to refine access. The pulp chamber space should be thoroughly irrigated with sodium hypochlorite solution and canal orifices identified using a straight probe or DG16 endodontic explorer. It is useful to remember that dentine is yellow/brown in colour, while the floor of the

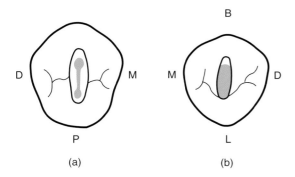

Fig. 9.13 Access cavity outline for upper (**a**) and lower (**b**) premolar teeth.

pulp chamber is grey. Stop and take radiographs if the canal(s) cannot be readily located.

Further refinement of the access may be performed following canal identification to enable straight-line access to the canals (Fig. 9.15). In addition, troughing may be performed using a small long-neck bur or ultrasonic inserts to remove dentine overlying canal orifices when looking for difficult canals such as second mesiobuccal canals in upper molar teeth (Fig. 9.16). Early progress into such canals is frequently hindered by an abrupt exit from the pulp chamber. Careful removal of overlying dentine permits easier access to these canals, which, prior to enlargement coronally, may only allow small files to pass for 2 mm before impacting on the outer canal wall.

Straight-line radicular access and preparation of coronal two-thirds

Root canals are infinitely variable in their shapes and sizes. This variation has more effect on canal preparation than the instrumentation system used. Larger canals allow easy placement of instruments and irrigating solutions, whereas smaller ones require pre-enlargement coronally prior to

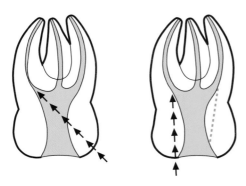

Fig. 9.15 Modification of coronal and radicular access to create straight-line access.

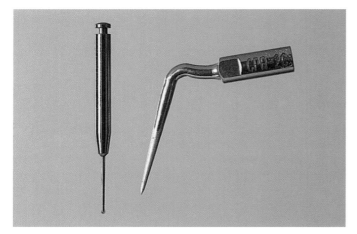

Fig. 9.16 LN bur and ultrasonic tip used for dentine removal on the pulp chamber floor.

the canal exploration. Preliminary assessment of the canal can be made with the smallest and most flexible instruments. Frequently the operator will not be able to determine the working length initially as files may be binding coronally.

Pre-enlargement is achieved by watchwinding file sizes 10–35 in series, gradually opening up narrow canal orifices to a size sufficient to take a Gates-Glidden bur or Orifice shaper. The pre-enlargement can then be developed further to produce straight-line radicular access, taking care to work the drill away from furcal regions of roots. A file should stand upright in the tooth and pass undeflected into the apical one-third of the canal once adequate straight-line radicular access has been achieved.

The advantages of preparing the coronal two-thirds first are listed in Box 9.4.

Coronal interferences influence the forces a file will exert within a canal. This is of particular importance in curved canals where files may prepare more dentine along the furcal (danger zone) compared with the outer canal wall. It is important to be aware of this, to limit the size of enlargement in curved canals and direct files away from the furcal wall to avoid a strip perforation (Fig. 9.17). Gates-Glidden burs may be used to relocate a canal away from the danger zone, but care should be taken to avoid over-enlargement. Gates-Glidden burs nos 6 and 5 should only be used on the walls of the access cavity, and no. 4 no deeper than the canal orifice. The no. 3 may be used to the mid-canal region and the no. 2 to the beginning of the canal curvature, or to near full bur length in a straight canal. The no. 1 is quite fragile, but may be used at ultra-slow speeds provided it is loose in the canal.

Box 9.4 Advantages of preparing the coronal two-thirds first

- The bulk of pulpal and related irritants are removed, reducing debris accumulation apically
- The bacterial count in the more coronal aspects of the canal is reduced
- Files and irrigating needles/solutions may be introduced deeper into the canal
- Files pass through irrigant as they move apically
- The increased space allows files to fit passively in the canal, making extrusion of infected material into the periapical tissues less likely
- Tactile sense and control when using files in the apical third are increased because the flutes do not bind coronally
- Precurved files remain curved, can be easily inserted and freely pass down the canal
- A greater volume of irrigant is present, enhancing pulp digestion and antimicrobial activity
- Larger files may be used for the working length radiograph
- Working length is more accurate because there is a more direct path to the canal terminus

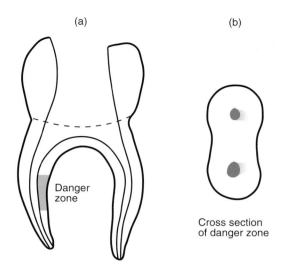

(a)   (b)

Danger
zone

Cross section
of danger zone

Fig. 9.17 (a) Lateral view of the danger zone where care needs to be taken in order to avoid strip perforation. **(b)** Cross-sectional view of the danger zone.

It is important to ensure that the apical region of the canal is not blocked with dentine debris or pulp tissue when using a crown-down technique. For this reason, small files with or without chelating agents are used to prevent blockage and ensure canal patency. Although apical preparation develops throughout canal enlargement, it is not completed until the end of the procedure when greater control is possible over the files in this most delicate region of the root canal.

Length determination

It is essential that care is taken over identification of the correct canal length. Clinically, the aim is to identify the apical constriction, which is the narrowest point of the root canal; apical to this the canal space widens to form the apical foramen. Frequently, however, an apical constriction is not present and thus a more useful landmark may be the apical foramen.

The most common way of determining canal length is using the working length radiograph. A file is placed in each canal at what is estimated to be the working length. This estimate of length is obtained by studying the preoperative radiograph (after adjustment for elongation or foreshortening) and using knowledge of the average lengths of teeth. Allowances obviously need to be made for fractured teeth and incisal wear. Tactile feel may also help in establishing the approximate working length, provided pre-enlargement has been performed. A bisecting angle radiograph may be taken; alternatively, the film may be held using a pair of Spencer Wells artery forceps or an Endo Ray film holder (the latter two techniques allow for radiographs more resembling a paralleling technique to be performed). The file position is checked on the radiograph

and adjusted as necessary. It is recommended that a repeat radiograph should be exposed with the file reset if it is more than 2 mm from the desired position.

Recently, electronic apex locators (Fig. 9.18) have been developed which greatly assist in the placement of the first length determination file (Box 9.5). These devices have a lip clip and a probe, which is touched against the file shaft. As the file approaches the foramen, the resistance or impedance changes and a visual display indicates when the file has touched the periapical tissues. It is usual to recheck the reading with different file sizes (08, 10, 15, 20 depending on canal size) to confirm its accuracy. The file position is then checked by exposing a radiograph and adjusted as necessary. The combination of electronic apex locators and radiographs is a reliable way of determining canal length. Care must be taken to ensure that the pulp chamber is dry and that there is minimal fluid in the root canals. Otherwise the fluid may short-circuit the apex locator through the gingival tissues and cause a false reading. This is a particular problem in heavily restored or crowned teeth.

Apical preparation

Considerable debate exists as to where to complete the apical preparation. Studies have shown that in vital cases

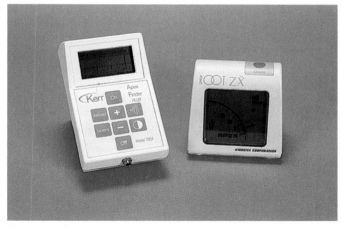

Fig. 9.18 Electronic apex locators: the Raypex (left) and the Root ZX (right).

Box 9.5 Apex locator usage
1. Use a file that is large enough to touch the canal wall in the apical region
2. Dry the pulp chamber and most of the root canal prior to use
3. Check absence of a short-circuit with metallic restorations
4. Working length is 0.5–1 mm short of 0.0 reading on apex locator
5. Confirm length on radiograph

(when it is unlikely that infection has spread to the apical 2 mm) the best success has been achieved when finishing 2 mm from the radiographic apex. In non-vital cases, however, bacteria, their by-products and infected dentine debris may remain in the apical few millimetres which may prejudice apical healing. Retrospective research has demonstrated that in these situations improved success is achieved when root canal preparation is finished at or within 0.5 mm of the radiographic apex.

In larger, straight canals, the apical portion is prepared using a slight rotational action of the file to an appropriate size after straight-line access has been confirmed. The original canal diameter is the major determinant of apical preparation size. The apical part of curved canals is generally kept small, usually a size 30, or in very curved canals a size 25. Stainless steel instruments larger than size 25 rapidly lose flexibility and will attempt to cut straight ahead. Repeated use of a small file will result in a canal preparation larger than the file, in other words the canal is still being enlarged.

Once the apical size has been determined and prepared, a greater flaring of the canal is accomplished by using successively larger instruments, each one about 0.5–1 mm shorter than the previous one. The distance of stepping back is determined by the degree of canal curvature. Alternatively, a greater taper hand file may be used in a reverse balance force mode to flare the junction of the apical and middle thirds. Greater tapered files, in view of their increased taper, are more likely to bind coronally, and final apical preparation should always be completed with 0.02 taper instruments. Care must be taken not to advance greater taper files too far down the root canal at any one time as this will result in binding and stress along their length, greatly increasing the risk of fracture especially at the tip.

Canal patency must be maintained at all times. This is accomplished by irrigating after each successively larger file, and then recapitulating with a file smaller than the one that prepared the apical portion of the canal (no. 15 is frequently used). Irrigation is used between each file to remove debris as well. Failure to recapitulate will result in canal blockage. Frequently, blockage can be difficult to clear and attempts to do so may result in a ledge or even perforation (Fig. 9.19).

Apical patency is considered controversial but is becoming increasingly accepted, particularly in retreatment or necrotic cases, provided the file is only just taken out of the root. There is no indication to use large files vigorously out of the root canal. A patency file is a small flexible instrument (08, 10) which will move passively through the terminus of a root canal without binding or enlarging the apical foramen. The aim is to prevent apical blockage, which will in turn reduce the incidence of ledge formation and transportation of the root canal. The use of a patency file also helps to remove vital (if this is desired) or necrotic pulpal remnants from the end of the canal. To

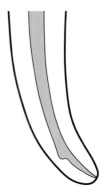

Fig. 9.19 A ledge in the apical third of canal preparation. This usually occurs as a result of using files that are too large or canal blockage.

use a patency technique, therefore, infers an intention to clean to the full canal length.

It is important that adequate resistance form is created at the end of the root canal preparation in order to reduce the risk of overfilling. There are two ways of achieving this: either producing an apical stop (intentional ledge) approximately 1 mm short of the radiographic root edge (Fig. 9.20a), or producing an apical seat (a shape that tapers back from the foramen), itself blending with the rest of the canal preparation (Fig. 9.20b). An electronic apex locator is a useful adjunct to the working length radiograph when creating an apical seat as part of the patency technique.

The use of excessively large files in curved canals may produce an hourglass shape termed a zip and elbow (Fig. 9.21). The choice of apical preparation is a personal one. Proponents of a patency technique would claim more of the canal is cleaned, whereas opponents emphasise the increased danger of extruding pulp tissue (infected or non-infected), dentine chips or obturation material from the root canal.

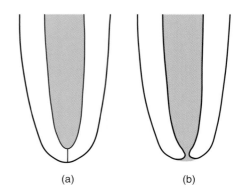

(a)   (b)

Fig. 9.20 **(a)** An apical stop. **(b)** An apical seat.

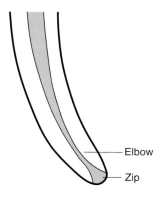

Fig. 9.21 Zip and elbow formation.

Rotary nickel titanium instrumentation techniques

It is important to appreciate that these instruments are for canal enlargement not canal negotiation. Increased taper rotary nickel titanium (NiTi) instruments are particularly effective when used in a crown-down manner. These are used either large size to small size or larger taper to smaller taper (Box 9.6). These new techniques are a major develop-ment, but care needs to be taken in their use to avoid file separation. Nickel titanium has good shape memory, so it is difficult to see when files are fatigued. Any instruments that show the least sign of damage should be discarded, as should ones used in very calcified or severely curved canals.

Rotary nickel titanium instrumentation techniques are evolving continuously as a greater understanding is gained of how best to use these instruments safely (Box 9.7). Pre-enlargement, coronal flaring and a crown-down approach are now recognised as important factors for getting the best results and limiting instrument failure. Each rotary instrument may be dipped in a lubricant prior to use, and they should be preceded by irrigation and a small hand instrument. This moves irrigating solutions deeper into the canal system and maintains the canal path. Apical preparation should be completed at the end. The increased taper instruments produce canal flaring as they advance down the canal. The sequence (Box 9.6) is repeated as necessary until the 20/0.06 reaches full length; two or three complete recapitulations may be necessary. It is important to finish the preparation by hand as this allows gauging of the apical size of the canal and checking that apical taper is present.

Increased taper rotary instruments with varying tip sizes have the advantage that they may be used to produce a range of sizes of apical preparation and may also be stepped back to produce more flare if desired. Greater taper (GT) files that have the same tip size may under-prepare the apical region of canals. It is therefore essential to use a subroutine with hand instruments to check the adequacy of preparation as previously described for the hand GT files (p. 100). The ProTaper series has files for shaping the coronal two-thirds and finishing the apical third. These instruments are available in different tip sizes and have variable tapers along their length.

Box 9.6 Rotary canal instrumentation sequences

Rotary canal instruments are used either large to small, or larger taper to smaller taper. Three instrumentation sequences are described below. In these techniques, straight-line access should be present and the canal should be patent. Apical size and canal taper are determined using hand instruments.

Orifice shapers and 0.06 ProFiles (Gates-Glidden burs may be substituted for Orifice shapers)
Orifice shaper 60/0.08
Orifice shaper 50/0.07
Orifice shaper 40/0.06
ProFile 35/0.06
ProFile 30/0.06
ProFile 25/0.06
ProFile 20/0.06

Rotary GT instrumentation (all size 20 at tip)
Rotary GT 0.10
Rotary GT 0.08
Rotary GT 0.06

ProTaper Shaper and Finisher files
- S1 to length of exploratory file, brush laterally when resistance met
- S2 (or Sx if wished to relocate canal)
- Establish electronic apex locator length
- S1 and S2 to EAL stop brushing, finishing 1 mm short
- Then confirm working length
- F1 to EAL 0.0–0.5 mm, gauge with hand files
- F2, F3 as required, may be stepped back at 0.5 and 1 mm intervals

---

Box 9.7 Guidelines for the use of rotary nickel titanium instruments

- Speed should be limited to 150–300 rpm in an electric handpiece
- Instruments must be used with a light touch, such as would not break a narrow lead propelling pencil
- A touch/retract/touch/retract technique is recommended; never keep the instrument at the same point in the canal
- Advance files no more than 1 mm at a time
- Limit the use of each file to approximately 4 seconds
- Damaged files should always be discarded
- It is important to be cautious in certain situations:
  - calcified canals (ideally it should be possible to place a size 20/0.02 taper file to length prior to using rotary files in the apical third)
  - canals having sharp curvature in the apical region
  - two canals that join into one smaller canal at a sharp angle
  - large canals that suddenly narrow

Lightspeed instruments are used to create an apical stop, with canal taper being produced using the instruments in a step-back manner. They have the disadvantage of not imparting a taper to the canal automatically because of their design, but the narrow cross-sectional area of their shaft makes them very flexible. Lightspeed instruments are useful for apical preparation, but there are more effective rotary instruments for imparting a taper to the root canal preparation.

The rotary nickel titanium instrumentation technique looks to be a promising development in canal preparation. However, it is important to be cautious in certain situations and to practise the technique extensively in extracted teeth in order to get a feel for the instruments.

ONE-VISIT ROOT CANAL TREATMENT

Root canal therapy may be performed in one visit if time allows and the canals can be dried. However, it is important that procedures are not rushed and compromised just so that treatments can be performed in one visit. One-visit root canal treatment is particularly appropriate for vital cases such as irreversible pulpitis (Box 9.8).

An advantage of doing a procedure in two visits is that an intracanal dressing of calcium hydroxide can be placed. This compound has a high pH and will further help to reduce the bacterial flora. Care needs to be taken to ensure that a sound coronal seal of 3–4 mm of temporary dressing material is present to prevent recontamination of the canal between visits. It is also usual to place a small pledget of cotton wool prior to placing the temporary dressing in order to prevent it dropping into the canal between visits or during subsequent removal.

ROOT CANAL OBTURATION

The objective of root canal obturation is to provide a hermetic (fluid-tight) seal of the canal from coronal to apical. Complete as opposed to apical seal is considered important because recontamination occurs as a result of coronal leakage, especially from saliva. If the remainder of the coronal seal (temporary or final restoration) is inadequate, contamination of the root canal filling will occur eventually leading to failure.

Box 9.8 Single- versus multiple-visit treatment

- Single-visit treatment is appropriate for vital non-infected cases
- Infected cases benefit from an intervisit dressing of $Ca(OH)_2$
- Coronal seal must be maintained to prevent recontamination between visits

---

Requirements before root canal filling

Chemomechanical preparation must be complete, the root canal dry and the tooth asymptomatic before a root filling is inserted. Any serous exudate from the periapical tissues indicates the presence of inflammation. It is advisable to recheck the canal length in situations of persistent seepage as this may frequently result from over-instrumentation and damage to the periapical tissues. If there is persistent seepage, calcium hydroxide should be used as a root canal dressing until the next visit.

Properties of root filling materials

A root canal filling material should:

- be easily introduced into the root canal
- not irritate periradicular tissues
- not shrink after insertion
- seal the root canal laterally, apically and coronally
- be impervious to moisture
- be sterile or easily sterilised before insertion
- be bacteriostatic, or at least not encourage bacterial growth
- be radio-opaque
- not stain tooth structure or gingival tissues
- be easily removed from the canal as necessary.

A sealer should:

- satisfy the above requirements of a root filling material
- provide good adhesion to the canal wall
- have fine powder particles to allow easy mixing, or be a two-paste system
- set slowly.

Types of root filling materials

The root filling materials available are as follows:

- solid and semisolid materials (e.g. gutta-percha and silver points) – silver points are not recommended as they do not seal the canal laterally or coronally and may cause tooth or gingival staining
- sealers and cements (e.g. Tubliseal, AH Plus, Pulp Canal Sealer, Roths Sealer, AH 26)
- medicated pastes (e.g. N2, Endomethosone, Spad, Kri) – these are not recommended as they may contain paraformaldehyde, which is cytotoxic.

Gutta-percha filling techniques

Both cold and warm techniques (except where indicated) will produce acceptable clinical results if used correctly; however, personal preference usually determines the final choice (Box 9.9).

Cold lateral condensation

The objective of cold lateral condensation of gutta-percha is to fill the canal with gutta-percha points (cones) by

Box 9.9 Gutta-percha filling techniques

Cold condensation
- Single cone (not recommended as it does not seal laterally and coronally)
- Cold lateral condensation

Warm condensation
- Warm lateral condensation
- Thermomechanical compaction
- Vertical condensation
- Thermoplasticised gutta-percha
- Carrier-based techniques

condensing them laterally against the sides of the canal walls (Fig. 9.22). The technique requires a tapered canal preparation.

A spreader is selected that reaches to within 1 mm of the working length. Two types of spreader are available for condensing gutta-percha: long-handled and finger. The advantage of a finger spreader is that it is not possible to exert the high lateral pressure that can occur with long-handled spreaders, which reduces the possibility of root fracture. A master point is selected that allows a friction fit in the apical portion of the root canal. When this is marked, it is called 'tug back' (like pulling a dart out of a dart board). However, this may be difficult to achieve with small size gutta-percha points, and therefore it is usual to accept a friction fit in narrow canals. If it is not possible to place the point to working length, select one that passes to full length and trim 0.5 mm off the end using a scalpel (this has the effect of making the point slightly larger). Retry the point and adjust as necessary. The length of the point is marked at the reference position and a check radiograph is exposed.

Sealer is mixed according to the manufacturer's instructions and introduced into the canal by coating the apical third of the master point. This is placed into the root

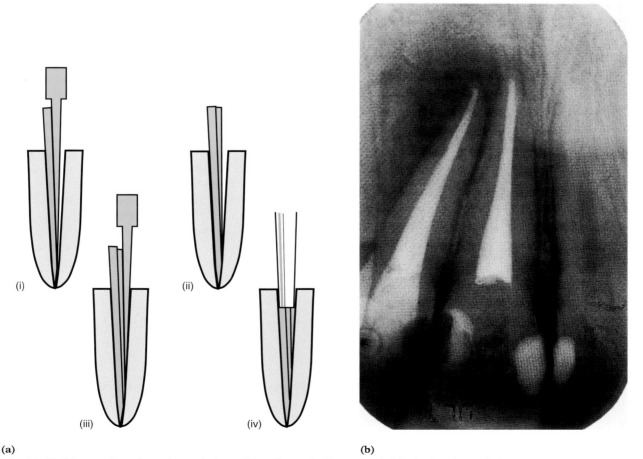

(a)   **(b)**

Fig. 9.22 **(a)**, (i)–(iv) Lateral condensation technique. **(b)** Radiograph of two canals filled using this technique.   103

canal slowly to aid coating of the canal walls and reduce the likelihood of sealer passing into the periapical tissues. If two or more canals are obturated with gutta-percha, undertake one at a time unless they meet in the apical third.

Once the master cone is seated, a spreader is placed between it and the canal wall using firm pressure in an apical direction (lateral pressure may bend or break the spreader or fracture the root). This pressure, maintained for 20 seconds, will condense the gutta-percha apically and laterally, leaving a space into which an accessory point is placed. An accessory cone the same size or one size smaller than the spreader is used. Rotate the spreader slightly, remove it, and immediately place the accessory cone. Repeat the procedure until the root canal is filled. The finger spreader condenses each cone into position; however, the final cone is not condensed as this would leave a spreader tract and contribute to leakage.

The gutta-percha is cut off 1 mm below the cemento-enamel junction or gingival level (whichever is the more apical) using a hot instrument, and vertically condensed with a plugger. It is important not to leave root filling material coronally as it may stain the crown of the tooth. The access cavity should now be sealed, the rubber dam removed and a postoperative radiograph taken (Fig 9.22b).

Warm gutta-percha techniques

Warm lateral condensation will soften the gutta-percha and make it easier to condense, possibly resulting in a denser root filling. The spreader may be heated by placing it in a hot bead steriliser before insertion into the canal. Alternatively, the friction of ultrasonic vibration may be used to introduce heat into the root filling.

Thermomechanical compaction involves the use of a compactor, which resembles an inverted file, placed in a slow-speed handpiece. The frictional heat from the compactor plasticises gutta-percha and the blades drive the softened material into the root canal. Care must be taken only to use this instrument in the straight part of the canal in order to avoid gouging of the walls. A modification of the technique has been described as an adjunct to lateral condensation. First, gutta-percha is laterally condensed in the apical half of the canal to provide apical control, and then a compactor is used to plasticise and condense the gutta-percha in the straight coronal half of the canal.

Vertical condensation of warm gutta-percha involves applying heat to the gutta-percha, condensing it down the root canal from coronal to apical (the downpack) and then filling the remaining space (the backfill). The procedure aims to seal the terminus of the canal with an accurate cone fit, and the downpack then forces sealer and gutta-percha along the lines of least resistance. Significant changes have been made to the armamentarium recently,

simplifying the technique and making it more operator friendly.

The original technique of vertical condensation used two types of instrument: a pointed heat carrier that was warmed to cherry-red heat in a Bunsen burner, and a flat-ended plugger that was used cold to condense the thermoplasticised gutta-percha. The introduction of electric heat carriers (Touch and Heat) afforded more control over the length of time that heat was applied and recently the introduction of a more sophisticated thermostatically controlled heat carrier, the System B, has further simplified the technique. Two variations in warm condensation of gutta-percha exist: the classical interrupted technique, and the recently introduced continuous-wave method.

The downpack for both methods is commenced by using the heat carrier to sear off the gutta-percha master cone at the canal orifice (Fig. 9.23). Immediately following this, a cold, loosely fitting plugger is introduced to condense around the periphery of the gutta-percha and seal the canal coronally. A sustained push is now applied to the centre of the gutta-percha, causing the sealer and warm gutta-percha to follow the path of least resistance down the main canal and along any lateral or accessory canals. This sustained push is termed a wave of condensation.

In the *classical interrupted technique*, a series of waves of condensation are utilised as follows. The heat carrier is reapplied 3–4 mm into the gutta-percha and removed with a small bite of gutta-percha attached. The filling is then condensed as described previously to form a second wave of condensation. This cycle is repeated until 5 mm from the canal terminus, or up to the end of the straight part of the canal, and a sustained application of apical pressure is made as the gutta-percha cools.

In the *continuous-wave method*, the downpack consists of one continuous wave of condensation, rather than several interrupted waves. The appropriate plugger (one of four sizes that fits to within 5–7 mm of the canal terminus) is selected to match the taper of the canal, and is activated for 2 or 3 seconds as it passes down the canal and condenses the gutta-percha to just short of its binding point. The plugger is then held, applying vertical pressure for 10 seconds prior to reactivation, which allows the plugger to drop to its binding point prior to removal together with excess gutta-percha.

The downpack of both techniques results in obturation of the apical third, filling of lateral and accessory canals and an empty coronal two-thirds. Backfilling of the canal is achieved by delivering increments of thermoplasticised gutta-percha and condensing them.

Thermoplasticised gutta-percha is conveniently delivered using the Obtura gun (Fig. 9.24). Small increments are placed and condensed in order to keep shrinkage to a minimum. It is also useful in cases of internal resorption where the gutta-percha flows into canal irregularities as it is condensed. Care must be taken to ensure that there is

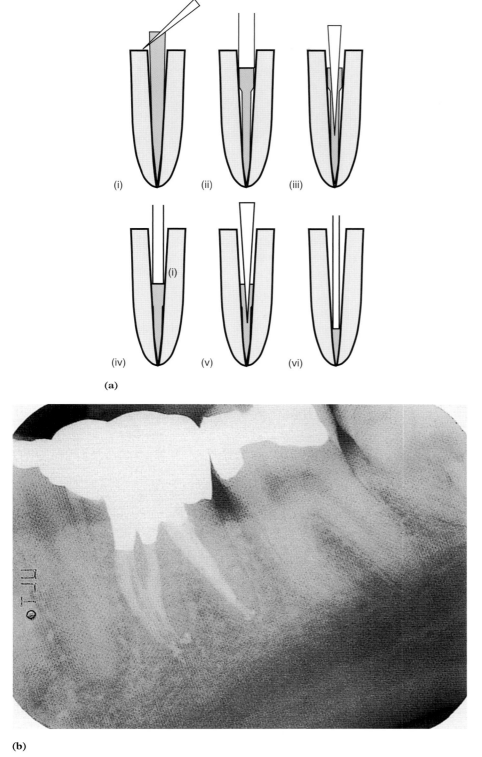

(i)　(ii)　(iii)

(iv)　(i)　(v)　(vi)

(a)

(b)

Fig. 9.23 (a) Vertical condensation technique. (b) Radiograph showing how vertical condensation helps to obturate complex canal anatomy.

adequate apical resistance form to ensure that excess gutta-percha is not pushed out of the canal system.

Carrier-based systems consist of a solid central core usually made out of plastic (although originally constructed from stainless steel or titanium) which is supplied with a covering of gutta-percha. The size of the carrier required is checked using a size verification device. The carrier is placed in the oven provided and heated until the gutta-percha is soft. Sealer is placed in the canal, the carrier is pushed home to the desired length, and any excess is cut off in the pulp chamber at orifice level. Carrier-based

105

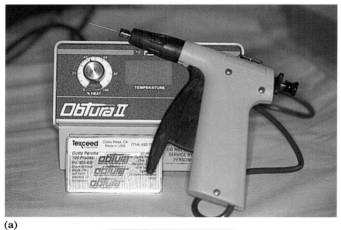

(a)

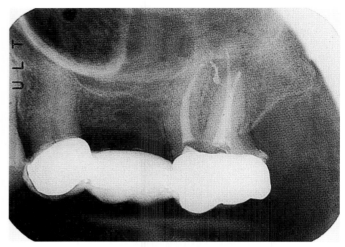

Fig. 9.25 Radiograph showing excess obturation material opposite a lateral canal.

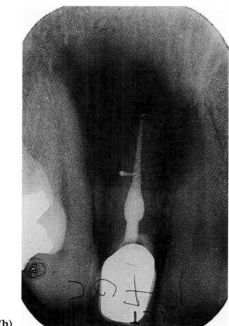

(b)

Fig. 9.24 (a) The Obtura 2 gutta-percha gun. (b) Internal resorption case filled with Obtura 2.

systems produce excellent results in experienced hands but have the disadvantage of a solid central core that can complicate restoration, especially post-placement.

Under- and overfilling

A small amount of cement may be seen apically after obturation, especially when using warm gutta-percha techniques. Cement may also be seen opposite large accessory, or lateral, canals (Fig. 9.25). It is therefore important that a relatively inert sealer is used. Proponents of vertical condensation argue the distinction between overfilling and vertical overextension of underfilled canal systems; that is, filling materials may be overextended or extruded beyond a canal system that has not been sealed internally. Underfilling of a canal system could also indicate that it has not been debrided satisfactorily. In such situations, necrotic

pulp tissue, bacteria and their by-products would be expected to lead to failure. Overfilling infers that the whole canal system is obturated but that excess material has been placed beyond the confines of the root canal, and represents a quite different situation. The aim of vertical condensation is not to produce extrusion of filling material. Nevertheless, this can occur and histological studies have shown that these overfills do produce an inflammatory response even though patients do not report discomfort.

Occasionally gross apical overfills of gutta-percha may be observed following lateral or vertical condensation. Such overfills indicate lack of apical control and require canal re-obturation as it is unlikely that it will be adequately sealed. Similarly, canals with voids should normally be reobturated unless the spaces are very small.

Root fracture

The obturation of a root canal may rarely produce a root fracture. Periodontally involved teeth or thin roots/over-instrumented canals are particularly at risk. Such an event is usually catastrophic for the tooth, except in the case of multi-rooted teeth where it may be possible to amputate a root or hemisect the tooth. Root fractures may be avoided by using passively fitting pluggers/spreaders and not applying excessive obturation forces.

The remainder of the seal

It is important after completing canal obturation to ensure that there is an adequate coronal seal over the root filling, as coronal leakage has been shown to be an important cause of failure. This can be achieved by placing a layer of bonding resin or glass ionomer over the floor of the pulp chamber and canal orifices. However, a suitable core should be placed as soon as possible (Fig. 9.26).

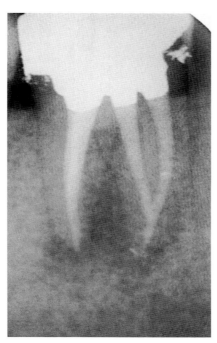

Fig. 9.26 Molar tooth with amalcore completing the root canal seal.

ASSESSMENT OF ROOT CANAL TREATMENT

Success and failure of root canal therapy

Clinical and radiographic observation is required for at least 1 year following endodontic treatment but preferably for 4 years. Success of root canal therapy is indicated by:

- no loss of function
- absence of pain and swelling
- no sinus tract
- radiographic evidence of a normal periodontal space around the tooth.

If a radiograph reveals that a lesion has remained the same or has only diminished in size, then the treatment is not considered a success. In such situations, observation for 4 years is advised. If total repair has not occurred by that time, the treatment is considered a failure (Box 9.10).

The cause of failure may lie either inside (intraradicular) or outside (extraradicular) the root canal system.

Intraradicular causes of failure include:

- necrotic material being left in the root canal
- contamination of an initially sterile root canal during treatment
- persistent infection of a root canal after treatment
- loss of coronal seal and reinfection of a disinfected and sealed canal system
- bacteria left in accessory or lateral canals.

Extraradicular causes of failure include:

- persistent periradicular infection
- radicular cysts
- vertical root fractures.

Box 9.10   Indications of failure of root canal therapy

- A lesion occurring subsequent to root canal treatment
- A pre-existing lesion increases in size
- A lesion has remained the same or only decreased in size over the 4-year observation period
- There is pain, swelling or loss of function
- A sinus tract is present
- Signs of continuing root resorption or hypercementosis are present

---

Further causes of failure may be iatrogenic in nature, in particular when post space has been created without consideration of the intra- and extraradicular anatomy (Fig. 9.27). Such cases may result in root perforation or root fracture at the tip of the post.

Bacteria play an important role in failure. It is therefore essential that teeth for root canal retreatment can be isolated with rubber dam, in order to prevent leakage of saliva and confine hypochlorite irrigation.

Management of failed root canal treatment

Failure, depending on its aetiology, may be dealt with in one of three ways: root canal retreatment, periradicular surgery or extraction. Extraction is usually indicated for root fractures in single-rooted teeth or in cases of gross caries where the tooth is non-restorable. On occasions, it may be possible to resect a fractured root in multi-rooted teeth or perform crown lengthening when gross caries is present in order to make isolation and future restoration possible.

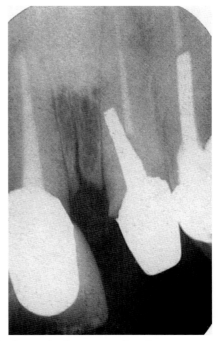

Fig. 9.27 Radiograph of a post perforation.

107

Root canal retreatment

Root canal retreatment is usually considered in preference to surgical intervention, despite the latter being a quicker solution, as surgery will only seal over uncleaned canal space, which will eventually leak. Additional problems with a surgical approach include the effects of compromising root length and bone support on prosthetic or periodontal grounds. If it is considered that access to the root canals cannot be gained without risk of compromising the tooth's prognosis then surgery is indicated.

The aim of root canal retreatment is to eliminate micro-organisms that have either survived previous treatment or re-entered the root canal system. The feasibility of root canal retreatment depends on the operator's ability to gain access to the root canal system and, in particular, the apical third. Careful assessment of the preoperative radiograph should be made with regard to whether or not a post has been used, what type it is, the type of root filling material (paste, gutta-percha, silver point), and potential problems such as curves, perforations or ledges.

In a retreatment procedure, access is usually complicated by the presence of coronal restorations, retentive devices in the root canals and root canal filling materials. Additional magnification and lighting are especially useful

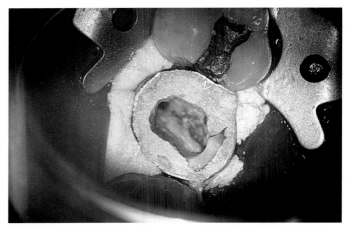

Fig. 9.28 Copper band used to support restorative material helps isolation in a retreatment case.

in root retreatment procedures. Loupes and a headlamp will provide good visibility of the pulp chamber floor and canal orifices. Working in the middle and apical thirds of the root canal, however, requires an operating microscope to see clearly.

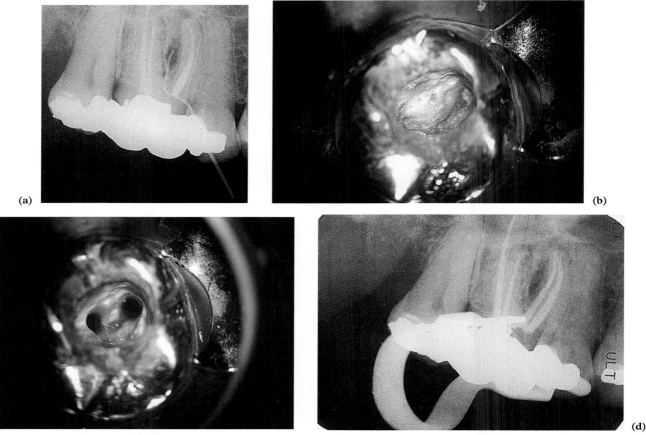

(a)

(b)

(c)

(d)

Fig. 9.29 (a) Radiograph showing persistent lateral lesion associated with upper first molar mesiobuccal root. (b) Mesiobuccal region of pulp chamber. (c) Completion of canal preparation. (d) Radiograph showing re-obturated mesiobuccal root.

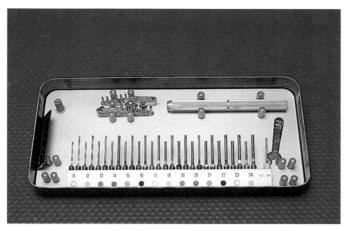

Fig. 9.30 Masserann post removal kit.

The quality of the coronal restoration must be considered when gaining access. Evidence of leakage coronally around the restoration margins usually indicates that it should be removed prior to performing root canal retreatment. Removal of the restoration has the advantage of:

• ensuring removal of all caries

• allowing a thorough check to be made for cracks
• providing excellent access for identifying missed canals.

In cases of extensive breakdown, it may be necessary to place a copper band and build up a small core prior to embarking on treatment in order to ensure a seal around the margins of the dam, avoid compromising asepsis and establish a four-walled access cavity to contain irrigant solutions (Fig. 9.28).

It is usual to encounter a core under a coronal restoration in root canal retreatment cases. The most common non-tooth-coloured materials include amalgam and cermet cements. These can be removed using surgical length round tungsten carbide burs in the high-speed handpiece followed by long neck burs used at slow speed (Fig. 9.29).

When the floor of the pulp chamber is approached, ultrasonic tips offer a safer alternative to burs for dispersing material remaining over furcal areas and in the orifices of root canals. Tooth-coloured cores are more awkward to remove as they may be difficult to distinguish from dentine. Careful observation of the dried access cavity floor will usually allow differentiation between the dentine and the restorative material. In addition, the texture of the

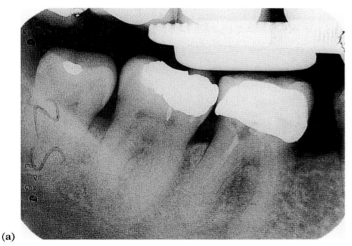

(a)

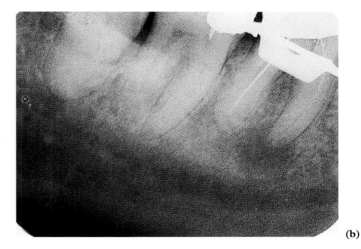

(b)

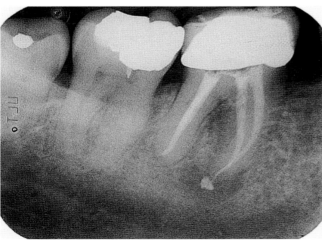

(c)

Fig. 9.31 (a) Preoperative radiograph of lower molar containing hard root canal paste. (b) Interim radiograph to check progress, mesial root canals ledged. (c) Final radiograph following negotiation of canal past the ledge and obturation.

restorative material is rougher than the dentine and this can be detected using an endodontic explorer. The access cavity should be thoroughly evaluated at this stage with regard to its extent and the possibility of discovering previously untreated canals.

The removal of a post should not be attempted if the force to remove it could result in root fracture. Ultrasonic vibration may be used initially to try to break the cement seal. It is important not to use ultrasound at too high power as this may produce microcracks in the root or excessive heat, especially if a coolant is not used. In some situations, ultrasonic vibrations may result in the post becoming free within the canal. If ultrasonic vibration is unsuccessful, it is necessary to use a device to pull out the post and core. This can usually be accomplished in anterior teeth using a post extractor.

The fracture of a post within a root canal can pose a major problem, and care should be taken to try not to further weaken, fracture or perforate the root. Such situations should first be tackled by troughing around the post to remove the luting cement using a small long-neck bur or an ultrasonic tip. As progress is made up the root canal, the smaller suborifice tips may be used.

Use of ultrasonic tips will remove many fractured posts without having to resort to additional means such as the Masserann kit (Fig. 9.30). In this system, a suitably sized trepan is directed along the side of the post in the space created by the ultrasonic tips. A smaller trepan may then be used to grip and remove the fractured portion (additional ultrasonic vibration applied to the trepan may be useful at this point). If the post is of the screw type, it may be unscrewed after the use of ultrasound to weaken the cement seal either by placing a groove in its end or by grasping it with a tight fitting trepan.

Access to the apical third of the root is usually restricted by the presence of materials used to obturate the canal. Those most frequently used include pastes, gutta-percha and silver points. A thorough evaluation of the access cavity should be performed, modifying it as necessary to give straight-line access to the root canals prior to attempting removal of the filling materials.

Soft pastes can usually be easily penetrated using short, sharp hand files and copious irrigation. The use of an ultrasonically powered file with accompanying irrigation can be helpful in these situations, especially for removing remnants of paste from root canal walls, which may remain despite careful hand instrumentation. Rotary nickel titanium instruments may also help with removal. Hard pastes can be particularly difficult to remove (Fig. 9.31) and usually need to be drilled out with a small long-neck bur, or chipped out using an ultrasonic insert as described previously. These procedures can only be used in the straight part of the canal and it is important to employ magnification and lighting, as the risk of going off-line and perforating is high. Irrigation with EDTA and sodium hypochlorite should be employed together with frequent

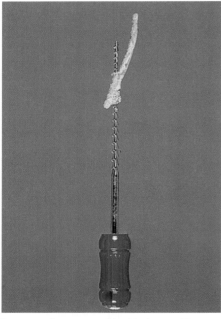

Fig. 9.32 Gutta-percha removed by Hedstrom file.

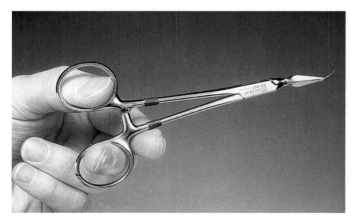

Fig. 9.33 Steiglitz forceps used for silver point removal.

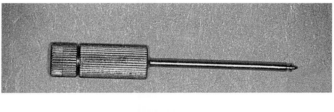
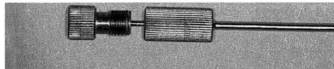

Fig. 9.34 Masserann extractor which may be used for gripping silver points or fractured instruments.

drying to ensure good visibility, especially deep within the canal.

Poorly condensed gutta-percha root fillings may be removed by rotating one or two small Hedstrom files (Fig. 9.32) around or between the root canal filling points, pulling and removing them intact. If this is unsuccessful, removal of the root canal filling should be considered in stages, removing first the coronal and then the middle and apical thirds. Gates-Glidden drills may be used coronally in the straight part of the canal. These are available in a range of sizes and have a safe cutting tip that reduces the risk of perforation, provided that too large a size is not used. Care should be taken with these drills, because, if too fast a speed is used, they may inadvertently screw into the canal and cause considerable damage (a suitable speed is around 1000–1500 rpm). Other rotary instruments that may be used for the removal of gutta-percha include those made from nickel titanium, which are extremely efficient in this respect. They may be used with care at higher speeds (up to 700 rpm) than for canal preparation.

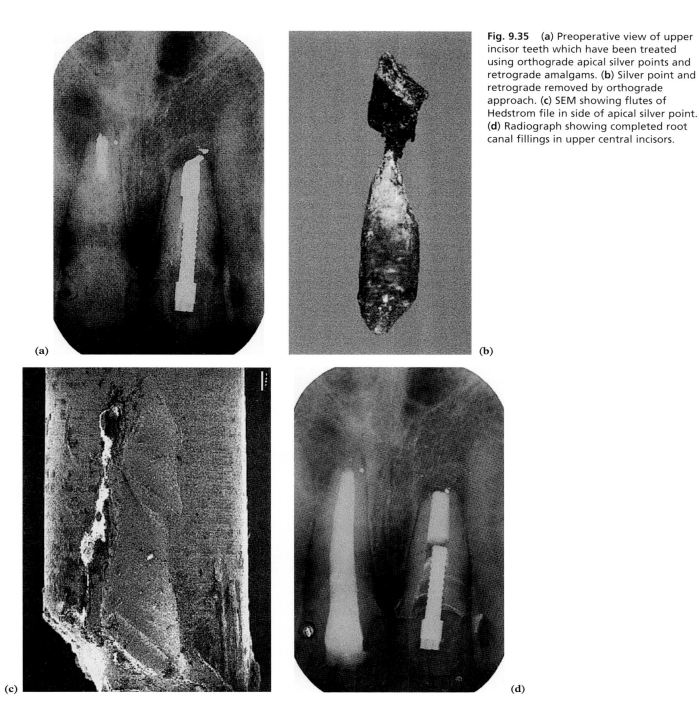

(a)

(b)

(c)

(d)

Fig. 9.35 (a) Preoperative view of upper incisor teeth which have been treated using orthograde apical silver points and retrograde amalgams. (b) Silver point and retrograde removed by orthograde approach. (c) SEM showing flutes of Hedstrom file in side of apical silver point. (d) Radiograph showing completed root canal fillings in upper central incisors.

If gutta-percha removal is being attempted around a curvature, it is important to use a solvent such as chloroform, oil of cajaput or oil of turpentine to soften the gutta-percha, aid mechanical removal and reduce the chance of transporting the main axis of the canal. Chloroform is the most effective solvent for dissolving gutta-percha.

The seal of silver point root canal fillings is rarely as good as the radiographic appearance would suggest, and in many cases relies on the cement used. If this washes out, then corrosion will occur leading to failure of the root canal filling. The approach to removal depends on whether the point extends and can be seen to extrude within the pulp chamber. In such situations, many silver points can be removed easily by grasping with Steiglitz forceps or pin pliers and levering (Fig. 9.33). If the points cannot be removed easily, ultrasonic vibrations can be applied to the forceps holding them.

If the silver point has been cut off at the canal orifice, it is usually not possible to grip it. In such situations, an ultrasonic tip may be used to cut a trough around the point; care needs to be taken not to touch the point as the silver is much softer than the steel used in the manufacture of the ultrasonic tip and preferential removal of the point will occur. A Masserann extractor (Fig. 9.34) can be used to grip the point and remove it once a trough approximately 2 mm deep has been prepared.

Sometimes it may be necessary to work an ultrasonic spreader tip down the side of a point placed deep in a root canal. Removal in these situations may be facilitated by placing a Hedstrom file along the side of the point and pressing it into the soft silver in order to help pull it coronally (Fig. 9.35). Occasionally it may help to apply ultrasonic vibrations to the Hedstrom file prior to pulling.

Instrument fracture. The separation (fracture) of root canal instruments is a procedural hazard in root canal therapy. File fracture may be minimised by:

- maintaining a good quality control programme
- discarding any damaged instruments
- not forcing instruments
- using instruments in the correct sequence
- not rotating stainless steel instruments more than a quarter turn clockwise.

The removal of fractured instruments has traditionally been performed using Masserann trepans and extractors together with ultrasonic vibration. New developments in ultrasonic tip designs, the use of magnification and lighting, and in particular the operating microscope have simplified instrument removal (Fig. 9.36). Loupes and a headlamp will help in the removal of superficially placed instruments. If working deep within the canal, it is advisable to use the operating microscope, especially if using ultrasound.

It may be possible to bypass a separated instrument which cannot be removed. This becomes more difficult apically as the canal is usually rounder in cross-section in this region. If this is not possible, the canal should be shaped, irrigated and obturated to the level of the fractured instrument, as in vital uninfected cases success rate will frequently not be affected (Fig. 9.37). However, if the root canal system is infected then the fractured instrument may preclude thorough debridement of the root canal system. In such situations, prognosis is compromised.

Frequently after removal of filling materials or broken instruments, a ledge will be noted in the side of the root canal. This may usually be bypassed by placing a sharp bend at the tip of a small file. The ledge may then be smoothed using a linear filing motion. Shaping and irrigation of the canal system can then be completed prior to canal obturation. Canals may also be blocked; in such situations, the access cavity is refined and a small sharply curved file is used to pick around the blockage. Frequently the coronal part of the blockage is denser and once this is penetrated rapid progress may be made to the apex. On occasions it may not be possible to unblock a canal and care must be taken not to over-instrument and create a perforation.

The success of root canal retreatment is good (94–98%) when it is being undertaken to achieve a technical improvement in potential failures. When periradicular pathology is present, the success rate is much lower (62–78%). Retreatment itself can bring its own problems: perforation, separated instruments and compromised cleaning and obturation of the canal system. It is important that patients are informed of such factors prior to embarking on this procedure.

Apical surgery

Apical surgery is an alternative to root canal retreatment. However, conventional orthograde root canal treatment is preferred to surgery if at all possible, even if it is considered that surgery may be necessary. It must be remembered that the main cause of failure is inadequate debridement and bacterial contamination of the root canal

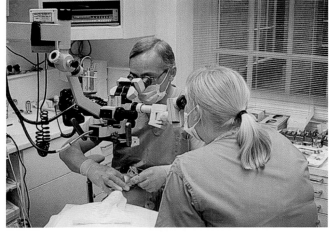

Fig. 9.36 Photograph of operating microscope.

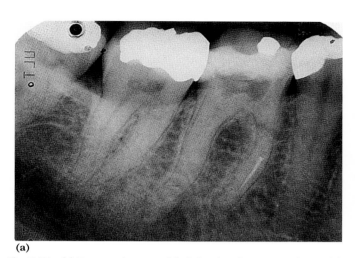
(a)

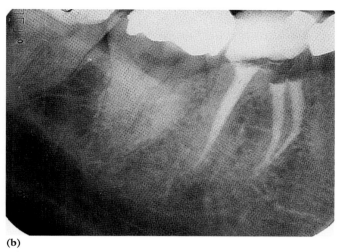
(b)

Fig. 9.37 (a) Fractured rotary nickel titanium instrument in mesial root of a lower molar. (b) Radiograph following instrument bypass and obturation.

system; hence the importance of root canal retreatment whenever possible. On occasions, however, retreatment of a tooth may involve the removal/destruction of expensive crown and bridgework. In such situations, a patient may opt for a surgical as opposed to an orthograde approach. This should only be undertaken if the patient understands that dismantling of restorations may be necessary in the future, should the surgery fail.

Ideally, surgery should only be performed on cases that are considered hopeless. Such situations may include large posts, sclerosed canals and broken instruments. Further important indications for periradicular surgery include obtaining tissue for a biopsy or examination of the root surface to check for root cracks/fractures.

Restoration of teeth (complex restorations)

INTRODUCTION

Traditionally, more extensive restorations on teeth were performed using non-adhesive techniques. The materials of choice were gold, porcelain and metallic ceramics. These were placed either intra- or extracoronally and relied on the preparation having near-parallel walls, assisted by a luting cement to fill the marginal gap and help with the retention process. With the development of new materials and techniques for bonding to the tooth, there has been a blurring of the methods used, and accordingly restorations may rely on a multitude of factors for retention which incorporate both mechanical and adhesive principles.

REPLACEMENT OF LOST CORONAL TOOTH STRUCTURE

Indirect restorations are frequently placed on teeth which have lost substantial amounts of tooth structure. Retention and resistance form are lost as the height of the tooth preparation is reduced in relation to the intended occlusal surface position of the final restoration. A foundation or core build-up restoration may be required to supplement retention and resistance form. The strength required of a foundation restoration will vary, depending on the location of the tooth in the dental arch, as well as on the design of the surrounding tooth preparation. Apart from acting as a transitional restoration in the management of a damaged tooth, a core build-up restoration must withstand crown preparation and impression-taking and contribute to the retention and support of a provisional crown before the definitive crown restoration is placed (Fig. 10.1).

When retention and resistance depend significantly on the core build-up, the strength of the foundation restoration and its retention to the underlying tooth tissue can directly influence the survival of the restoration. Some core materials lack sufficient strength and/or adhesion to tooth tissues to serve this function. Posterior teeth are exposed to greater forces than are anterior teeth and the direction of load differs. Teeth that have to serve as

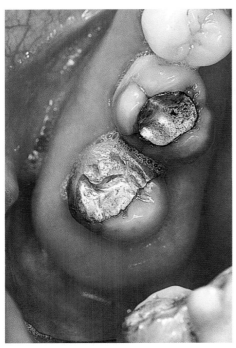

Fig. 10.1 Core build-up of lost coronal tooth structure.

abutments for fixed or removable prostheses are subject to increased stress.

The restoration of severely broken down teeth is an increasing problem for the restorative dentist, as more patients retain their natural teeth into older age. Clinical studies demonstrate an increased incidence of tooth fractures in teeth with large restorations compared with sound or minimally restored teeth.

Whilst advances in adhesive restorative materials and techniques may result in more predictable retention of restorations with compromised retention, the success of these techniques is still to be confirmed by clinical trials. Such techniques may be operator-sensitive as the success of an indirect restoration depends on the ability of the cement or resin lute to prevent dislodgement of the restoration from the tooth preparation; the latter must possess adequate retention and resistance form. Whilst resistance form is considered more critical than retention form, it is impossible to separate these two features. Retention will prevent dislodgement of the restoration along a direction parallel to its path of insertion, whilst resistance prevents dislodgement in any other direction. Minimal taper and maximum preparation height are critical features for good retention. The fit of the restoration, any surface treatments which facilitate adhesion, and the nature of the cement lute are also important variables. If adequate retention and resistance form can be developed from natural tooth structure, the strength of any core or foundation restoration is less critical and minor depressions or undercuts in the tooth preparation can be restored with adhesive restorative materials.

CHOICE OF CORE MATERIAL

Clinically, there are times when the remaining tooth structure is so reduced that the margins of the crown must be placed at or just below the core. It is under these conditions that the choice of core material may be critical.

Core build-up materials for direct placement include:

- dental amalgam
- resin composite
- reinforced glass ionomer cements
- resin-modified glass ionomers/compomers (polyacid-modified resin composites)

Each candidate core material has advantages and disadvantages. Box 10.1 lists desirable properties for a core material.

Dental amalgam

Amalgam has adequate mechanical properties for many core build-up situations. It is radio-opaque and has been shown to have superior cariostatic properties to composites. It has high thermal conductivity and coefficient of thermal expansion. It is not adhesive to tooth structure, although methods of bonding amalgam using resin adhesives are available, and glass ionomer/resin ionomer cements show promise. Conventional dental amalgams set too slowly to allow tooth preparation during the same visit as core build-up. Modern fast-setting spherical alloys may allow preparation 20–30 minutes after placement. Silver amalgam has been reported to be the most reliable direct core build-up material under simulated clinical conditions because of its high compressive strength and rigidity (Fig. 10.2).

Box 10.1   Desirable properties for a core material

- Compressive strength to resist intraoral forces
- Flexural strength to prevent core dislodgement during function
- Biocompatibility with surrounding tissues
- Ease of manipulation
- Ability to bond to tooth structure, pins and posts
- Capacity for bonding with luting cement or having additions made to it
- Coefficient of thermal expansion conductivity similar to dentine
- Dimensional stability
- Minimal water absorption
- Short setting time to allow tooth preparation and core placement to be carried out during the same visit
- No adverse reaction with temporary crown materials or luting cements
- Cariostatic potential
- Low cost
- Contrasting colour to tooth tissue unless being used for anterior cores

---

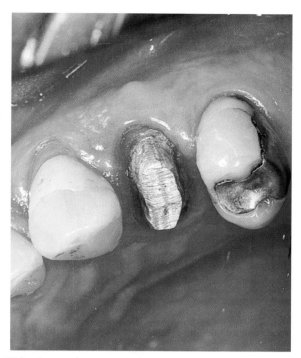

Fig. 10.2   An amalgam core.

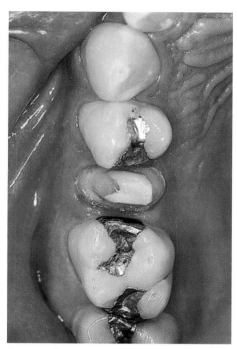

Fig. 10.3   A composite core.

Resin composite

Composite core materials are becoming increasingly popular for core build-ups. Provided adequate moisture control is obtained, these materials may be reliably bonded to tooth substance, and their command set nature allows immediate tooth preparation. An incremental technique is required to ensure complete polymerisation unless specific light-activated core composites are used.

Most resin composite core materials possess similar compressive and tensile strengths to amalgam cores. Only radio-opaque composites should be considered as core materials. The high coefficient of thermal expansion of composite cores and their greater potential for water uptake are negative aspects of these materials. In addition, eugenol-based temporary cements may soften their surface or impede bonding of resin-based luting cements. Composite is best as a direct core material when substantial coronal tooth structure remains for bonding and where reliable moisture control may be obtained. Several composite core materials contain fluoride which is released in trace amounts for up to 5 years but no clinically relevant cariostatic property has yet to be established for these materials (Fig. 10.3).

Glass ionomer cements

Conventional glass ionomer restoratives are popular with many dentists as core materials because of their adhesive properties and ease of handling. They are relatively slow-setting and their early resistance to moisture is poor. Many products are not radio-opaque. Although they may be considered to have adequate compressive strength for use as core build-up materials, their flexural strength and fracture toughness are low. Conventional glass ionomer cements are therefore only suitable where there is substantial tooth substance remaining to support the material and where adequate resistance form may be obtained on natural tooth tissue. Cermet cements do not provide advantages over conventional glass ionomers and often have poor adhesion to tooth structure. More recently-introduced condensable glass ionomer cements may prove a better alternative as these materials can be bonded more reliably and are stronger.

Resin ionomers and compomers

Resin-modified glass ionomers (RMGIs) and polyacid-modified resin composites (compomers) are attractive candidates for core materials because they offer the advantages of both glass ionomers and resin composites. These materials offer improved flexural strength in comparison to conventional glass ionomers whilst the high coefficient of thermal expansion of composite has been reduced. Light activation offers speed of set. Some concerns have been expressed about the risk of fracture of all-ceramic crowns when resin ionomers or compomers are used as core build-up materials and/or luting cements, and there is in vitro evidence to support this. Glass ionomers, resin-reinforced glass ionomers and most compomers are significantly weaker than tooth structure. They should be limited to situations where only minimal tooth structure is missing, and where increased tooth strength and abutment retention are not required.

PREOPERATIVE ASSESSMENT (Table 10.1)

Restorability of tooth

The extent of caries and the existing restorations should be assessed. When teeth are prepared for crowns there is often amalgam remaining in proximal boxes, class V areas and other regions. All previously placed materials should be removed (unless the operator has recently placed the restoration and is sure it is reliably retained to sound tooth tissue), allowing teeth to be rebuilt without the risk of an insecure foundation or previous pulpal exposure remaining undetected. If more than 50% of the coronal tooth structure is remaining and there is no requirement for increased tooth preparation strength, then a bonded compomer or resin ionomer base may be used to restore the tooth to the ideal preparation form. If ≥50% of the coronal tooth structure has been lost and there is not a minimum of 2 mm sound tooth structure circumferentially gingival to the tooth preparation, a high-strength (bonded amalgam or composite) core build-up is required to increase tooth strength and aid crown retention/ resistance form.

Mechanical retention in teeth may be increased by:

- grooves
- boxes
- dovetails
- converting sloping surfaces into vertical and horizontal components
- reducing/covering undermined cusps.

The use of pins and posts should only be considered as a last resort as they will further weaken already compro-mised teeth. In clinical situations, flat one-surface cavity designs occur infrequently and it is often possible to create steps or varying levels within a preparation increasing retention and resistance to occlusal forces. Other methods of increasing retention and resistance without having to resort to pins include circumferential slots, amalgapin channels or 'pot-holes' and peripheral shelves.

Spherical alloys are best suited to condensing into small retentive features of a cavity preparation and suitable small-diameter condensers are required. Slot-retained restorations are more sensitive to dislodgement during matrix removal than pin-retained restorations. Occasionally, when minimal tooth structure remains for mechanical retentive features, pins may be required to supplement retention. The amount of remaining coronal tooth structure (not undermined) is assessed after removal of caries and old restorations. Unsupported tooth structure may need to be removed if the build-up is to serve as a direct permanent load-bearing restoration. Retention of thin slivers of unsupported tooth structure may, however, be appropriate if the build-up is to serve as a foundation for a crown.

Pulpal/endodontic status

Prior to core build-up, an assessment should be made of the pulpal status of the tooth in question. If the pulp is exposed or there are signs/symptoms of irreversible pulpitis, endodontic treatment should be performed. In the case of an endodontically treated tooth, the quality of the treatment should be assessed radiographically (Fig. 10.4). If the treatment is considered inadequate, a decision will need to be taken as to whether there is potential for retreatment or whether the tooth would be better extracted.

Table 10.1 Pattern of tooth destruction and type of restoration indicated

| Pattern of tooth loss | Extent of tooth loss | | | |
	Minimal	Moderate	Moderate to severe	Total loss of coronal tooth structure
Central/internal (i.e. occlusal dentine caries)	Amalgam or composite (PRR)	Cement base and amalgam	Pin core and crown	N/A
Peripheral/external (i.e. tooth surface caries)	Amalgam, composite or RMGI	Amalgam, composite or RMGI	Crown	N/A
Above combined	Amalgam, composite or RMGI	Amalgam (large tooth) or cast gold onlay (small tooth)	Pin core and crown	Pin core and crown (molars) or root canal therapy and core + crown (premolars)

PRR, pin-retained restoration; RMGI, resin-modified glass ionomer.

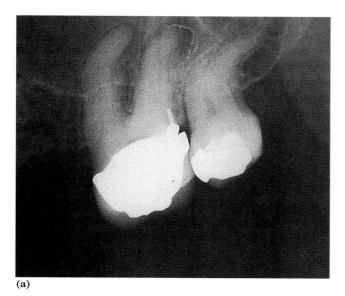

(a)

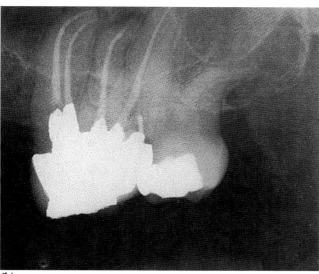

(b)

Fig. 10.4 Assessment of RCT molar tooth for crown.

Periodontal/occlusal assessment

The periodontal status of the abutment should be assessed. If there is inadequate sound tooth structure apical to the preparation margin for satisfactory retention and resistance form, surgical crown lengthening may have to be considered. The occlusal relationships should be assessed, but not all teeth requiring build-up will subsequently need to be crowned and the occlusal relationship and the potential functional stresses on the tooth will influence this decision.

Greater strength is required for crowns in the following cases:

* patients with bruxism or clenching habits
* teeth that support crowns with heavy canine or incisal guidance
* abutments for fixed and removable prostheses.

PIN RETENTION FOR CORE FOUNDATIONS

The increased strength of the latest dentine/enamel bonding agents, coupled with the revived use of retentive slots, pot-holes, grooves and channels, has led to a reduction in the use of pins. However, pins may be useful for providing retention to the core, although they should be used carefully. There tend to be more disadvantages associated with their use, and incorrect placement can lead to pulpal or root surface perforation. Other problems include crazing/tooth fracture or failure of the pin to seat fully, leading to looseness or fracture of the pin (Fig. 10.5).

Guidelines for the use of pin retention for core foundations

* Use one pin per missing cusp or marginal ridge, up to a maximum of four.
* Use large-diameter pins whenever possible.
* Use the minimum number of pins compatible with adequate retention (pins weaken amalgam).
* Pins should extend 2 mm into dentine and restorative material.
* Keep 1 mm of dentine between the pin and the enamel–dentine junction.
* Pins should be placed away from furcation areas and parallel to the external tooth surface.
* Coating of pins with adhesion promoters such as Panavia and 4-META materials improves fracture resistance of composite and amalgam cores.
* Pins rarely need to be bent.

FOUNDATION RESTORATIONS FOR ENDODONTICALLY TREATED TEETH

For endodontically treated anterior teeth with moderate to severe coronal destruction, cast gold post and cores are the restorative method of choice (Fig. 10.6; see also Box 10.2).

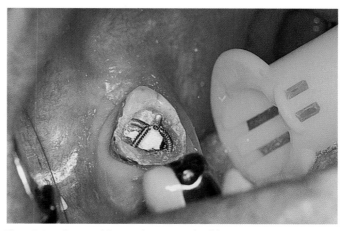

Fig. 10.5 Pins used in amalgam core build-up.

119

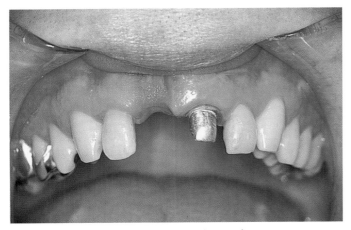

Fig. 10.6   Gold post and core on anterior tooth.

Root-filled molar teeth often perform satisfactorily with direct cores retained by extension into the pulp chamber together with a portion of the root canals. Core retention can be increased by bonding and/or placement of one or more prefabricated intraradicular posts (Fig. 10.7).

Endodontically treated premolar teeth may be restored either with custom cast post and cores or prefabricated posts used with direct core build-ups. Direct pattern post cores allow better control over the fit and the shape of the final core. They result in a better-fitting final crown restoration because they are cemented before crown preparation and impression-taking. The disadvantage is that additional clinical time is spent at the chairside in com-

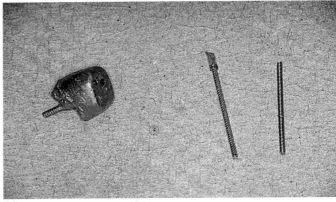

(a)

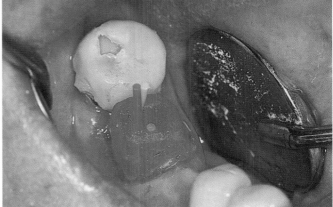

(b)

Fig. 10.7   (a) Prefabricated intraradicular posts. (b) In situ on posterior RCT molar.

parison to an indirect technique. However, an accurate impression of the prepared post space that extends deeply into the canal of an endodontically treated tooth is also a challenge. Many post crowns fail because posts are made too short, and frequently the full length of the prepared post hole is not employed in the final restoration (Fig 10.8).

For optimal post preparation:

- use a length equal to or greater than the length of the final clinical crown
- maintain a minimum of 4 mm apical gutta-percha seal.

Shorter posts are undesirable because they:

- are less retentive
- produce unfavourable stresses within the root
- predispose to fracture
- result in loss of cementation.

A flat seat should be created at the occlusal end of the tooth preparation to prevent possible wedging effects, and as much coronal and radicular tooth structure as possible should be preserved. Parallel-sided posts are more retentive than custom-made tapered posts; however, when a parallel-sided post is used in a thin tapered root there is an increased risk of perforation laterally towards the apex (Fig. 10.9). Parallel-sided posts with tapering apical sections

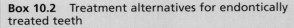

Box 10.2   Treatment alternatives for endontically treated teeth

Anterior teeth
- Acid-etch retained composite
- Cast gold post/core
- Composite core/prefrabicated post with and without pin(s)

Posterior teeth
- Amalgam restoration (with or without cuspal overlay 2–3 mm) or acid-etch composite (semi-permanent) restoration. No post or pins
- Amalgam restoration using pulp chamber retention (molars only). The 'coronal-radicular amalgam core' (Amalcore)
- Pin-retained amalgam (molars only). One functional cusp missing
- Prefabricated post- and/or pin-retained amalgam (molars only) where the crown has two or more cusps undermined or missing
- Cast gold post and core where there are molar abutments or premolars with undermined/missing cusp(s)
- Prefabricated post (+ pin) retained amalgam or composite core where the crown is placed on premolar teeth with undermined cusp(s)

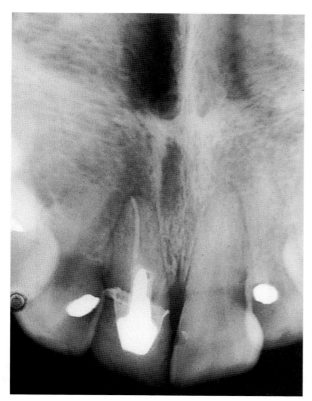

Fig. 10.8   A post that has been made too short.

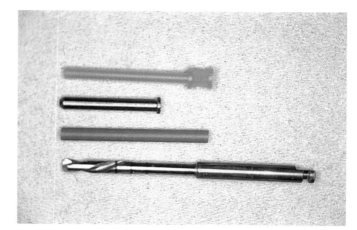

Fig. 10.9   Commercially available parallel-sided posts.

are commercially available (TYNAX, Whaledent). Post width should be the minimum to allow for a close fit between post and root canal dentine wall in the coronal and apical 3 mm of the post hole.

Small-diameter posts are best made from wrought alloys or heat-treated type 4 cast gold alloys, otherwise there is an increased risk of displacement or distortion. Wider posts lead to excessive destruction of tooth tissue and reduce the strength of the radicular dentine. The thickness of the remaining dentine is crucial to avoid root fracture. A post and core can transfer occlusal forces intraradicularly, predisposing the tooth root to vertical fracture. The role of the final crown restoration in protecting the post-restored endodontically treated tooth is very important. Clinical experience and laboratory studies have shown that extension of the cast crown restoration at least 2 mm apical to the junction of the core with the remaining tooth structure provides extracoronal bracing and prevents fracture of tooth structure. This 'hugging action' of a subgingival collar of cast metal has been described as the ferrule effect (Fig. 10.10).

This element is more important than the design of the post if tooth fracture is to be avoided. In vitro fatigue studies have shown that failure of the cement seal of a crown occurs first on the tension side of the tooth, especially when the ferrule effect is small and the post is off-centre. Clinical studies indicate a higher root potential for root fracture when cemented crowns do not provide a ferrule effect (Table 10.2).

CROWNS

The placement of an indirect restoration requires preparation of a cavity with undercut-free cavity walls to allow a path of withdrawal and insertion of the completed restoration. This allows a pattern or impression to be removed from the cavity. The finished restoration should be capable of insertion into the tooth without the generation of stress. Preservation of remaining tooth structure is important because the restoration relies on the strength and integrity of the remaining prepared tooth substance for retention. The restoration can be used to protect and reinforce the remaining tooth structure to some extent, but the less remaining enamel and dentine, the greater the risk of mechanical or biological failure.

Indirect restorations must be cemented or bonded into place to provide retention and cavity margin seal. The degree of retention available for a non-adhesive indirect restoration depends upon the surface area of the opposing

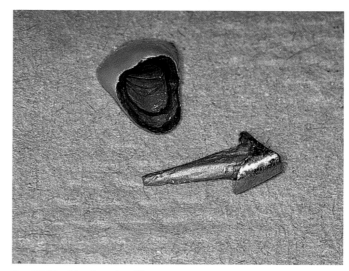

Fig. 10.10   The ferrule effect.

121

Table 10.2 Compensating for inadequate retention/resistance form in cast restorations

Extent of tooth loss	Clinical situation	Operative procedure	Final restoration
Moderate to severe	Short preparation or excessive taper One or two cusps missing but ≥ 50% coronal tooth structure remains Wall thickness/length ratio >1:1	Modify isthmuses/boxes Add grooves/pinholes Modify sloping surfaces into horizontal walls/horizontal planes Surgical crown lengthening	Non-standard partial or full veener
Severe	Loss of > 50% crown wall Thickness/length ratio <1:1 Short preparation for a long crown	Apply necessary pulpal protection Pin amalgam or composite core Surgical crown lengthening	Standard full veneer
Total loss of coronal tooth structure	All cusps undermined/lost Supragingival height < 1 mm	As above plus elective endodontics and post/core for premolars	Standard full veneer

vertical walls of the cavity and their degree of convergence. Only when the restoration is adhesively luted with a resin-based luting cement combined with an enamel/dentine adhesive is the luting agent a major contributor to retention.

Indirect restorations may be:

- intracoronal (inlays)
- extracoronal (crowns)
- a combination of intra- and extracoronal (onlays).

Restorations may be:

- wholly metallic (precious or non-precious alloys)
- ceramic/composite
- a combination of the above (metal-ceramic crown).

Crowns may cover all available surfaces of the tooth (full veneer crowns), or they may be partial veneer (e.g. three-quarter or seven-eighths crowns).

The stages in the clinical procedure involved in an indirect restoration are usually as follows:

1. Decision as to restoration type (full or partial coverage; intracoronal or extracoronal), materials and method of luting (conventional cementation or bonding with a resin-based luting material)
2. Discussion with patient before tooth preparation stage as to type of restoration and aesthetic implications
3. Tooth preparation (this may require prior occlusal adjustment or diagnostic wax-up to facilitate production of provisional restoration)
4. Fabrication of temporary/provisional restoration
5. Impressions and occlusal records
6. Shade selection
7. Try-in
8. Cementation or bonding.

PREOPERATIVE PLANNING

Before considering embarking on indirect restorations, patients should be assessed to ensure that their peri-

odontal condition has been stabilised and their caries risk is low.

The restorative assessment of the individual tooth involves:

- sensitivity/vitality tests
- long cone periapical radiograph
- examination of the quality of any existing restorations
- assessing whether the remaining tooth structure after preparation will have sufficient strength
- assessing the need for crown lengthening prior to treatment
- occlusal considerations.

The occlusal assessment should involve consideration of the tooth position relative to the opposing as well as the adjacent teeth, as this will influence preparation design. If there are occlusal interferences, these may place such a crown under high functional stresses and will require removal at a prior visit. The surfaces of the crown will need to be duplicated so that either the group function or canine guidance occlusion is maintained.

The tooth may be a key unit in the arch, i.e. partial denture abutment, and the shape of the surface should be modified to allow the subsequent placement of the denture. In such situations, mounted study casts are a useful aid in planning the preparation design as well as carrying out the occlusal assessment.

Any tooth preparation for a crown should follow the appropriate biomechanical principles (Box 10.3), and when planning replacement of a failed indirect restoration, it is important to identify the cause(s) of failure so that this may be corrected at the time of preparation.

Common causes of failure include:

- poor preparation design/shape resulting in lack of retention and/or resistance form
- insufficient reduction or lack of support/thickness for ceramic or composite
- undercut preparations
- failure to identify and/or correct occlusal problems
- poorly fitting restorations resulting from poor impression procedures or faulty laboratory technique

> **Box 10.3**   Biomechanical principles of tooth preparation
>
> * Preservation of tooth structure and pulp vitality
> * Obtaining adequate retention and resistance form
> * Obtaining adequate structural durability of the restoration
> * Obtaining adequate marginal integrity
> * Preservation of periodontal health
> * Appropriate aesthetics

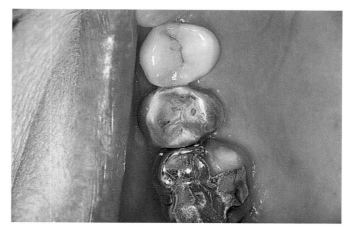

Fig. 10.11   Cast gold veneer crown at UL5.

* inappropriate prescription/planning; no preventive regime
* incorrect shade.

CHOICE OF MATERIAL FOR INDIRECT RESTORATIONS

There are four types of material that can be used for indirect restorations:

* gold
* porcelain
* indirect composite
* metal ceramic.

Gold

This is generally considered to be the most satisfactory extracoronal restorative material. It has a hardness similar to enamel, and occlusal and axial contours can easily be built up in the wax prior to casting. Cast gold alloy restorations include single and multiple surface inlays. The latter may include partial or complete coverage (onlays) of the occlusal surface. Extracoronal gold restorations include full veneer crowns and three-quarter crowns, in which only one surface of the tooth (usually the buccal) is left uncovered (Fig. 10.11).

Gold can be used in thin sections but it is not aesthetic. One millimetre of tooth reduction is required occlusally, with the exception of the functional cusp bevel where 1.5 mm is necessary. The choice of restoration and preparation design will depend upon the exact details of each clinical situation.

Indications for use

* In situations of severe occlusal stress
* Following endodontic treatment of posterior teeth
* Full or partial coverage of posterior teeth where there has been significant loss of coronal dentine
* In situations where other materials are not suitable for establishing proper proximal and/or occlusal contacts
* For restoration of adjacent and/or opposing teeth to avoid problems arising from use of dissimilar metals.

Contraindications

* Evidence of active caries/periodontal disease
* Economic and social factors
* Aesthetics
* Where patient management requires short visits and simple procedures.

Porcelain (ceramic)

This is a brittle material which is liable to fracture in thin section unless appropriate fit surface treatment is performed (etching and silanisation) and the restoration is adhesively luted with a resin-based cement (porcelain veneers and dentine-bonded ceramic crowns). A minimum margin reduction of 0.8 mm is required with 1.5–2.0 mm incisally/occlusally. Crown margins are prepared just below the gingival margin (intracrevicularly) if aesthetics dictates that this is necessary (Fig. 10.12).

Adequate retention for non-adhesive ceramic crowns depends on near-parallelism of opposing walls, particularly in the gingival third of the preparation. Porcelain crowns are relatively weak restorations and are restricted to anterior teeth unless a high-strength ceramic (Inceram, Procera, or Empress II) is used.

Indications for use

* Large inadequate restorations on anterior teeth, provided there is enough tooth substance for a strong preparation
* Severely discoloured anterior teeth
* Over an existing post and core substructure.

Contraindications

* Teeth which do not allow ideal preparation form to support the porcelain
* Teeth with short clinical crowns
* Edge-to-edge occlusion

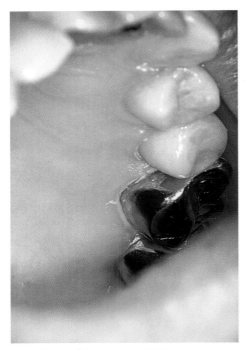

Fig. 10.12 An all-porcelain crown at UL5.

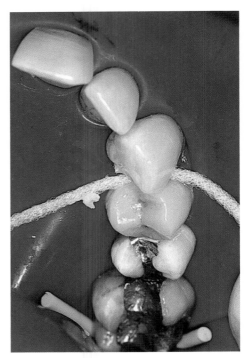

Fig. 10.13 An indirect composite onlay at UL4.

• When opposing teeth occlude on the cervical fifth of the palatal surface.

Porcelain jacket crowns are finished to a shoulder or butt joint margin design unless the preparation is to be bonded (dentine-bonded crowns). All-ceramic crowns are preferred to metal ceramic crowns on post-crowned teeth where there is a risk of trauma. In this case, the weaker porcelain jacket crown fractures rather than the stress being transferred via the post core leading to root fracture.

Indirect composite

Laboratory composites with improved strength and wear resistance are now commercially available and are increasing in popularity. Coupled with improvements in resin-based luting cements and dentine bonding systems, indirect composite restorations (with or without fibre reinforcement) may be considered appropriate for single unit inlays, onlays and crowns (Fig. 10.13).

Laboratory composites are generally preferred to porcelain restorations for inlays, whereas the latter offer more permanent form stability in onlay and crown situations. Some prefer a material which is less wear-resistant and as such is sacrificial in nature to a highly wear-resistant ceramic restoration which may ultimately cause excessive wear of the opposing dentition.

Metal ceramic

Metal ceramic crown restorations offer a combination of strength and good aesthetics. Additional tooth preparation (1.5 mm) is required to allow for both the metal sub-structure and metal overlay. These crowns are frequently over-contoured due to inadequate tooth reduction. Heavy tooth preparation to achieve adequate thickness for both materials may result in an increased incidence of pulp death. If this is a risk then a bevelled shoulder or cervical chamfer may be preferred to the conventional full 1.5 mm axial reduction in cases where the tooth preparation has to be extended down onto root surface or where there is a large pulp. Metal occlusal coverage is generally preferred to maximise retention and resistance form and to minimise tooth reduction. Metal occlusal contacts are easier to create and adjust. Porcelain occlusal surfaces are more aesthetic but demand additional tooth reduction and create the risk of excessive occlusal wear of opposing tooth surfaces (Fig. 10.14).

Indications for use

• Anterior teeth where there is insufficient space for an all-ceramic restoration
• Repeated failure of porcelain jacket crowns (identify reason first)
• Posterior crowns where aesthetics is important and full or partial veneer gold crowns are contraindicated on this basis.

Contraindications

• Where excessive wear of teeth opposing porcelain occlusal surfaces may be expected. Either a sacrificial indirect

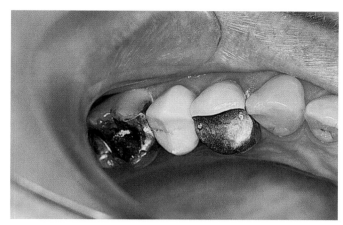

Fig. 10.14 Metal ceramic crowns on posterior teeth with (left) and without (right) occlusal porcelain coverage.

composite approach is preferred or permanent night-time protection with a Michigan splint may be indicated

- Where pulpal damage risk is high, particularly in a young patient. Dentine-bonded ceramic crowns have provided a more conservative viable option in many of these cases.

TOOTH PREPARATION GUIDELINES FOR INDIRECT RESTORATIONS

All preparations should have the maximum height and minimum taper for optimal resistance and retention form consistent with the clinical situation. To achieve this and to permit an adequate thickness of restorative material without over-contour, the surface of the preparation should mimic that of the intended restoration.

Features of preparations for indirect restorations

- Undercut-free preparation – there must be one point above the preparation from which all the margins and internal line angles can be seen.
- A single path of insertion over as great a distance as possible – this is achieved by preparing opposing walls to be near-parallel to give maximum retention. The position of the adjacent teeth should be considered as they may overhang the margins of the prepared tooth. The path of insertion is therefore dictated by the adjacent teeth.
- Resistance form needs to be provided by restoration to displacing forces which are usually occlusal in origin.
- The opposing walls in the gingival half of the preparation should be made near-parallel. The occlusal third to half will usually be more tapered as a result of the two planes of labial reduction required to provide sufficient room for the restorative material within the original tooth contours.
- With short clinical crowns there is an increased risk of failure because of the short insertion path. Preparation

length can be increased by crown lengthening, and resistance form may be improved by the use of grooves, slots or boxes and by converting sloping surfaces into vertical and horizontal components.

- Occlusal reduction should follow cuspal outline to maximise retention and minimise tooth reduction. For porcelain fused to metal crowns and for gold crowns these distances are 2 and 1 mm, respectively.
- The finished margin position and type are determined by the gingival contour, the nature of the restorative material, the presence or absence of a core margin and the choice of luting agent. Whenever possible, the margin should be supragingival following the natural gingival contours. Finish margins should ideally extend at least 1 mm past core margins to rest on sound tooth tissue.

Types of finish margins (Box 10.4, Fig. 10.15)

Chamfers and shoulders give definite finish margins which may be identified on preparations, temporary crowns and dies. Occasionally, knife-edge preparations may be indicated for full veneer crowns where there are deeply subgingival margins (however, periodontal surgery may be more appropriate here), bulbous teeth or pins close to the preparation margin. Metal ceramic crowns may be constructed with metal collars, especially on long preparations on posterior teeth. Lipline on smiling may indicate whether this is a practical proposition. A chamfer or knife-edge finish may avoid excessive tooth reduction in this situation.

Preparation stages

The following sequence is usually adopted:

- Occlusal reduction using depth grooves as a guide to the amount of tooth reduction. Grooves are only of use when the shape of the restoration is intended to match the original tooth.
- Gross buccal and palatal/lingual axial reduction. The preparation is kept near-parallel cervically and the labial reduction is made to mimic the contour of the final restoration in two, or occasionally three, planes. The preparation is extended as far interproximally as possible without risking contact with adjacent tooth structure.
- Initial interproximal reduction is achieved with a narrow tapered diamond. A sliver of tooth substance/restoration may be left to protect the adjacent tooth at this stage.

Box 10.4 Types of finish margins
- Full veneer crown – chamfer
- Metal ceramic crown – buccal shoulder/palatal chamfer normally
- Porcelain jacket crown – shoulder

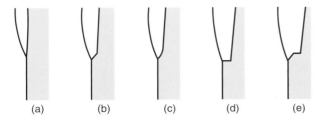

Fig. 10.15 Types of finish margins. (**a**) Knife edge; (**b**) bevel; (**c**) chamfer; (**d**) shoulder; (**e**) bevelled shoulder.

• Complete axial reduction can determine final finishing line position. Finish margins at least 1 mm past any existing restorations and just below the gingival margin labially if required for aesthetics.

INDIRECT ADHESIVE RESTORATIONS

Tooth-coloured inlays (Box 10.5)

The increasing expectation of patients that restorations be tooth-coloured has led to an increasing interest in direct and indirect composite and ceramic restorations in posterior teeth. Ceramic and composite inlays are generally considered to be appropriate for larger rather than smaller cavities, given that direct placement resin composite restorations may provide good service in small- to medium-sized cavities.

Computer-aided design and manufacture techniques (CAD-CAM, e.g. Cerec, Siemens, Germany) are capable of producing accurately fitting inlays from blocks of ceramic material. These techniques have the distinct advantage of producing the inlay at the chairside in a short time (approx. 15–20 minutes), thereby obviating the need for placement of a temporary restoration and a second visit for placement.

Composite inlays are constructed from a variety of composite types and are 'supercured' using a mixture of heat and pressure, and heat and light.

Clinical technique for adhesive inlays

Despite the differences in the physical properties of composite and ceramic inlay materials, the suggested cavity preparation designs may be similar. The concepts described

---

Box 10.5 Examples of tooth-coloured ceramic inlay materials

• Feldspathic porcelain
• Reinforced ceramics (such as Fortress: Chameleon Dental, KS, USA)
• Pressed ceramics (such as Empress II: Ivoclar-Vivadent, Leichtenstein)

---

above for adhesive preparations may be employed. This type of restoration will normally be appropriate to larger rather than smaller cavities, and will often be a replacement for a failed amalgam or gold restoration. The aesthetic inlay cavity will therefore often have an approximal 'box' and occlusal key. The taper for the preparation should be greater than that employed for gold inlay preparations, i.e. at least 6°, given that the inlays are weak before cementation, and try-in or removal from a near-parallel preparation may result in fracture of the inlay (Fig. 10.16).

No bevels should be placed on the occlusal aspect of the cavity, as thin sections of composite or ceramic may be prone to fracture under occlusal loading. All cavity margins should be in enamel and they should be supragingival to permit moisture control during placement of the inlay. Cavities should be at least 2 mm deep occlusally. All line angles should be rounded.

Clinical and laboratory technique for aesthetic inlays are outlined in Table 10.3. Using these techniques, a satisfactory aesthetic result is possible (Figs 10.17 and 10.18).

The dentine-bonded crown

The dentine-bonded crown is a comparatively recent addition to the clinician's armamentarium. It has been described as a full-coverage ceramic restoration which is bonded to the underlying dentine (and any remaining enamel) using a

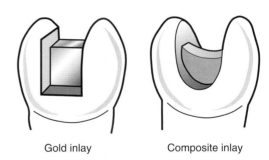

Gold inlay   Composite inlay

Fig. 10.16 Comparison between typical inlay cavities for gold and composite inlays.

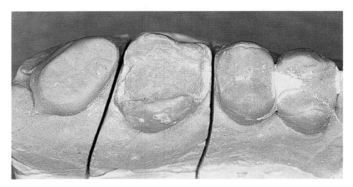

Fig. 10.17 Cavity preparation for a composite inlay to replace a failed gold inlay (patient requested tooth-coloured restoration).

Table 10.3   Clinical and laboratory techniques for aesthetic inlays (stages 1 and 2)

Operation	Rationale
Stage 1 Impression technique	As for a gold inlay
Laboratory instructions	Request for etching of the fitting surface of ceramic inlays with hydrofluoric acid to provide a micromechanically retentive fitting surface
	The fitting surface of composite inlays are sandblasted as the achievement of a micromechanically retentive fitting surface is more difficult
	A silane bond enhancer should be applied to both ceramic and composite inlays both in the laboratory and also prior to cementation
Temporary restoration	The temporary restoration should be constructed in a light or chemically cured provisional material and cemented with a eugenol-free temporary luting material.
Stage 2 Remove temporary and clean cavity with pumice	Removes contaminants such as eugenol
Handle inlay with care, try into cavity: do NOT check occlusion	Inlay is weak prior to cementation
If satisfactory fit, clean inlay fitting surface with phosphoric acid for 15 seconds	Fitting surface may have been contaminated with salivary pellicle
Apply silane bond enhancer to inlay fitting surface and allow to evaporate	Silane will improve adhesion of resin to ceramic inlay by circa 20%
Isolate, preferably under rubber dam	Saliva and/or blood contamination will reduce bond strength
Apply matrix, or organise alternative means for removal of excess luting material at gingival margin, such as floss and Superfloss	Excess luting material will cause gingival irritation
Mix luting material and apply to cavity	Application of luting material to inlay may result in fracture of inlay
Place inlay slowly and carefully	Rapid insertion of the inlay may result in its fracture
Remove excess luting material from accessible surfaces with sponge pellets or equivalent, and interproximal excess with a probe or floss if a matrix has not been placed	Removal of excess luting material is much more difficult when it has been cured
Cover margins with anti-air-inhibition gel	This will allow full polymerisation of the lute and prevent removal of the uppermost layer when finishing margins
Light cure from all directions in excess of manufacturer's suggested timing	It is not possible to overcure a composite and light is absorbed by the inlay, especially if a dark shade has been chosen. Physical properties of dual-cure materials are better when light-cured
Finish margins, check occlusion in all positions, and polish	Smooth margins will not retain plaque

resin composite-based luting material, with the bond being mediated by the use of a dentine bonding system and a micromechanically retentive ceramic fitting surface. Appropriate ceramics include feldspathic porcelain and aluminous porcelain, but any reinforced ceramic (e.g. Empress: Ivoclar-Vivadent, Leichtenstein) may also be appropriate provided that it is possible to etch its fitting surface with hydrofluoric acid or a hydrofluoric/hydrochloric acid mixture to produce a micromechanically retentive fitting surface. The bond between ceramic and resin luting material is enhanced by application of silane to the fitting surface. As with ceramic inlays, these crowns are weak until bonded to the underlying tooth. Indeed, since feldspathic porcelain is often used as the outer ceramic layer in many restorative modalities, such as metal-ceramic or aluminous porcelain, in the dentine-bonded crown technique, the tooth acts as the core, bonded to the ceramic by way of the dentine bonding agent and luting material (Fig. 10.19).

Advantages and disadvantages of dentine-bonded crowns are as follows:

Advantages
• Good fracture resistance

127

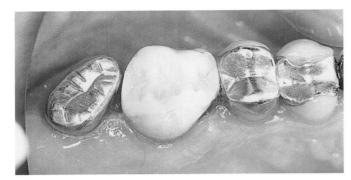

Fig. 10.18 Composite inlay at placement visit.

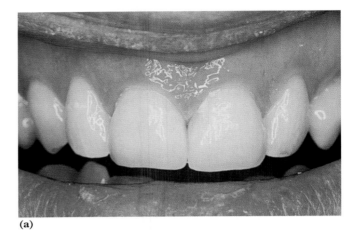

(a)

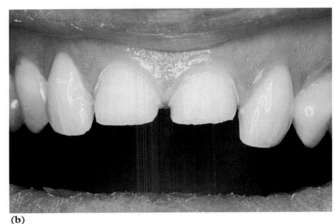

(b)

Fig. 10.19 (a) Dentine-bonded all-ceramic crowns constructed in feldspathic porcelain on central incisor teeth. (b) Preparation for crowns illustrated in (a) shows minimal shoulder and less tooth reduction than for conventional crowns. (Reproduced by courtesy of George Warman Publications, of Dental Update.)

- Achievement of good aesthetics
- Minimal axial preparation results in less pulpal irritation (occlusal/incisal reduction is as for a porcelain jacket crown)
- Reduced potential for microleakage
- Use in situations where preparation taper is large or crown height poor
- Luting material is virtually insoluble in oral fluids
- Use in patients who are sensitised to any constituent of casting alloys
- Correctly finished, they should not cause irritation of the periodontal tissues
- No marginal gap as this is filled with the luting material.

Disadvantages

- Problems of isolation for the bonding procedure if deep subgingival margins are present
- The luting procedure is more time-consuming than for conventional crowns, resulting in a higher chairside cost
- Lack of extensive long-term clinical data on effectiveness.

Dentine-bonded crowns are indicated:

- as replacements for failed, conventional crowns
- in cases of tooth wear
- as alternatives to metal-based alloys.

They are not suitable where isolation is not possible, such as deeply subgingival margins or in patients with uncontrolled caries or severe parafunctional habits.

The placement technique for dentine-bonded crowns is outlined in Table 10.4. This has been considerably simplified by the introduction of self-adhesive resin luting materials such as RelyX Unicem (3M ESPE, Seefeld, Germany) which obviate the need for separate etching and bonding stages.

PORCELAIN LAMINATE VENEERS

The advent of new tooth-coloured restorative materials and techniques within the last three decades has led to increased consumer orientation towards aesthetic dentistry (Fig. 10.20).

Three main discoveries have led to the evolution of the porcelain laminate veneer (PLV):

- etching of enamel
- introduction of Bis-GMA resins and the subsequent development of resin composite luting materials
- surface treatments which provide a micromechanically retentive ceramic fit surface.

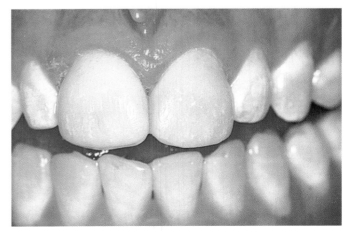

Fig. 10.20 Porcelain laminate veneers on anterior teeth.

Table 10.4   Dentine-bonded crown placement technique

Operation	Rationale
Remove temporary and clean preparation with pumice	Removes contaminants such as eugenol
Handling crown with care, try into preparation; do NOT check occlusion	Crown is weak prior to cementation
If satisfactory fit, clean fitting surface with phosphoric acid for 15 seconds	Fitting surface may have been contaminated with salivary pellicle
Apply silane bond enhancer to fitting surface and allow to evaporate	Silane will improve adhesion of resin to crown by about 20%
Isolate, preferably under rubber dam	Saliva and/or blood contamination will reduce bond strength
Organise means for removal of excess luting material at gingival margin, such as floss and Superfloss	Excess luting material will cause gingival irritation
Apply dentine-bonding agent in thin layer to dentine surface	Provides adhesion of resin luting material. Thin layer essential as pooling at internal line angles will prevent seating of crown
Mix luting material and apply to crown	Must be handled carefully
Place crown slowly and with care	Rapid placement may result in fracture of thin margins
Remove excess luting material from accessible surfaces with sponge pellets or brushes, and interproximal excess with a probe and/or floss; run Superfloss through at gingival margin	
Cover margins with anti-air-inhibition gel	This will allow full polymerisation of the lute and prevent removal of the uppermost layer when finishing margins
Light cure from all directions in excess of manufacturer's suggested timing	It is not possible to overcure a composite and light is absorbed by the crown, especially if a dark shade has been chosen. Physical properties of dual-cure materials are better when light-cured
Finish margins, check occlusion in all positions, and polish	Smooth margins will not retain plaque

These major discoveries, coupled with the continued evolution of laboratory techniques (platinum matrix build-up technique for porcelain laminates; refractory investments; new ceramics with optimised properties specific to porcelain laminates) and materials/clinical procedures (porcelain etching gels; stable silane solutions; veneer bonding composites/specific instrument kits for tooth preparation and establishment of appropriate preparation criteria), have made porcelain laminate veneers a well-established and predictable treatment modality.

Indications

Porcelain laminate veneers can be used in a variety of clinical situations. For example, colour defects or abnormalities of the enamel, such as the following, can be masked:

- Intrinsic staining or surface enamel defects caused by:
  - physiological ageing
  - trauma
  - medications (tetracycline administration)
  - fluorosis
  - mild enamel hypoplasia or hypomineralisation
  - amelogenesis imperfecta
  - erosion and abrasion

- Extrinsic permanent staining not amenable to bleaching techniques.

In addition, discoloured non-vital teeth that otherwise might require post crowns can be veneered (perhaps after internal bleaching has been attempted). Whilst PLVs may afford a more conservative alternative to post crowns in these situations, these restorations may appear darker in time as the root-filled tooth is liable to colour change. External bleaching through the palatal surface of the natural tooth (or internal bleaching) may reverse this situation (Fig. 10.21).

Porcelain laminate veneers may also be used to correct peg-shaped lateral incisors, to close proximal spacing and diastemas, to repair (some) fractured incisal edges, and to align labial surfaces of instanding teeth. Any closing of diastema must take the overhanging porcelain/occlusal guidance relationship into consideration, since this involves the risk of fracture. Converting a canine to the shape of a lateral incisor (in the case of a missing lateral) usually requires a partial veneer crown (reverse three-quarter) preparation. When major changes to the shape of the teeth are planned, it is advisable that a diagnostic wax-up on a study cast is carried out first. Alternatively, mock-up facings of composite or porcelain may be made on a cast

129

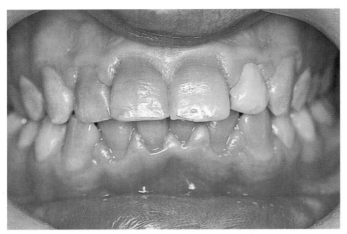

Fig. 10.21 Discoloured teeth that will benefit from porcelain laminate veneers.

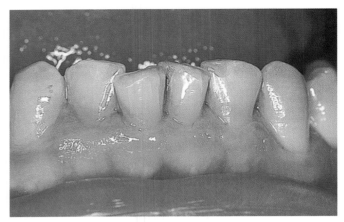

Fig. 10.23 Severely rotated teeth not suitable for porcelain laminate veneers.

of the unprepared teeth for chairside and/or intraoral evaluation by the operator or patient (Fig. 10.22).

Contraindications

Veneers are contraindicated when there is a poorly motivated patient with a high caries rate and appreciable amount of periodontal destruction. Recession, root exposure (with discoloration) and a high lip line are other contraindications.

PLVs are normally contraindicated if the preparation does not preserve at least half of the surface area remaining in enamel or if it has to be extended onto cervical root structure. A more extensive restoration such as a metal-free dentine-bonded ceramic crown or a conventional high-strength porcelain jacket crown may be more appropriate in these situations.

Labially positioned, severely rotated or overlapped teeth will prove difficult to restore with veneers (Fig. 10.23), as will teeth in which there is loss of substantial amounts of structure, including labial enamel, and those with inter-proximal caries or unsound/leaking restorations. The presence of small labial or proximal restorations may not contraindicate veneers.

When lower incisor teeth meet in close apposition to the palatal surfaces of opposing maxillary incisors, the occlusal forces are less favourable and the available bonding area is often considerably reduced. Where it is seen that veneers are more difficult to place, they should only be considered when all other alternatives are unacceptable to the patient.

Another situation in which PLVs may not be appropriate is when teeth are severely discoloured. Opaque porcelains and luting cements can be used but the end result may be a dull, 'lifeless' over-contoured restoration with poor cervical appearance because the veneer can only be extended onto the enamel-covered crown surface. It is difficult to achieve a good aesthetic result on a single, very discoloured tooth with a PLV and, in such cases, a crown restoration may be more appropriate.

Design considerations

Teeth can be veneered without any preparation (e.g. an instanding upper lateral incisor) but this is generally not favoured as it will result in over-contouring (complicating plaque control) and the restoration may be difficult to locate accurately on cementation. Indications for a 'non-preparation' approach include patients who are averse to having any tooth preparation (they must have the implications of this fully explained to them in advance and this must be recorded in the notes).

Removal of surface enamel makes resin–enamel bonding more effective. The presence of small labial or proximal restorations may not contraindicate veneers. They may be incorporated into the preparation and they should be replaced before or during veneering to ensure caries removal, effective bonding and good marginal seal. Restoration with glass ionomer cement rather than composite resin may be indicated.

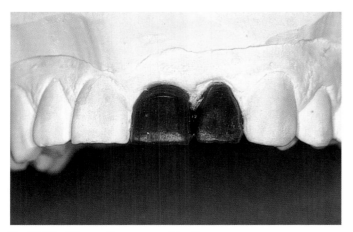

Fig. 10.22 Diagnostic wax-up of teeth.

Tooth preparation

Labial reduction

A polyvinyl siloxane putty template of the tooth prior to preparation may be used to help the clinician measure the amount of reduction. Depth orientation grooves may be prepared using commercially available depth-limiting burs specially designed for PLVs. Alternatively, hemispherical depth orientation dimples may be prepared using a 0.5 mm radius round diamond bur (Fig. 10.24).

Great care must be taken to avoid perforation of thin cervical enamel (sometimes it is better to leave the cervical region minimally prepared or unprepared because the enamel is so thin). Lack of sensitivity during preparation (without local anaesthetic) is not a reliable indicator in this respect. Although small areas of the preparation can involve dentine without adversely affecting retention, it is best to avoid this if possible. Dentine bonding agents may be used to bond the resin luting cement to dentine but this is not ideal, particularly at the preparation margins. Labial reduction should finish with a chamfer margin at the proximal 'stop', thus preserving the contact area.

Cervical margin placement

Porcelain laminate veneers generally allow supragingival margins to remain visible (because of their optical properties) and tooth preparation allows a good emergence profile to be maintained. Supragingival or equigingival margins should normally be preferred for the following reasons:

- they are less likely to involve cervical dentine
- the margins are accessible for finishing and polishing
- plaque control is simplified
- assessment of marginal fit is easier
- moisture control during bonding is simplified.

About 0.3–0.5 mm of enamel should normally be removed (0.3 mm cervically) and the preparation should end proximally just short of the contact point(s) and level with the gingival margin (or supragingivally if the lip line permits) in enamel. A 0.3 mm chamfer creates a finish line which is easy to identify and reproduce in the laboratory. It allows correct tooth contour to be established cervically. It facilitates veneer placement and reduces the risk of margin fracture at try-in. Greater reduction, up to 0.7 mm in depth, may be required to mask heavy tetracycline discoloration, and if the lip line is high, the preparation may also have to be extended intracrevicularly to achieve satisfactory aesthetics. The surface produced by conventional medium grit diamond burs is adequate, as composite/enamel bonding is facilitated by the rough surface. A finishing bur is, however, preferred for margin refinement.

Proximal reduction

Although undercut areas should not be introduced in the preparation, care should be taken that the veneer extends adequately in the proximal subcontact areas (cervical to the contact points) to avoid an unsightly band of exposed tooth structure remaining (especially mesially). A labial or labio-incisal path of insertion helps to prevent this. The aim is to place the margin beyond readily visible regions. Provided the tooth does not have proximal restorations, placement of the proximal 'stop line' should be guided by aesthetic considerations. It is essential to extend the margin of the veneer beyond the visible area.

This is especially important when the colour of the tooth differs greatly from that of the veneer. Assessment of correct proximal margin placement should be determined from frontal and/or side-on views. Proximal extension of the veneer to the lingual proximal line angle may be

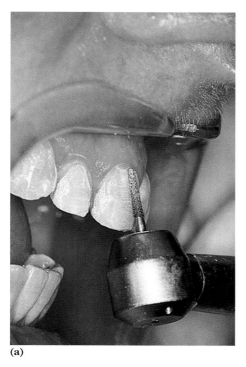

(a)

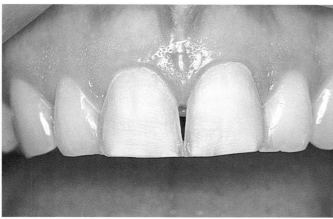

(b)

Fig. 10.24 (a, b) Labial reduction for porcelain laminate veneer.

required to achieve a favourable restoration contour when there are diastemas to be masked or when there is caries or an existing restoration proximally.

Incisal coverage

The veneer is extended to or taken over the incisal tip depending on the need to rebuild or lengthen this area (taking into account occlusal constraints). An incisal bevel is the preparation of choice when the tooth to be veneered is of the correct length and the anticipated functional occlusal loads will be low. If the occlusion permits, the incisal edge of the tooth should not be routinely covered as the preparation is then more conservative and does not alter the patient's natural incisal guidance/tooth contacts. However, when the incisal edge of the tooth is not over-laid, the occlusal third of the PLV is often very thin (0.3 mm or less). If there is edge-to-edge occlusion or evidence of incisal wear then there is a greater risk of chipping or incisal fracture of the veneer from occlusal load (Fig. 10.25).

In addition, when the teeth are thin, the difference in resilience between the prepared natural tooth and the PLV can, under occlusal load, lead to cracking or fracturing of the ceramic. A similar consideration applies if extensive composite restorations are present.

Complete coverage of the incisal edge with a minimum thickness of 1 mm of ceramic (preferably 1.5 mm) will offer the following advantages:

- It restricts incisal fracturing in cases of heavy occlusal load.
- It facilitates changes in tooth shape/position.
- It facilitates handling and positioning of the PLV at try-in and during bonding.
- It allows the veneer margin to be placed outside the area of occlusal impact.
- It facilitates achievement of good aesthetics in the final restoration.

An incisal edge overlap preparation is used when tooth lengthening is indicated, when it is necessary to cover/ protect part of the palatal surface, or when the incisal edge is poor aesthetically due to minor chipping etc. Incisal reduction must provide a minimum ceramic thickness of at least 1 mm. A thicker layer should be used for canine teeth and lower incisors. The lingual margin placement for a lower incisor may be extended one-third of the way down the lingual surface, transforming the veneer in effect into a partial crown. With this type of preparation the ceramic will be exposed mostly to compressive stresses and less to flexural stresses. Despite the small preparation surface area, the failure rate is relatively low. The degree of extension onto the lingual/palatal surface will depend upon the particular clinical situation. The lingual finish margin should be prepared as a hollow ground chamfer to a depth of 0.5–0.7 mm. This margin should be located away from centric stops or areas of direct occlusal impact.

Impression

A silicone impression taken in a full arch stock impression tray is adequate. Alternatively, a twin-mix single-stage addition-cured silicone impression taken in a special tray may be used. Occlusal stops should be placed on teeth away from those prepared. Retraction cord placement is rarely necessary and, if required, may indicate overpreparation.

Simply blowing with an air syringe should reveal the margin in the final preparation. Gingival retraction, however, is required to record the root emergence profile when the cervical margin is placed equigingivally or sub-gingivally for aesthetic or other reasons. Non-medicated retraction cords (small braided cords – Ultrapak No. 1 or No. 2, Ultradent) are preferred to reduce any risk of gingival recession. Any undercuts created by the cervical embrasure spaces may be filled in lingually with softened wax to avoid the risk of the impression tearing.

Temporary cover

This is rarely indicated for minimal veneer preparations and, when required for a single veneer, can be accomplished with light-cured composite resin build-up. The tooth preparation is coated with a layer of water-soluble separator (glycerin), light-cured composite restorative is applied and excess removed from interproximal spaces before curing. After light curing, the hardened material may be removed for shaping and polishing. It may be cemented to the tooth surface with a layer of composite after the preparation has been spot-etched centrally (Fig. 10.26).

Pairs of veneer preparations may be made at the chair-side or in the laboratory on a quick-setting plaster cast poured from an impression. Multiple temporary veneers may be made at the chairside with the aid of a transparent vacuum-formed plastic mould prepared from a model in the laboratory. A light- or chemically cured provisional composite resin may be used to make the provisional veneers. After trimming and adjustment, the veneers may

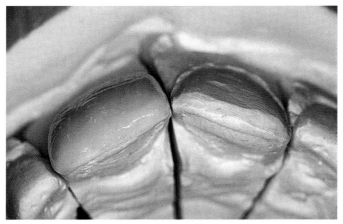

Fig. 10.25 Incisal preparation for porcelain laminate veneer.

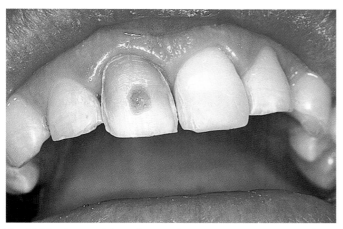

Fig. 10.26 Spot-etching of UR1 prior to temporary coverage for porcelain laminate veneer.

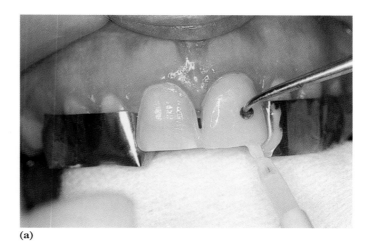

(a)

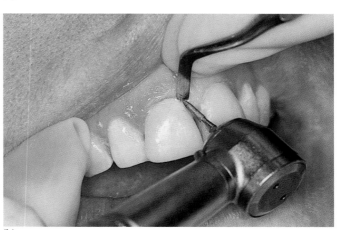

(b)

Fig. 10.27 Luting (a) and finishing (b) of porcelain laminate veneer.

need to be relined to improve marginal fit. These temporary prostheses are generally not separated but are cemented in one piece. A eugenol-free temporary cement or zinc phosphate may be used for this purpose or a resin-based temporary cement (Temp Bond Clear, Kerr). When there is incisal coverage or the veneer has had to be extended interproximally or converted to a partial cover dentine-bonded crown (reverse three-quarter), there is a greater need for a provisional restoration to satisfy patients' aesthetic demands and to reduce the risk of tooth sensitivity.

Laboratory aspects

Porcelain veneers may be fabricated on platinum foil matrices, or using refractory dies. With both techniques the fit surface of the fired porcelain veneer is grit-blasted with 50 micron Al_2O_3. The veneer fit surface is then etched with a hydrofluoric acid etch gel and a silane solution is applied to it. It is important, if possible, to get most of the desired final shade from the porcelain restoration itself rather than the luting cement.

Try-in

Clean prepared teeth with a pumice/water slurry, rinse and dry. If necessary, clean interproximally with finishing strips. Care is needed to avoid trauma to the gingival margin and bleeding. The tooth is isolated (cotton wool rolls, suction) and airway protection (gauze or throat pack) is placed.

The individual veneers are checked for fit and contour. (If multiple, try in together). *Do not* seat veneers forcefully but adjust as required with diamond burs (veneers are fragile at this stage and final minor adjustments are best left until after bonding). If porcelain margins are exposed, silane and bond resin have to be reapplied in the laboratory before proceeding (Fig. 10.27).

Choose the correct shade of composite luting cements (use the shade of veneer itself as a guide). Use water or glycerin if required for initial aesthetic try-in (an air gap will adversely affect the shade evaluation). Only if essential, use a trial mix of luting composite applied to the veneer fit surface (having wetted the tooth surface with water) for shade assessment. Switch off the operating light beforehand! Wipe out excess resin with cotton wool and place the veneer in an appropriate solvent (ethyl alcohol) to remove remaining unpolymerised luting cement.

Cementation or bonding

Obtain strict moisture control with cotton wool rolls, saliva ejectors and sponges, etc. Gingival retraction cord may also be required. Adjacent teeth are protected with soft metal matrix (Dead soft matrix material, Den Mat) or mylar strips folded over uninvolved contacts to secure in place or use wedges.

Acid etch with phosphoric acid gel for 30 seconds, rinse for 20 seconds, and dry until a frosted appearance is evident. (If areas of exposed dentine are present, use an enamel/dentine bonding system in accordance with the manufacturer's instructions.)

Apply unfilled bond resin and blow thin. Do not light cure! It is essential that excess bond resin is not allowed to pool in interdental or cervical areas where it may prevent complete veneer seating.

Place the chosen shade of composite resin luting cement as a thin layer over the veneer fit surface (avoid incorporating air bubbles) and seat the veneer onto the tooth with slow continuous pressure until fully in place. Remove gross excess cement from the margins with a probe (or a brush tip dipped in unfilled resin). Run Superfloss interproximally in a labial to palatal direction to remove interproximal excess. If the veneer is correctly seated, 'tack' it into place with a 10–20 second period of light irradiation incisally. Remove more excess resin taking care not to drag out cement from under the margins. Complete light curing by overlapping light guide tip applications (60 seconds each) in incisal, labial and proximal areas.

Cement adjacent veneers one at a time (always check for correct seating beforehand!).

Finishing

Gross excess cement can be removed with hand instruments such as scalers and composite finishing burs. Remove residual excess from the margins with water-cooled composite finishing burs which may also be used for fine trimming of porcelain margins. The gingiva is protected by retraction with the blade of a 'flat plastic' hand instrument and the proximal area is finished with composite finishing strips. The contact point should be checked so that it allows floss to pass between smoothly. The finished result is shown in Figure 10.28.

The final polish of margins is undertaken with impregnated polishing discs and cups (Enhance-Dentsply), polishing pastes (Prisma-Gloss/Dentsply) and/or composite polishing discs (Soflex 3M). A final check is made on the occlusion and the PLV is adjusted to remove premature contacts in all excursions.

Review and maintenance

The patient is reviewed 1 week later to ensure that all excess resin cement has been removed and that correct plaque control procedures are being employed. The marginal integrity is checked for signs of marginal leakage, colour, aesthetic acceptability and gingival health at regular recall. The occlusion is inspected for interferences and

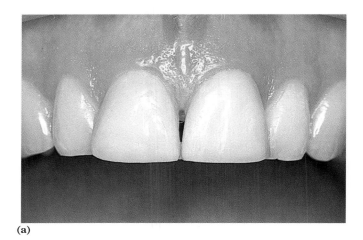
(a)

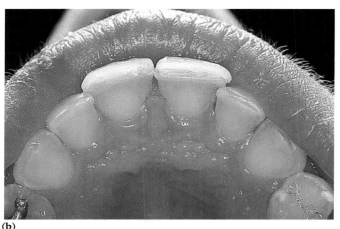
(b)

Fig. 10.28   Final finishing of veeners.

adjusted if required. It is known that properly executed porcelain veneers rarely fail due to bond failure. However, a mouth guard should be provided for contact sports players to avoid damage.

SUMMARY

Complex restorations are clinically rewarding but they do require careful treatment planning to ensure their longevity in the mouth. This aspect of restorative dentistry ensures that the patient has a functional restoration which is mechanically sound but also biologically compatible.

11

Treatment of tooth substance loss

INCIDENCE OF TOOTH SUBSTANCE LOSS

There is a paucity of data on the incidence of tooth substance loss (TSL) in the population, but anecdotal evidence suggests that in some countries, such as the UK, it is increasing among all age groups, while in others, such as the USA, the problems are not so severe, at least within the younger age groups. In general, the TSL which affects the younger age groups tends to be erosive, as a result of overconsumption of carbonated beverages, while in the older age groups, TSL is more likely to be multifactorial. The prevelance of tooth wear from different studies in children is shown in Table 11.1.

REASONS TO TREAT TOOTH SUBSTANCE LOSS

Treatment of TSL may be required for a variety of reasons:

- The patient may request it because of poor aesthetics of the worn teeth or because of sensitivity or pain.
- There may be infections associated with teeth which have become non-vital as a result of severe TSL.
- Patients may also complain of difficulty in eating because of reduced masticatory function.
- There may be temporomandibular joint (TMJ) disorders.
- There may be problems in phonation.

Although the patient may not complain of any symptoms or notice problems, the clinician may suggest treatment because the TSL is progressing and the dentition requires protection from further tooth loss by restorations. The dentist may also suggest treatment because of reduced function, temporomandibular joint (TMJ) disorders or compromised aesthetics.

From the above, it is apparent that there will be cases in which the patient is unaware of the problem because of its slow rate of progression. In general, therefore, except in cases of erosive TSL in young patients, treatment can be planned at a relaxed pace.

A definition of pathological tooth wear is given in Box 11.1.

Table 11.1 Summary of prevalence studies of tooth wear in children

	Age (years)	% affected
Hind & Gregory (1994)	1–4	20
Millward et al (1994)	4–5	38
Chadwick et al (2006)	5–6	52
UK Child Dental Health Survey (1993)	11	25
Bartlett et al (1998)	11–14	57
Milosevic et al (1994)	14	30

Box 11.1 Pathological tooth wear as defined by Smith & Knight (1984)

- Pulp exposure
- Loss of vitality due to tooth wear
- Exposure of tertiary dentine
- Exposure of dentine on buccal or lingual surfaces
- Notched cervical surfaces
- Cupped incisal or occlusal surfaces
- Wear in one arch more than the other
- Inability to make contact between worn incisal or occlusal surfaces in any excursion of the mandible
- Restorations projecting above the tooth surface
- Wear producing persistent sensitivity
- Reduction in length of incisor teeth so that the length is out of proportion to the width

---

Box 11.2 Causes of erosive tooth wear (Watson & Burke 2000)

Extrinsic erosion
(caused by acid originating outside the body; generally the pH is 2.5 or less)
- Environmental – wine tasters, swimmers, acid fumes (unlikely since the advent of industrial legislation)
- Dietary – soft drinks, acidic food
- Medications – vitamin C, mouthwashes
- Lifestyle – sports drinks, ecstasy (drug), frothing

Intrinsic erosion
(due to stomach acid reaching the teeth, with a pH of 1; this acid is typically 100 times stronger than in extrinsic erosion, and therefore much more destructive)
- Gastric reflux:
  - Sphincter incompetence: oesophagitis, hiatus hernia, pregnancy, diet, drugs, neuromuscular disease
  - Increased gastric pressure: obesity, pregnancy, ascites
  - Increased gastric volume: after meals, gut obstruction, spasm
- Vomiting:
  - Psychosomatic: stress-induced, bulimia nervosa, anorexia nervosa
  - Gastrointestinal disorders
  - Drug-induced: primary, secondary, xerostomia
- Regurgitation
- Rumination

THE HISTORY

In all cases, it is essential that a full history is taken and a complete examination carried out with the aim of making a definitive and accurate diagnosis (Box 11.2). Patients should be asked to give details of their concerns and symptoms, if any, and for how long the symptoms have been present. A patient complaint of sensitivity to cold and heat may indicate rapid loss of tooth substance, as secondary dentine is not being laid down as quickly as the TSL is occurring. This may suggest that early intervention is indicated before the pulp becomes irreversibly damaged. Chipping of incisal enamel is another factor that patients may notice. The rapidity with which this is occurring may also indicate the rapidity of the TSL. Most commonly, the patient's presenting complaint will be of poor aesthetics relating to shortened teeth, incisal translucency and/or chipping, or functional problems such as difficulty in chewing. Ascertaining the patient's reason for attendance should give an indication of eagerness for treatment and what particular factors should be addressed. The history should also give an indication of possible patient compliance, given that patients who are unaware of their dental problems are unlikely to be willing to undergo an extensive course of treatment. In such cases, the problems should be carefully explained and an appointment made to review the patient's attitude. Should the patient's compliance be in any way suspect, minimal treatment only should be offered at the outset.

The patient's medical history should be taken carefully, with special reference to medical conditions associated with TSL. These include gastric ulceration, hiatus hernia, oesophagitis, gastro-oesophageal reflux and, indeed, any medical condition which predisposes to gastric regurgitation. The patient should be asked about indigestion and heartburn, both of which may indicate a tendency for gastric reflux. However, the condition may be subclinical, in that the patient may be unaware of the occurrence of gastric reflux. Rumination is often confused with regurgitation. In this habit, recently eaten food is forced from the stomach by strong contractions of the abdominal muscles. The food is chewed again and re-swallowed, often many times, thus providing the opportunity for erosion of the teeth. Surprisingly, this strange behaviour is fairly common and the habit can last a lifetime.

Pregnancy may indirectly be associated with TSL, given the possibility of repeated vomiting as a result of morning sickness.

A number of medications may be associated with TSL, including chewable vitamin C, hydrochloric acid for achlorhydria and some iron-containing preparations. The use of the drug ecstasy reduces salivary flow. The mixture of dry mouth, vigorous 'raving' and rehydration with acidic drinks is linked to erosion.

Diets high in fibrous foods and citrus fruits may also predispose to TSL, as may diets which are high in carbonated beverages such as cola drinks. Some patients 'swish' the cola drink around their mouths, which is likely to increase the overall erosive effect, by increasing the time that the drink is held in the mouth. In cases where diet is suspected as being contributory to TSL, the patient should be asked to keep a diet diary for a number of days. Excessive alcohol consumption may result in vomiting and/or gastritis, both of which could be contributory factors to TSL.

In the past, the patient's occupation was considered to be of relevance (e.g. erosion was found to be associated with the acidic environment of a car battery factory). However, contemporary industrial employment legislation is likely to preclude the occurrence of such erosive conditions. More recently, erosion in a wine taster has been reported, and also in members of an Olympic swimming team, due to the acidic nature of the chlorinated water in which they were swimming. However, while these isolated cases are of interest, they are not principal causes of TSL.

Occasionally the cause cannot be identified. Given the secretive nature of some eating disorders (such as anorexia nervosa), and the possibility that alcoholism may also be a causative factor in some erosive cases, discussion of the cause of TSL may be difficult with some individuals. Nevertheless, a caring approach may help patients to discuss their problems. Often the patients appear to be more willing to discuss these problems with the dental nurse, and there may therefore be some merit in leaving the patient with the nurse once the subject has been brought up. In this respect, the pattern of TSL in bulimic patients is well defined and possibly pathognomonic, with TSL typically affecting the palatal surfaces of the upper incisor, canine and possibly premolar teeth (Fig. 11.1) and the occlusal surfaces of the mandibular molars and premolars. Amalgam restorations which are present in these teeth may appear 'proud' of the remaining tooth substance, given that the amalgam is less soluble in gastric acids than tooth substance (Fig. 11.2).

Abrasion may occasionally be identified as a cause of TSL, e.g. from pen chewing and, in seamstresses, from holding pins between the anterior teeth. However, it should be noted that the abrasive action of toothbrushing is increased dramatically when it is carried out within 30 minutes of the teeth having been subjected to an erosive attack by citrus juices or food, or by regurgitation of gastric acid.

While erosion has been considered to be the most prevalent reason for TSL, attrition associated with

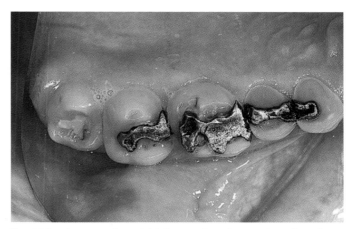

Fig. 11.2 A restoration which is proud on the tooth surface due to erosive tooth substance loss of the surrounding hard dental tissues.

clenching and/or grinding habits is a cause of TSL in a proportion of patients. These patients may or may not be aware of their habits, but may complain of symptoms such as tender masticatory musculature on waking. Some may have TMJ problems.

Identification of all potential causative factors of TSL is desirable prior to treatment. Wear appears to occur intermittently and there may be active and inactive periods. An assessment of the rapidity of progression is of value in assessing the need for treatment and its urgency. As a general rule, increasing sensitivity of a tooth or group of teeth is an indication that wear is progressing faster than the deposition of reparative dentine. Also, chipping of incisal edges of anterior teeth is a sign that TSL is undermining the enamel in these areas. These are often reasons for patients to express anxiety and request treatment.

THE EXAMINATION

An assessment of status is essential and should include a full clinical examination, radiographs, mounted study casts and intraoral photographs. Often special investigations such as 24-hour monitoring of potential gastric reflux may be indicated, but this, for example, should only be undertaken with the assistance of a gastroenterologist. The number and position of missing teeth should be noted, as too should the position of over-erupted teeth. In cases where there is a loss of posterior support, the number of teeth in occlusal contact should be counted in order to ascertain the need for provision of posterior support by prosthodontic means. The tooth surfaces affected by TSL should be noted and may be graded by the use of an index of tooth wear such as that discussed earlier (Ch. 3).

Despite the fact that, for TSL to occur, teeth must be well supported and firm, the clinician must not assume that all firm teeth are free from periodontal

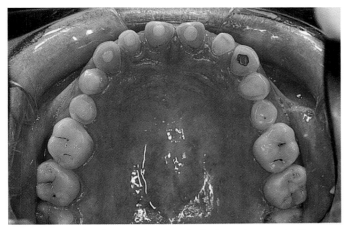

Fig. 11.1 Tooth substance loss in a bulimic patient, typically affecting the palatal surfaces of the upper incisor, canine and possibly premolar teeth.

disease. A full periodontal assessment is therefore important. Given the importance of assessing the vertical component of the occlusion, the freeway space should be measured. Radiographs will provide an indication as to the amount of reparative dentine and the proximity of the pulp (in teeth affected by TSL) to the tooth surface. The radiographs may also show teeth in which pulpal damage has led to pulpal death and an associated area of periapical radiolucency. Extraoral examination may reveal muscle hypertrophy, which may be as a result of bruxism, or enlarged parotid glands, which may be associated with bulimia.

TREATMENT OF TOOTH SUBSTANCE LOSS

The principles for treatment of caries were developed over a century ago and, until recently, remained largely unchanged (see Ch. 6). By contrast, the principles for treatment of TSL have been suggested comparatively recently and have been developed as a result of treatment experience rather than scientific evaluation.

A number of difficulties compound the problem of treating teeth which are already affected by TSL. Principal among these is the mechanism by which continuous tooth migration/eruption and alveolar bone growth compensates for occlusal and incisal TSL. By this means, occlusal face height is maintained. As a result, despite considerable TSL, there may often be little interocclusal clearance, as demonstrated in Figure 11.3. However, in other cases, the freeway space may be maintained, despite severe TSL. It has also been suggested that cementum is deposited at the root apex of teeth involved in the compensatory mechanism.

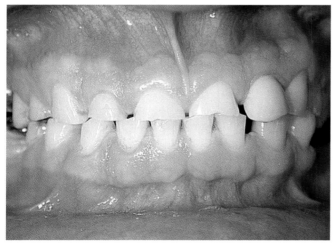

Fig. 11.3 Patient with considerable tooth substance loss, but little interocclusal clearance.

Classifications for treatment of TSL

Tooth substance loss may be classified simply into:

* localised
* generalised.

Only rarely are large numbers of teeth affected by TSL and normally it will be localised to a small number, usually in one arch. In general, when only a small number of teeth are affected, these alone should be treated. However, the cause of the TSL should also be determined, where possible, so that the patient may be advised about preventive measures.

Generalised TSL is usually the result of several contributory factors, e.g., the bruxist who also consumes excessive quantities of carbonated beverages, especially at bedtime, or the bulimic who consumes excessive carbonated beverages and who brushes his/her teeth with an (abrasive) toothpaste shortly after vomiting. These patients will often require extensive restorative treatment, dependent on the factors discussed below.

A widely accepted classification of TSL, which then forms a basis for treatment, is to assess the appearance of the patient and the need to increase the occlusal face height. The classification categories are as follows:

1. Appearance satisfactory
2. Appearance not satisfactory: no increase in occlusal face height required
3. Appearance not satisfactory: increase in occlusal face height required:
   (i) sufficient space available
   (ii) insufficient space available.

For cases in category 1, the treatment indicated is counselling, restoration of edentulous spaces where appropriate, control of any bruxist or clenching habits, adjustment and elimination of any occlusal interferences and routine dental work. For cases in category 2, the treatment indicated is as for category 1, plus conventional restorative measures to deal with the aesthetic problems. The treatment of cases classified into category 3 is more complex. At the outset, the clinician must decide whether the patient can tolerate the increase in occlusal vertical dimension.

Treatment of category 1 patients

Prevention is an essential aspect of the management of tooth wear. Accordingly, for patients in whom the appearance is satisfactory and there is little or no loss of occlusal vertical dimension, treatment may be limited to the following.

Counselling

These patients should be apprised of the cause of their TSL and how further progress of the condition may be limited. It may well be that their rate of disease progression is slow and they should be told this. For patients in whom the cause of the TSL is erosive, dietary advice should be given, and these patients should be left in no doubt that further TSL will occur if strict dietary guidelines are not adhered to (Box 11.3).

For patients in whom the TSL is a result of regurgitation of gastric acid, such as those with gastric ulcers or hiatus hernia, the dentist and patient should collaborate with the patient's general medical practitioner in an effort to reduce the effects of reflux. This will generally include avoiding foods which cause regurgitation and the use of an antacid mouthwash (e.g. bicarbonate of soda) immediately after regurgitation or vomiting to neutralise the acid in the mouth. Patients suffering from bulimia or anorexia may receive help and advice from self-help groups which have been set up in many major towns and cities. Patients may also benefit from chewing sugar-free chewing gum and from topical application of bicarbonate-containing toothpastes.

For TSL patients in whom parafunctional habits are thought to play a part, treatment is by provision of a splint or night bite-guard to be worn while sleeping. Hypnotherapy may also be of value.

Conventional restorative treatment

Localised areas of TSL, where dentine is exposed, may be restored in order to prevent further wear of the exposed dentine surfaces (Fig. 11.4). Reduced posterior support, which has been considered to be a contributory factor in TSL, should be treated by provision of dentures, bridges or implants.

Monitoring

Monitoring is an important aspect of the treatment of category 1 patients. This may be carried out with the aid of mounted study casts and intraoral photographs, and by making the patient aware that symptoms such as tooth sensitivity or chipping of enamel at incisal edges may be an indication of progressive TSL. Dated reference casts (study models) can be used at follow-up visits for macroscopic comparison with the teeth in order to monitor wear. These

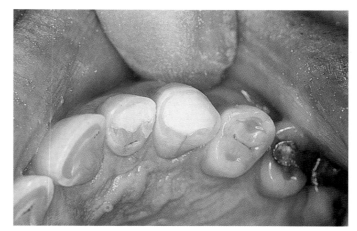

Fig. 11.4 Localised areas of tooth substance loss, where dentine is exposed, may be restored by conventional means.

casts are best given to the patient for safe keeping. Long-term models should be cast with die-stone, as they themselves are prone to wear with repeated handling. If a silicone index was originally taken, it can be placed on the latest casts for easy viewing of potentially worn sites (Fig. 11.5, Box 11.4).

Treatment of category 2 patients

These patients require similar treatment to category 1 patients, as well as conventional restorative measures, such as crowns or resin composite restorations, to overcome aesthetic problems. Dentine-bonded all-ceramic crowns are particularly appropriate as they require minimal (~1 mm) tooth reduction axially. This is of particular importance in teeth which are already affected by TSL. Such crowns are aesthetically good, promote gingival health by well-finished margins and do not contain metal.

Box 11.3 Advice for patients with an erosive element to TSL

- Reduce the amount and frequency of intake of acidic drinks, such as carbonated beverages or citrus fruit drinks
- Avoid 'frothing' or swishing these drinks
- Avoid brushing the teeth for at least 30 minutes after drinking
- Chill the drink – the erosive potential of cold drinks is less than that of warm drinks
- Avoid drinking such drinks before bedtime or during the night

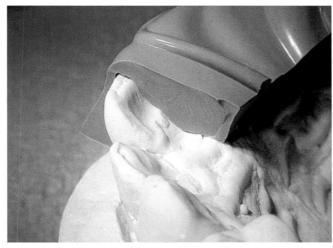

Fig. 11.5 Use of a silicone index on a patient's teeth.

Treatment of category 3 patients

Treatment of these cases may be complex. An increase in the occlusal vertical dimension (OVD) may be required to obtain space for the proposed restorations. Dahl considers that patients readily accommodate to an increase in the OVD of up to 2 mm (Briggs et al 1997). If an increase in OVD of greater than that amount is indicated, a diagnostic splint or overlay appliance should be constructed in order to ascertain the patient's ability to cope with the change in OVD. Such an appliance will often require adjustment at regular intervals until the patient is comfortable with the height. Alternatively, the increase in OVD may be achieved by applying acid-etch-retained resin composite provisional build-ups to the occlusal surfaces of the patient's posterior teeth. Again, these may be adjusted at regular intervals until the patient is comfortable. There is little evidence that moderate changes in the OVD lead to TMJ or muscle dysfunction problems provided that the occlusion is correctly managed.

Space for restoration(s) may be obtained in one of the following three ways, or by a combination of each:

A. By achieving a generalised increase in OVD by crowning or building up most or all of the teeth in one arch
B. By orthodontically intruding teeth which require restoration
C. By exploiting the difference between retruded contact position (RCP) and intercuspal position (ICP).

Patients in group A should be provided with a diagnostic restoration as described above prior to proceeding with definitive restorations. There are no rules about whether the crowns which increase the OVD should be placed in the upper or lower arches, or both: it is for the clinician to decide which teeth are most in need of full-coverage restorations.

Patients in group B may be treated using what is termed the 'Dahl principle'. In this category, only a small number of anterior teeth require restoration, but space is not available because of the compensatory mechanisms previously described, and preparation of the teeth may either reduce the teeth to an unmanageable degree or risk pulpal damage. In the original concept, designed for the treatment of patients whose upper anterior teeth had suffered palatal TSL, a removable prosthesis was constructed to cover the palatal surfaces of the anterior teeth. This caused disclusion of the posterior teeth, but these ultimately erupted into position, leaving a space between the anterior teeth into which a restoration could be placed. The treatment was further refined by the use of a fixed prosthesis, usually constructed in cobalt chromium (Fig. 11.6), and most recently by the placement of resin composite or ceramic veneers to achieve the resultant movement (Fig. 11.7). It is thought that the space between the anterior teeth is obtained as a result of compensatory over-eruption of the posterior teeth and intrusion of the anterior teeth.

As tooth substance is lost (group C), there may be flattening of the occlusal surfaces of the posterior teeth. This, in turn, may lead to the patient adopting a more anterior ICP and cause an increase in the horizontal space between the RCP and the ICP. It may be possible to exploit this space in a small number of cases where room is required for the restoration of anterior teeth.

TYPES OF RESTORATION

In cases where extensive numbers of full-coverage posterior restorations are required, these may be constructed in metal ceramic or gold, the latter requiring less reduction of tooth substance (of special importance in teeth which may have already been subjected to some TSL). Metal occlusal surfaces may also produce less wear of the opposing dentition, but patients are less likely to accept these, especially in the lower arch, for reasons of aesthetics. In cases of shortened crown height, additional retention may be achieved by the use of boxes and grooves. These will not only improve the retention, but also the resistance form. If all that is required is the building up of the occlusal surfaces of the posterior teeth, and the teeth are relatively sound, it may be possible to use adhesive ceramic or composite onlays.

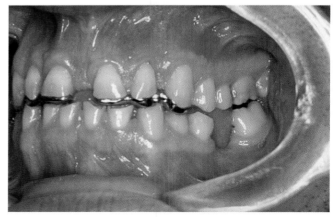

Fig. 11.6 A 'Dahl' appliance.

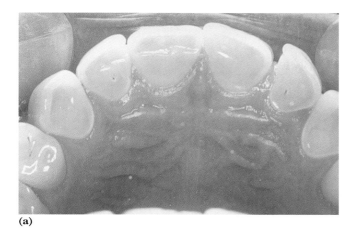

(a)

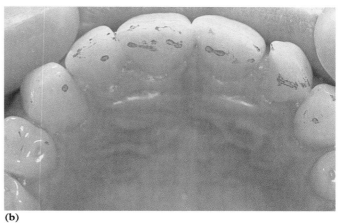

(b)

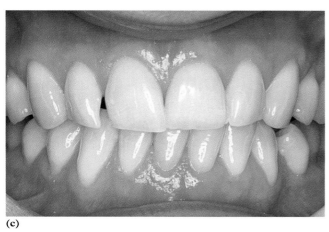

(c)

Fig. 11.7 Use of the 'Dahl principle' to obtain vertical space by orthodontic movement of teeth. **(a)** Erosive TSL affecting palatal aspect of maxillary anterior teeth. **(b)** Composite placed over exposed dentine using a dentine bonding agent. This effects an increase in OVD of approx. 2 mm. **(c)** Disclusion of the posterior teeth occurs. These teeth will erupt into contact in 1–3 months.

For anterior teeth, the choice of restorative material depends, to some extent, on the amount of tooth substance remaining. A shortened crown will be unlikely to achieve the necessary retention for a non-adhesive restorative procedure such as a metal ceramic crown cemented with a 'traditional' cement. In such cases, it will be necessary either to undertake a crown-lengthening procedure or to use an adhesive crown, such as a dentine-bonded crown. If the latter is used in cases where the tooth is shortened due to TSL, the completed restoration is also likely to be shorter than is ideal from an aesthetic viewpoint, and the patient may elect to undertake crown-lengthening surgery to achieve an improvement in aesthetics by improving the crown length to width ratio (Fig. 11.8).

It should be stated that the addition of retentive features such as grooves may enhance resistance form and protect the bond in adhesive techniques. The preparation for dentine-bonded crowns should not be extended subgingivally because of difficulties in isolation at the fit appointment, but for non-adhesive crowns, full use of the gingival crevice may be necessary to achieve the optimal retention. It is the considered view of the authors that devitalisation of the pulp and root canal treatment for reasons of retention should not be resorted to unless there are no other

viable alternatives, in view of the reduced rates of success of post-retained crowns, when compared with other full-coverage restorations. It should also be stressed that the retention of each individual crown is of importance and that no additional retention is gained by splinting a series of crowns which, individually, have compromised retention. The use of adhesive, dentine-bonded crowns in cases of TSL appears to be increasing, due to the ease by which retention may be achieved, the need for only minimal additional tooth preparation and the good aesthetic result which may be achieved. Further research is required to determine the long-term success of these restorations in such cases.

Finally, for patients whose TSL has a bruxist element, it is essential that this is controlled before treatment, or that the patient agrees to wear a night bite-guard or splint following the restorative process (Fig. 11.9). Furthermore, such patients should be made aware that their bruxist habit is likely to reduce the longevity of their new restorations. Patients whose teeth have been affected by TSL at an early age should also be made aware that their restorative cycle has commenced at a much earlier stage than would have occurred if normal physiological mechanisms had been the cause of their TSL. They should be told that

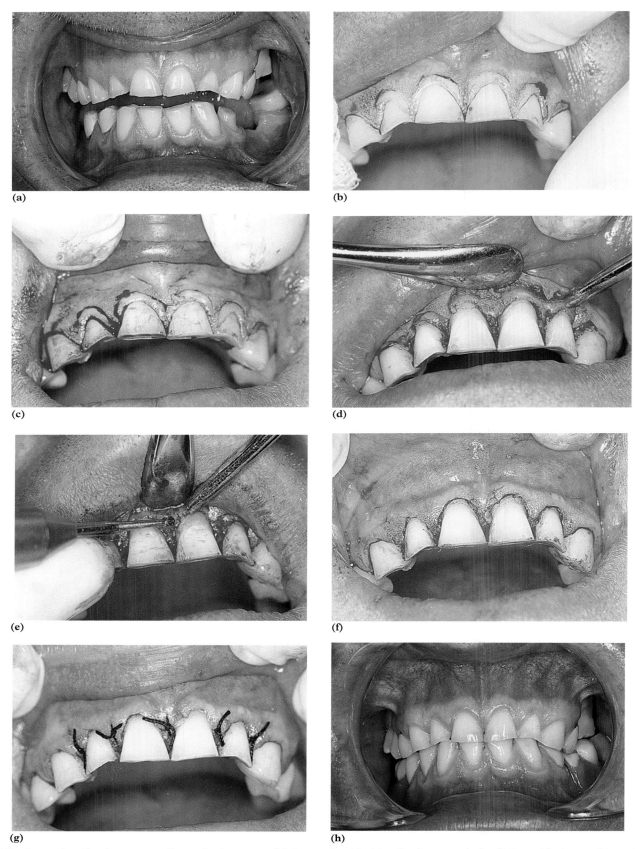

Fig. 11.8 Crown-lengthening surgery. Case prior to surgery (**a**); inverse level incision (**b, c**); removal of soft tissue (**d**); 1 mm of bone is removed (**e**); the flap is repositioned (**f**) and sutured (**g**); the final result (**h**).

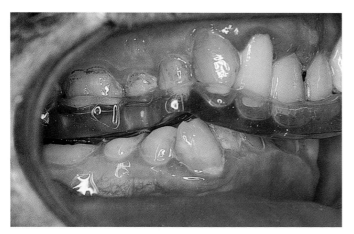

Fig. 11.9 Occlusal guard to protect teeth from nocturnal grinding.

SUMMARY

The treatment of TSL can be complex and it is first necessary to determine the cause of the problem. This will only be found by the taking of a careful and sometimes sensitive history and carrying out a careful examination. The best form of treatment is to stabilise the tooth loss and prevent the situation becoming worse. Only when the TSL is under control can it be treated. The more complex cases can be very time-consuming and involved and often require consultation with a clinician with specialised training in this area.

this cycle of restorative care will continue throughout their life, and that this should be budgeted for in the same way as cars and household items which eventually require replacement.

12 The principles of tooth replacement

INTRODUCTION

The edentulous space which occurs following tooth loss may be filled using a fixed prosthesis, such as a bridge, or a removable prosthesis such as a partial denture. Loss of tooth substance can be managed by other advanced procedures such as overdentures or osseointegrated implants. In many cases intervention may not be required, if the patient has no overriding aesthetic or functional problems. The most common choice facing the clinician is whether to provide a fixed or a removable prosthesis and this important area is discussed below. Alternative methods of replacing teeth are discussed later on in the chapter.

FIXED OR REMOVABLE PROSTHESIS?

This choice will be influenced by many factors relating to the nature of the tooth loss and the wishes of the patient.

Teeth have many functions. Posterior teeth, for example, are required for chewing. Anterior teeth are required for biting, and they also have an aesthetic function. Teeth are also important for speech, as certain sounds, e.g. 'th' and

145

'sh', rely on contact between the tongue and the surfaces of the hard and soft tissues.

For a patient, the idea of a fixed prosthesis is usually more attractive than that of a removable partial denture which has to be taken out to be cleaned. However, although a patient's wishes are an important consideration, the clinical decision on the final prosthesis may be driven by dental concerns (Box 12.1). In some cases, where aesthetics is not a consideration and the occlusion is stable, a simple option is to leave the space unfilled and monitor the situation. A prosthesis in this situation will often add complication and interfere with periodontal care and should not be contemplated unless there is a strong clinical reason to do so.

Dental factors

The number and position of teeth that are lost will influence the clinical decision. Furthermore, the status of the abutment teeth on either side of the edentulous space will dictate the type of restoration to be placed. A single incisor tooth with sound abutment teeth will favour the provision of a fixed restoration such as an etch-retained bridge, whilst the loss of four anterior teeth will produce a large span that may be more suitable for a removable partial denture. The loss of a single tooth is often best treated with a fixed prosthesis or implant fixture in the

long term, with a removable prosthesis being present during the healing phase. Bridges are ideal for restoring small spaces within an otherwise complete arch where there are strong and well-supported teeth on one or both ends of the space. If the vertical height of the space has been diminished by the over-eruption of an unopposed tooth, it is sometimes possible to crown it to produce a more favourable occlusal plane (Fig. 12.1). Alternatively, the over-erupted opposing tooth can be intruded by a Dahl appliance. This involves the use of a removable or cemented appliance to encourage axial tooth movement (Fig. 12.2). As the numbers of missing teeth increase, the balance swings in favour of removable partial denture therapy. Some patients may be best treated by a combination of bridgework and removable prostheses. Furthermore, the concept of the 'shortened dental arch' should be kept in mind when considering treatment options (Fig. 12.3, Box 12.2).

The abutment teeth must have sufficient tooth structure to be able to withstand the extra forces placed on them.

Box 12.1   Factors that govern the clinical decision on type of prosthesis

Dental factors
- Abutment teeth present
- The number of teeth lost
- Position of the tooth loss
- Periodontal considerations:
  - tooth support
- Conservation status of the teeth:
  - strength of tooth tissue
- Root canal treatment proposed or required
- Quality of underlying ridge and bone
- Presence of soft or hard tissue pathology
- Occlusion considerations:
  - canine guided
  - group function
  - opposing teeth

Patient factors
- Patient's wishes and expectations of treatment
- Age
- Susceptibility to dental disease:
  - caries experience
  - periodontal experience
- Medical conditions
- Social factors:
  - diet
  - smoking history
  - cost involved

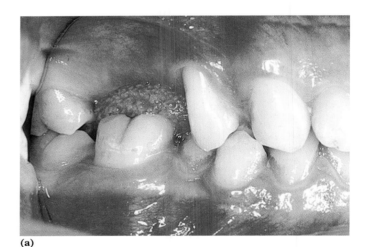

(a)

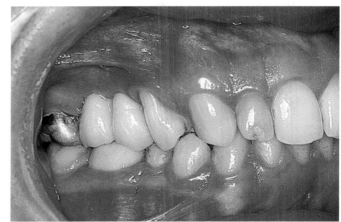

(b)

Fig. 12.1 **(a)** Over-erupted lower molar tooth opposing edentulous span. **(b)** Postoperative view after reduction and crowning of over-erupted molar to restore occlusal plane before restoration of space with fixed prosthesis.

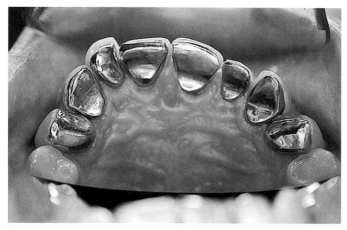

Fig. 12.2 Dahl appliance using gold onlays. (Courtesy of Mr A. Baxter.)

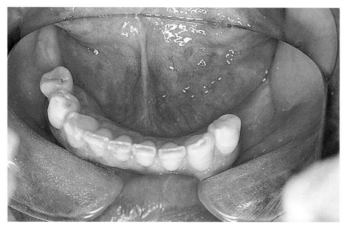

Fig. 12.3 This patient has a shortened dental arch from LR5 to LL4.

Box 12.2 Shortened dental arch

- Intact arches from 2nd premolar to 2nd premolar, in both jaws
- Functional occlusion
- Concentrate all resources on these teeth rather than on a lower standard of treatment for the remainder of the dentition

---

This is true whether the replacement restoration is fixed or removable. The periodontia must be healthy, even though reduced, before any restorative work is undertaken and the patient's plaque control must be good. The periodontal tissues must be healthy with little or no pocketing present and adequate bone support. The presence of periodontal disease can be determined by the usual screening parameters of low plaque and bleeding scores, and BPE scores of less than 2. Ideally the teeth should exhibit little or no mobility. The conservation status of the teeth should be satisfactory and any restorations should be sound with no caries present. A tooth with no restorations may preclude the placement of a fixed prosthesis, as considerable tooth removal may be required if crown preparation is required. However, it may allow the placement of an adhesive bridge. Proposed root canal treatment or the presence of a root-filled tooth needs careful consideration. Root canal treatment may lead to loss of tooth structure, which may weaken the tooth, and therefore other abutments may be required to take the increased load. Loss of alveolar bone following the removal of a tooth may lead to reduced ridge height. A removable prosthesis will often provide better aesthetics and soft tissue support by helping to replace this tissue loss. Furthermore, the presence of underlying soft or hard tissue pathology may require surgery, which may compromise the treatment plan.

The occlusion requires careful assessment during treatment planning. This often requires properly mounted study casts on a semi-adjustable articulator to fully appreciate the influence of the occlusion on the case being assessed. The loss of a canine tooth will be difficult to replace if the occlusion is canine-guided on excursive movements, whilst group function will involve several teeth. Articulated casts will also show the interocclusal clearance present, crown height, over-eruption or tilting of teeth.

When explaining the differences between a bridge (fixed prosthesis) and a denture (removable prosthesis) to a patient, the advantages of a denture must not be minimised. At the same time, the disadvantages of a removable denture with the large area of tissue covered need to be mentioned and, if possible, demonstrated on a model. Any display of metal from clasps or occlusal rests should be explained. The main advantage of a bridge is that it cannot be removed from the mouth. In addition, it usually only involves teeth adjacent to the space, thus simplifying plaque control. The major disadvantages are the time and cost involved, together with the problems associated with repair after damage. Other problems include cementation failure, tooth fracture and pulp death.

Although there are no absolute age barriers for the provision of crown and bridgework, such treatments are generally avoided in a very young patient because of possible risks to the dental pulp from extensive conservative procedures and the likelihood of subsequent trauma during childhood. Furthermore, incomplete eruption of the teeth often precludes satisfactory retention of retainers and continued eruption will gradually expose the gum margin of the tooth preparation, which may spoil the appearance of an anterior crown. Higher failure rates of conventional fixed prostheses have previously been reported (in young versus middle-aged patients) because of these factors. Caution should be exercised with elderly or debilitated patients who may find it difficult to withstand the rigours of extensive operative treatment.

Careful history-taking will quickly establish the patient's wishes and expectations of the treatment proposed. Past dental history, including an assessment of the patient's susceptibility to dental disease such as caries, and experience and attitude to periodontal care, will provide further insights to the complexity of the treatment that should be undertaken. Diet sheets are a useful way of identifying potential caries or erosive attack of the teeth. History of smoking will indicate a potential susceptibility to periodontal disease and is contraindicated in advanced treatment procedures (such as implant placement) due to poor post-surgical healing. Long-drawn-out procedures or treatment plans may not be possible with patients who have medical conditions which prevent regular attendance. The majority of patients become keenly interested in fixed bridgework when the advantages of such treatment for restoring edentulous spaces are explained to them. Those who lack interest or refuse to accept their role in the control of dental disease are not suitable candidates for indirect work. Very nervous patients may also be unsuitable on grounds of temperament.

Social factors which will influence attendance, such as distance to travel, employment considerations or family circumstances, must be considered. Finally, the costs involved will have a bearing on treatment options and it is always wise to plan for the least demanding option which brings about the most success and which is also cost-effective.

CLINICAL ASSESSMENT OF THE INDIVIDUAL SPACE TO BE RESTORED

The provision of a fixed or removable partial denture is written up in a detailed treatment plan contained within the patient's notes. In simple cases, such a procedure will often be the last item of treatment provision. However, in more complex cases, where there are multiple plastic restorations and possible provision of crowns, consideration of the fixed or removable prosthesis is made at an early stage in the treatment.

When the previous restorative treatment has been completed, the initial preparatory work consists of taking preliminary impressions and a design is drawn up using these preliminary casts. The vitality, periodontal support and health of the potential abutments should be assessed.

Radiographic investigation will aid in determining:

- the size and position of the dental pulp
- the gingival and pulpal extent of any caries or restorations
- the condition and level of the alveolar support
- the shape and length of the abutment root(s)
- the periapical status.

The patient's occlusion should be checked in intercuspal position and in lateral and protrusive excursions, to assess the clearance that can be achieved during tooth preparation. An assessment should be made of the occlusal forces likely to be borne by the prosthesis during function. Marked wear facets are often an indication of heavy para-

functional loads. This is an important visit and it is easy to make mistakes during the impression-taking and design stages which may influence the final restoration. High-quality casts which reproduce both hard and soft tissues will determine the accuracy of the design (Fig. 12.4).

Design

An occlusal record is required and this is made at a separate clinical visit. It will involve a retruded axis registration in wax combined with a face bow recording. If a number of teeth are missing then wax occlusal rims are required. The jaw relationship is recorded and the casts mounted on an articulator before the provisional design of restoration is made.

Registration of the jaw relationship

A specific jaw relationship is required for transfer to the articulator. This will be made for a contact relationship of the teeth, which may be either the intercuspal position (ICP) or retruded contact position (RCP). The ICP is the position of maximum intercuspation of the posterior teeth. It is characterised by simultaneous contact with no anteroposterior or lateral slide as the mandible closes. A patient will enter this position spontaneously and it is the closest relationship of the mandible to the maxilla. The RCP is a contact relationship of the mandible located up to 1–1.5 mm distal to the ICP. There is a forward movement from RCP to ICP with no deviation. If there are sufficient teeth present, the casts may be hand articulated without the need for occlusal rims, but a full registration will be required if there are insufficient teeth for stable positioning of the casts. This latter position will be needed if there is no natural tooth-to-tooth contact.

The registration is made with wax occlusal rims on a shellac base for the upper, and a wire strengthener for the lower. If there are insufficient numbers of missing teeth,

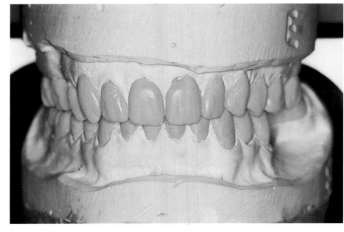

Fig. 12.4 Mounted study casts duplicating hard and soft tissues.

the registration is made using beauty wax which covers the occlusal surfaces with an aluminium palatal strengthener. If there is deviation on closure from the first initial contact to the ICP, the relationship is recorded at the point just before any tooth contact occurs. This will be on the retruded hinge axis. This pre-tooth contact registration allows the occlusion to be analysed on the articulator (Fig. 12.5).

Mounting on articulator

Diagnostic casts with the teeth registered in occlusion are mounted on an average movement or semi-adjustable articulator (Box 12.3). This is preferred to a simple hinge articulator which gives limited information on the movement of the jaw. An average movement articulator incorporates an average condylar guidance path which is set at approximately 30°. A face bow recording is used to orientate the upper occlusal plane to the condyles. This gives an accurate recording of the relationship that is then transferred to the laboratory where it is used to orientate the maxillary cast (Fig. 12.6).

> **Box 12.3   Articulators**
>
> Commonly used articulators include:
> * Hinge
> * Average movement
> * Semi-adjustable
> * Fully adjustable
>
> For treatment planning, average movement and semi-adjustable articulators are used in conjunction with a face bow recording.

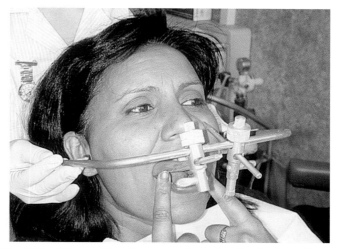

Fig. 12.6   Picture of face bow recording using the Dentatus face bow.

The maxillary cast is mounted in its correct position relative to the condylar axis by means of the face bow recording. The average movement articulator is limited in its reproduction of mandibular movements and for greater accuracy a semi-adjustable articulator is used. These articulators allow for a greater range of movement for the condylar and incisal guidance. They also allow for the bodily shift of the mandible (Bennett movement) during lateral excursion.

Fully adjustable articulators allow a greater amount of movement to take place and bring a greater degree of accuracy. The majority of cases can be analysed using semi-adjustable articulators and it is beyond the scope of this text to cover the fully adjustable articulator.

The design and production of the restoration is now made. This may be either fixed (bridge) or removable (partial denture).

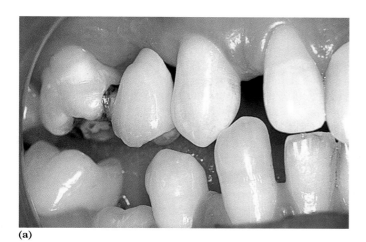

(a)

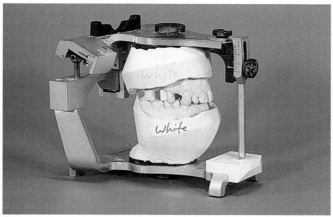

(b)

Fig. 12.5   (a) Initial contact (pre-tooth contact) on retruded arc of closure. (b) Accurate study casts mounted on an articulator are required for treatment planning of the edentulous space.

FIXED PROSTHESES (BRIDGES)

Study casts have added advantages when planning for a fixed prosthesis. These include making a more detailed assessment of the occlusion and undertaking trial procedures such as a diagnostic wax-up prior to embarking on the bridge procedure (Box 12.4).

Photographs can form a valuable record of the preoperative condition. The patient must be given an estimate of the total time involved in treatment as well as the probable length of appointments and the intervals in between. Serial study casts may also be of use in assessing the progress of tooth wear and whether the occlusion has stabilised. There are many clinical reasons for constructing a bridge, such as deterioration of the occlusion if a space is left unrestored. Teeth adjacent to the space may drift and cause premature occlusal contacts or loss of contact leading to food packing and the risk of caries and periodontal disease. Loss of function is not a serious issue if the gap is small. Although occlusal stability may initially be lost as a result of extraction and non-replacement, tooth movement may result in an occlusal relationship that becomes stable over time and is functionally acceptable. In cases of doubt, serial study casts will allow an assessment to be made as to whether there is occlusal stability. In some circumstances, orthodontic treatment will be required to realign teeth or to regain lost space before embarking on bridgework. In these circumstances, the bridge may serve an additional function of maintaining the result of the orthodontic treatment.

Improvement of appearance is an important reason for constructing an anterior bridge. In many cases, a well-constructed partial denture may prove superior to an anterior bridge from an aesthetic viewpoint. However, the greater comfort and stability provided by a bridge may outweigh the previous consideration. Finally, a most important indication for a bridge flows from the fact that all types of restoration may cause damage to the teeth and supporting tissues. A bridge may be superior to a denture because it covers less tissue and consequently has less potential for periodontal damage. Replacement of missing teeth with partial dentures may be a common source of periodontal disease when diet and plaque control are not adequate. However, there is a biological price to pay with a conventional fixed prosthesis, and long-term studies of crowned teeth show that in 0.5–10% of cases, pulpal necrosis and periapical lesions may develop following extensive crown procedures.

In preparing teeth for conventional bridge retainers, it is often necessary to remove substantial amounts of sound tooth tissue. Whilst an unrestored sound tooth makes the best abutment to prepare from a mechanical viewpoint, extensive cutting of tooth tissue can lead to loss of pulp vitality. The amount of tooth tissue to be removed may be greater than for individual preparations because mutual parallelism may be required between abutments that are out of alignment. In addition, space may be required within the retainer contours for a movable joint. The decision to provide a bridge must take these factors into account and the operator must be convinced that the risk of pulpal necrosis is minimal before proceeding with such treatment.

Types of bridge

Fixed-fixed

In this type of bridge, all joints are either soldered or cast in one piece, rigidly connecting all the abutment teeth (Fig. 12.7). It requires equal or good retention at either end of the edentulous span, and it must be possible to produce mutual parallelism of all retainers. This type of bridge is simple to construct and affords rigid splinting. It provides maximum retention and support for long spans and gives cross-arch splinting for larger bridges when the periodontal tissues are reduced. It demands heavy tooth preparation with the risk of overtaper when preparations are not mutually aligned and/or the span is long. Accurate construction and cementation may be difficult in cases with long spans. Significant framework distortion may occur when firing the porcelain veneer. For this reason it is recommended to avoid metal/ceramic bridges over four units in length. Catastrophic failures frequently occur when this type of bridge is incorrectly prescribed or poorly executed.

Fixed-movable

This type of bridge incorporates a stress-redistributing device which allows limited movement at one of the joints

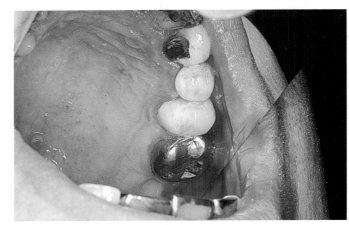

Fig. 12.7 Fixed-fixed bridge at UL3 to UL5.

Box 12.4 Advantages of articulated casts for bridgework

- Detailed assessment of the occlusion
- Preparations may be rehearsed on the study cast
- Diagnostic wax-up allows the patient to assess appearance prior to tooth preparation
- Waxed-up study casts can be duplicated and Vacuform matrices prepared for temporary bridgework to be made at the chairside
- Alternatively, a temporary bridge can be made in the laboratory on 'rough cut' preparations

between the pontic(s) and the retainer(s). The fixed end of the bridge has a rigid connector with the major retainer that is usually distal to the pontic (Fig. 12.8). The minor retainer houses the movable joint and does not require as much retention as the major retainer. The joint is normally of a slot and dovetail type. Because the abutment carrying the minor retainer can be depressed without the retainer being held rigidly to the rest of the bridge, there is no need for full occlusal coverage with this retainer. The movable joint gives support to the pontic against vertical occlusal forces and allows minimal movement in response to lateral forces. This prevents movement of one retainer transmitting torsional forces directly to another, leading to loss of cement seal. The 'cantilever' effect of the non-rigid design can place additional stress on the major retainer and a strong abutment is required and may be contraindicated for long spans. Where there is non-parallelism of the abutment teeth and a common path of insertion cannot be prepared, a fixed-movable bridge may be the solution.

In summary, fixed-movable bridges are more conservative and potentially more aesthetic than fixed-fixed bridges. They allow independent tooth movement and can use divergent abutments. Hybrid designs are possible and there is greater control of cementation. They are more complex to make and less rigid. A strong major retainer is required and span length is usually limited. The construction of temporary bridgework may be difficult.

Cantilever

A cantilever bridge has a pontic connected to a retainer at one end only. Hence leverage is imposed on abutment teeth. For this reason, multiple abutments are often used and this type of bridge is not employed when occlusal forces on the pontic will be heavy (Fig. 12.9). Thus distal cantilevers are rarely indicated. The retainers should be balanced for strength and retentive potential and must be joined rigidly. They are conservative, aesthetic, and

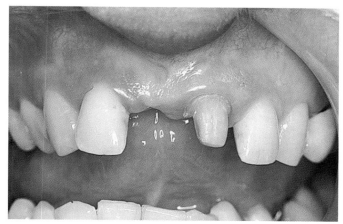

Fig. 12.9 Cantilever bridge with UL1 prepared for a crown retainer.

simplify plaque control and are indicated where occlusal forces are light. They require a strong pontic/retainer joint; there is only unilateral support and span length is limited.

Spring cantilever

This type of bridge supports a pontic at some distance from the retainer(s). It is both tooth- and tissue-supported and is only indicated in the maxilla. A metal bar, which fits in contact with the palatal mucosa, connects the retainer to the pontic (Fig. 12.10).

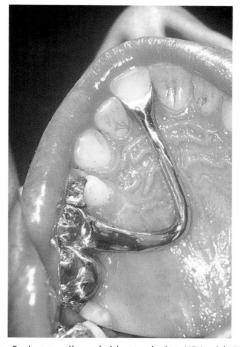

Fig. 12.10 Spring cantilever bridge replacing UR1 with FVC retainers at UR5 and UR6.

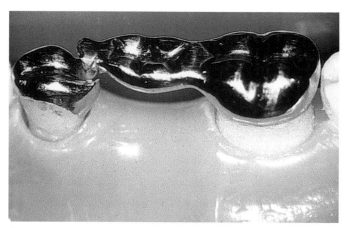

Fig. 12.8 Fixed-movable bridge with major retainer distal to pontic.

The spring cantilever bridge provides an aesthetic solution to the problem of replacing a missing upper incisor when the anterior teeth are spaced. The connecting bar should follow a wide curve to provide additional mucosal support and limit adverse leverage. The bar should be oval in cross-section and taper from the retainer to the pontic. It is not well suited for patients with steeply vaulted palates. Oral hygiene can be maintained by using dental floss to clean beneath the bar. This type of bridge involves permanent mucosal coverage and should therefore be used with discretion. Its use has fallen out of favour in recent years with the advent of more predictable implant treatment.

Compound

A combination of any two or more of the above designs may be referred to as compound or complex. As a general principle, it is best to use several small bridges to replace a number of missing teeth, rather than replace them all with one large complex or compound bridge. This will simplify replacement if a single bridge unit fails.

Treatment planning/preparatory work

Box 12.5 provides a useful checklist after the bridge design has been completed and prior to commencement of the clinical procedures.

Orthodontic considerations

It may often be necessary to correct malpositioned teeth adjacent to an edentulous space. When a tooth is tilted, it is difficult to obtain a common path of insertion with other abutments and it may also be difficult to prepare for a retentive retainer. Furthermore, if abutments are prepared in their tilted position, periodontal problems may occur between abutment and pontic, as plaque removal becomes difficult when interproximal spaces are inaccessible.

The space available for the pontic is important in the anterior region to allow good appearance. If space loss has occurred, it may be possible to correct it orthodontically. Alternatively, retainers may be constructed that are narrower mesiodistally than the original abutment teeth. Overlapping pontic designs can give a pleasing appearance in some situations. If the span length is excessive for a normal-sized pontic, alternative possibilities include orthodontic treatment, wider retainers, and alternative designs of bridgework such as spring cantilever.

Principles of tooth preparation

Optimal tooth preparation involves the triad of biological, mechanical and aesthetic principles (Box 12.6). The strength of a bridge is limited by the strength of its individual components. It is dependent on the materials used, their dimensions and the method of linkage to each other and to the supporting tissues. Regions of potential weakness are solder joints, connectors, and occlusal and incisal surfaces. The requirements of strength for any bridge will depend on the amount of masticatory force it has to resist over the length of the span. A bridge opposed by a denture has to resist much less occlusal force than one opposed by natural teeth. Aesthetics becomes increasingly important towards the front of the mouth. If the patient is prepared to show some gold, a more conservative retainer design may be possible (either conventional partial veneer or resin-bonded). Metal ceramic crowns can produce excellent appearance, but considerable tooth reduction is required labially and occlusally in order to accommodate the metal frame and the porcelain veneer. In situations where there is minimal occlusal stress, an all-porcelain metal-free bridge can provide the best appearance. The failure rate of such bridges has been reduced with modern adhesive materials and techniques. Fibre reinforced composites are also being introduced for metal-free adhesive bridgework. These may be used with direct (chairside) or indirect (laboratory fabricated) approaches. They are considered to be best in anterior fixed-fixed restorations where occlusal loading is less and support is provided at both ends of the span.

Box 12.5   Checklist prior to clinical bridge procedures

- All preparatory conservation work completed
- Good plaque control/periodontal condition
- Abutments tested for vitality
- Relevant radiographs available
- Occlusion assessed (adjustment required?)
- Diagnostic wax-up (Vacuform matrix required?)
- Selection of abutment(s)
- Doubtful restorations investigated and replaced
- Trial preparations on mounted casts
- Design of restoration (simple preferred)
- Integrate design to existing/anticipated treatment needs.

Box 12.6   Triad of principles for tooth preparation

Biological
- Conservative
- Supragingival margins
- Correct contours
- Tooth protection from fracture

Mechanical
- Retention form
- Resistance performance
- Resistance to deformation

Aesthetic
- Adequate porcelain thickness (buccally/occlusally)
- No or minimal metal display/show through

Bridge design

In choosing the design of bridge for a particular space, a number of decisions have to be made. Even for the replacement of a single missing tooth there are many possible variants in bridge design, including the number of abutments to be employed, the types of retainers to be used, the design of bridge to be selected and the choice of luting cement. Meta-analyses of the survival of conventional fixed prostheses show that whilst the survival probability is good at 5-year recall (4 or 5% failure), the failure rate increases after 10 years. At 15-year recall, failure rates are typically 25–30% and the principal mode of failure is by loosening or recurrent caries. When there is partial loss of cementation of a bridge, this may go unnoticed by the patient for some considerable time. This can result in extensive caries of the failed abutment, which can jeopardise the success of any replacement bridge or lead to loss of that abutment (Fig. 12.11).

When the abutment in question is a critical or terminal abutment, a replacement bridge may then become impossible, and hence the choice of bridge design and selection of retainers are crucial for long-term success. A common cause of bridge failure is the choice of abutments with crowns that are too small to provide sufficient retention. The clinical crown height should be sufficient to allow adequate retainer preparation. Any tooth with less than 4 mm crown height from marginal ridge to gum margin is questionable as an abutment. Slots, grooves, pins and adhesive cements may be used to increase retention in the case of short crowns, but their use complicates design and construction.

The longer the span, the greater the stress on the retainers will be and the greater the risk of cementation failure. Replacement of a missing molar requires more retentive preparation than for a lower incisor. Replacing an upper first premolar in a patient with group function occlusion will make more demands on bridge retention than for a situation where occlusal function on the pontic

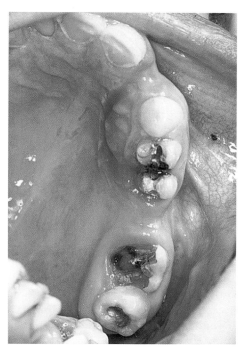

Fig. 12.11 Extensive caries revealed following removal of a complex bridge. The distal retainer required extraction.

only occurs in intercuspal position because of canine guidance. The extent of previous restorations, caries or endodontic treatment may have severely weakened the crown of a potential abutment. The extent of any caries on previous restorations must be known before the choice of retainer can be finalised. Failure to do so can result in a hasty design change during tooth preparation, which can lead to early failure. Whilst minor internal undercuts in a preparation can be obliterated with cement, larger losses of tooth tissue are best dealt with by incorporating features into the tooth preparation to compensate for inadequate retention/resistance form (Table 12.1).

Table 12.1	Compensating for inadequate retention/resistance form in cast restorations		
Extent of tooth loss	**Clinical situation**	**Operative procedure**	**Final restoration**
Moderate to severe	Short preparation or excessive taper One or two cusps missing but > 50% coronal tooth structure remains Width/length ratio >1:1	Use isthmuses/boxes Add grooves /pinholes Modify sloping surfaces into horizontal walls /horizontal and vertical components (terracing) Surgical crown lengthening	Non-standard partial or full veneer
Severe	Loss of > 50% crown Width/length ratio <1:1 Short preparation for a long crown	Pin amalgam or bonded Composite core Surgical crown lengthening	Full veneer
Total loss of coronal tooth structure	All cusps undermined/lost Supragingival height <1 mm	As above plus elective endodontics and post/core for premolars 1.5–2.0 mm circumferential ferrule	Full veneer

Root-treated teeth may require a post placed to aid retention of the core. The shape of an abutment crown may present retention problems when dealing with conical or short teeth. Retention of this type of retainer depends on placing grooves or slots in axial surfaces in addition to obtaining near-parallelism of opposing surfaces. Whilst the standard texts recommend taper angles of 2–6°, this is not routinely possible in clinical practice. A taper angle of 3° equates to a convergence angle of 6°. Mean convergence angles of bridge preparations from commercial laboratories range from 15° to 30° and hence a taper angle of 8° is more realistic. Long, narrow tooth preparations can have greater taper than short, wide preparations without sacrificing resistance. The latter require near-parallel walls if adequate resistance form is to be obtained. Special attention should be given to any tooth where the extent of caries of previous restoration has jeopardised pulp vitality. Investigations of crowned teeth reveal a twofold increase in pulpal necrosis where the tooth has a pin-retained core. When there is doubt about continued pulp viability, it may be wise to undertake elective endodontic treatment in advance of proceeding to abutment tooth preparation.

Choice of retainers

Factors which affect the choice of retainer include:

- the retention required
- bridge design
- amount of sound coronal tissue available
- strength of dentine after preparation
- extent of existing restorations
- occlusal protection required
- amount of metal display tolerable.

Supragingival margins are preferred wherever possible because they simplify bridge preparation, impression-taking and cementation, in addition to helping maintain periodontal health. Retainer margins may have to be placed subgingivally in order to cover existing restorations, gain adequate retention or hide metal display anteriorly. In such situations, the biological width must always be maintained. Tooth preparations should only ever be placed into the gingival sulcus and not encroach on the epithelial attachment. Inlays, partial and complete veneer crowns, and telescopic crowns, are the alternative retainers available to bridgework. Pins, posts and adhesive cements will all add to the retention.

Intracoronal inlays

In the case of the conventional bridge design, the use of intracoronal inlays without cuspal coverage is restricted to the minor retainer of a fixed-movable bridge. Studies have shown that when inlays are used without cuspal coverage as the retainers in a conventional fixed-fixed bridge, the failure rate is increased greater than 10-fold in comparison

to full crown retainers. This is because the abutment can be depressed in its socket while the retainer is supported by the remainder of the bridge. This can cause fracture of the relatively weak cement seal. However, inlay retainers have been shown to be more successful in resin-bonded bridgework. This is because of the better mechanical properties and adhesion of the luting resin cement to retainer and tooth. The MOD inlay with covered cusps (also called MOD onlay) is the minimum design of major retainer that should normally be considered for a posterior bridge. It has been argued that both approximal surfaces should always be covered for major retainers as subsequent caries of an uninvolved surface could endanger the bridge.

A more modern biological approach would be to secure adequate retention and resistance features by appropriate bridge design and material selection. Caries rate must be low and caries control excellent before any bridge is provided for a patient. Buccal and lingual extensions of an onlay preparation will aid the retention of this type of retainer even if only one proximal surface is involved (Fig. 12.12).

Partial veneer crowns

Partial veneer crowns are preferred to full veneer crowns where adequate retention and resistance form can be obtained, even when they are used as retainers for conventional bridge preparations. The advantages and disadvantages of partial veneer crowns as compared with more extensive full veneers are as follows:

Advantages
- Conservative
- Minimal gingival involvement
- Vitality testing possible
- Fit is readily assessed
- Cementation is easy
- Margins are accessible
- Versatile insertion path.

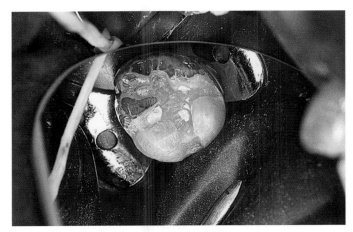

Fig. 12.12 Mesial half-crown preparation for long-span mandibular resin-bonded bridge. Note buccal and lingual slots and presence of varnish to facilitate removal of excess resin after bonding.

Disadvantages
- Less retentive (short/bulbous teeth)
- Less rigid (long spans/mobile abutments)
- Metal display
- Insertion path critical
- Root-filled teeth.

Telescopic crowns

Telescopic crowns are constructed in two parts: an inner sleeve is cast and cemented, and an outer full veneer crown is made to cover the inner sleeve. The outer crown is soldered to the other bridge units. This type of retainer can sometimes be used to overcome differences in the inclination of abutment teeth which cannot be solved by other designs of retainer. The amount of tooth tissue that would have to be removed from the mesial surface of a tilted lower molar abutment to ensure a path of insertion for a fixed-fixed bridge may lead to dramatic loss of retention. The use of a telescopic crown in this situation enables the mesial and distal surfaces of the tooth preparation to be prepared near-parallel for optimum retention whilst the path of insertion of the bridge is reproduced on the outer surface of the sleeve. In the case of multi-unit bridgework and splinting, the outer crowns may be placed with a temporary luting cement, allowing them to be removed subsequently for inspection or repair (Fig. 12.13).

Metal ceramic crowns

Metal ceramic crowns are frequently used as bridge retainers. They may be designed with metal or porcelain occlusal surfaces (Fig. 12.14, Table 12.2).

Clinical decisions

Many decisions about tooth preparation design can be made from trial preparations on articulated diagnostic casts. The best location for partial veneer margins and optimal path of withdrawal can be determined in this way. Mutual parallelism can be confirmed by preparing critical surfaces first. Adequate box dimensions for the connector of a fixed-movable bridge can be checked in advance (Fig. 12.15). Planned occlusal changes can be made by a trial adjustment of the mounted casts in advance of tooth preparation and a diagnostic wax-up can be employed to help assess potential aesthetics.

Conservative tooth preparations and the use of partial rather than complete coverage favour the employment of resin-bonded designs of bridgework. In the case of conventional tooth preparations, direct and indirect pulp capping should be avoided and elective endodontics considered if there is doubt about ongoing vitality following bridge preparation. Preparations should be prepared to a minimum practical taper avoiding unnecessary apical extension. A Vacuform matrix made from a diagnostic cast can assist in determining adequate depth of tooth preparation together with the use of occlusal and axial depth cuts.

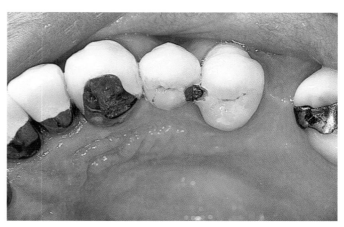

Fig. 12.14 Posterior metal ceramic bridge retainers at UL3 and UL5 showing partial and full porcelain cover.

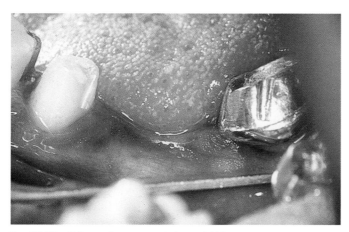

Fig. 12.13 Telescopic crown retainer at LL7.

Table 12.2 Indications for metal versus porcelain occlusal surfaces

Metal	Porcelain
Short teeth	Aesthetics is critical
Large pulp	Large teeth
Opposing enamel/metal occlusals	Heavily restored teeth
Parafunction	Opposing porcelain occlusal
Group function occlusion	Steep anterior guidance
Simple adjustment	Difficult adjustment
Average technical support	Excellent technical support

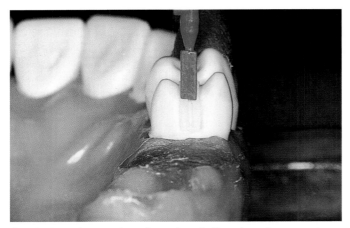

Fig. 12.15 Adequate box dimensions in Typodont three-quarter crown preparation to house male component of fixed-movable joint.

Estimating the amount of abutment root support

In 1926 Ante proposed that the combined peri-cemental area of the abutment teeth should be equal to or greater than the area of the tooth or teeth to be replaced. The work of Nyman, Lindhe and others has since shown that this statement is too rigid. The longevity of a bridge depends as much upon the quality of periodontal support as its quantity. In addition, appropriate occlusal design of retainers and pontics is important in preventing undue stress on periodontal tissues. Any bridgework should be designed so that it is in harmony with the patient's occlusion, and occlusal guidance created to protect the bridge during function. The number, length and shape of the abutment roots will indicate the support available for a bridge. In general, a canine may be an acceptable abutment for a lateral, but not vice-versa.

If the abutment tooth has lost half of its bone support in length, the effective loss is more than this because of root taper. Roots that are flattened or oval in cross-section offer greater rotation resistance than roots which are round in cross-section. Molars with fused roots offer less resistance than those with divergent roots. If roots are short and tapered, they will offer less resistance to the additional masticatory forces imposed by a bridge span. The traditional way of overcoming this problem was to increase the number of abutments. Rigid splinting of teeth in such circumstances often led to long-term failure because the retention and support available from the abutment teeth differed. The magnitude and direction of occlusal forces placed on a bridge abutment depends on the location of the tooth in the dental arch. Teeth vary in their amount of mobility in axial and buccolingual directions.

When a bridge involves teeth anterior and posterior to a canine, there is a higher risk of failure if a fixed-fixed design is used. Every effort should be made to choose alternative designs that do not invade both anterior and

posterior segments in a single bridge. This is shown in Figure 12.16, which illustrates a bridge replacing a missing lower first premolar. The second premolar had a short conical root which had lost bone support from previously treated periodontal disease. Both the second premolar and the first premolar were already crowned. The canine was sound. If a conventional fixed-fixed design using the canine and the second premolar as abutments had been chosen, this would have failed because of differential mobility. Splinting the canine to the second premolar and first molar in a four-unit fixed-fixed bridge would have protected the weak intermediate abutment to some extent from occlusal forces. However, this would have created problems with cementation where teeth have differential mobility and the failure rate of pier or intermediate abutments is high because of flexing of the span imposed by differential tooth movement under load. By choosing a fixed-movable design and employing a resin-bonded retainer for the major connector, it was possible to overcome this problem with a hybrid bridge.

Pontic design

The principles for optimal pontic design are as follows:

Biological
- No pressure on ridge
- Tissue surface cleansable
- Access to abutments.

Mechanical
- Rigid

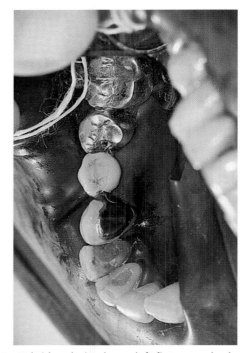

Fig. 12.16 Hybrid replacing lower left first premolar (see accompanying text for further details).

- Strong connectors
- Correct framework design.

Aesthetic
- Shade matched
- Adequate porcelain bulk
- Appears to 'grow out' of the ridge.

The angle of contact formed by the junction of the buccal and lingual or palatal surfaces of the pontic must be kept as wide as possible to discourage food stagnation. An acute angle between pontic and mucosa may lead to food trapping. Similarly, covering as much of a convex ridge surface as the original tooth did (a saddle design of pontic) will create problems with plaque control. Hence, a modified ridge lap form of pontic is preferred, wherever possible, for aesthetic pontics because it removes the concavity from the mucosal contact area (Fig. 12.17).

In the mandibular posterior region, where appearance is not usually an issue, a simple solution has been to use pontics that do not cover the mucosa and have a smooth rounded tissue surface. They are called hygienic, wash-through or sanitary pontics. The latter term may be for non-ceramic designs. However, if the distance between the tissue surface of the pontic and the residual ridge crest is small (<3 mm), it may encourage food trapping and a dome or bullet design of pontic where there is contact with the ridge surface is preferred. Interdental embrasure spaces should never be occluded and should always be accessible to cleaning by interdental brushes or floss threaders. All-gold pontics may be used to replace molars where appearance is not important. Metal ceramic pontics are suitable for anterior regions. Pontics for spring cantilever bridges may take the form of a porcelain jacket crown cemented to a core/diaphragm assembly at the terminal end of the bar

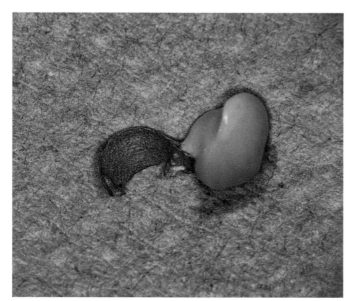

Fig. 12.17 Modified ridge lap pontic.

connector. This avoids having the pontic/cement junction next to the tissue.

RESIN-BONDED BRIDGES

A resin-bonded bridge consists of a cast metal framework that is cemented with resin composite to an abutment(s) which has preparation(s) confined either entirely or almost entirely to enamel. These bridges originated from direct composite bonding techniques which were used to provide short-term replacement of missing teeth. They used either natural crowns or acrylic resin or composite pontics. The limiting factor was the weakness of the resin composite (connector). Wire mesh, orthodontic brackets and metal pins placed interdentally have all been used in attempts to increase the life of these restorations. The more recent introduction of fibre-reinforced systems (glass fibres, Kevalar and ultrahigh-molecular-weight polyethylene fibres) has renewed interest in metal-free direct and indirect resin composite bridges. Advantages of the fibre-reinforced composite (FRC) bridge include:

- well suited to single-visit immediate tooth replacements
- frequently little or no tooth preparation required
- improved aesthetics
- transitional restorations and long-term provisionals
- suitable for the young and the elderly
- wear is kind to opposing teeth
- low treatment costs
- readily repaired.

Materials issues include fibre type, volume fraction, wave pattern, wetting agents and veneering composites, Clinical FRC bridges may be constructed using direct, semi-direct and indirect or laboratory fabricated approaches. Any reinforcing effect is only related to the position of the fibres in the restoration, thus making fibre volume fraction an important issue. The fibre should be placed in the most advantageous location and direction within the restoration to inhibit crack propagation. Existing design parameters for traditional metal-wing-retained adhesive bridges do not apply for FRC adhensive bridgework. Failure rates from studies to date are quite divergent and until further evidence accumulates, FRC bridges are best restricted to anterior transitional replacements in low stress situations. New high-strength ceramic systems may also have a role in the metal-free replacement of missing teeth with adhesive bridge techniques. Available evidence suggests thse are best restricted to simple cantilever anterior situations when a single tooth is missing.

Resin-bonded bridges were originally used for the replacement of individual missing anterior teeth in young patients where conventional bridgework was contraindicated because of pulp size, crown length or patient management problems. These patients often presented with sound abutment teeth but inadequate plaque control and little or no experience of operative treatment. Many of them participated in contact sports and removable partial dentures had often been the compromise solution in spite of their potential negative effect on periodontal health. Resin-bonded bridges became the preferred treatment and were used as interim or semi-permanent prostheses. Little, if any, enamel preparation was undertaken and the technique was essentially irreversible. Frequently they were described as non-preparation bridges. High failure rates were experienced with these initial designs of resin-bonded bridges. Meta-analyses revealed failure rates of 25% or more at 4-year recall. Subsequent more retentive designs involving tooth preparation to develop retention and resistance form gave a higher success rate. With appropriate choice of materials (non-precious alloy frameworks, chemically active resins), appropriate case selection and suitable preparation techniques, success rates of greater than 90% have been obtained with this design of bridge at 10-year recall. Optimal requirements for these bridges are outlined in Box 12.7.

Such bridges can be used as an intermediate restoration, avoiding the need for a removable prosthesis where expense or uncertain prognosis contraindicates other treatment. Resin-bonded bridges may also be used for the replacement of multiple teeth when an unusually large surface area of enamel is available for bonding and the occlusion is favourable.

All the clinical and laboratory stages involved in the planning, construction and cementation of a resin-bonded bridge are as critical as with a conventional bridge in order to ensure success. Whilst a resin-bonded bridge may be a conservative restoration for appropriate patients, there is a high risk of failure in unsuitable cases and careful patient selection is essential. Advantages and disadvantages of these bridges are outlined in Box 12.8.

Bridge design

Although fixed-fixed, fixed-movable, cantilever and spring cantilever designs have all been used, the preferred designs for resin-bonded bridgework are cantilever and fixed-movable. Debonding of one retainer of a fixed-fixed design is relatively common because of differences in retainer coverage and retention combined with variations in periodontal support and occlusal loading. Unilateral debonding of a fixed-fixed design may lead to rapidly progressive caries under the debonded retainer before the patient seeks treatment (Fig. 12.18).

If a single abutment simple cantilever bridge debonds, the patient will seek treatment immediately. Simple cantilever designs are preferred anteriorly, although fixed-movable designs may be required posteriorly for adequate support. The minor retainer of a fixed-movable design must have a positive rest with a non-rigid connector (Fig. 12.19). This design allows independent tooth mobility and there is therefore less torsional stress on the luting composite. The pontics are supported during function but are free to separate in the unseating direction. Such

---

Box 12.7   Requirements for resin-bonded bridges

- Space for an aesthetic pontic
- Sufficient area of surface enamel for bonding
- Abutment teeth unrestored or minimally restored
- Adequate occlusal clearance (0.5–1.0 mm in high stress areas) without exposing dentine
- Stable posterior occlusion
- Pontic is protected during function from opposing teeth
- Good isolation by rubber dam

Box 12.8   Advantages and disadvantages of resin-bonded bridges

Advantages
- Conservative
- Patient acceptability
- Reduced chairside time
- Economical
- Supragingival margins
- Simple impression
- Not temporary
- Versatile

Disadvantages
- Require sound aesthetic abutments
- Pontic and retainer space critical
- No trial cementation
- Unsuitable for long spans

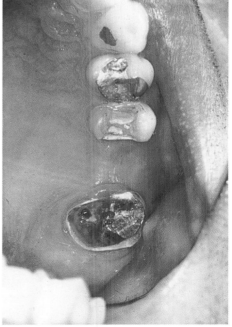

Fig. 12.18   Cementation failure at distal unit of a conventional fixed-fixed bridge. Extensive caries has resulted.

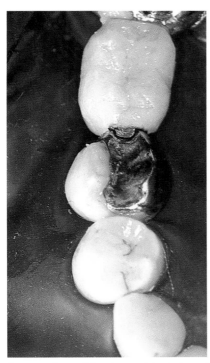

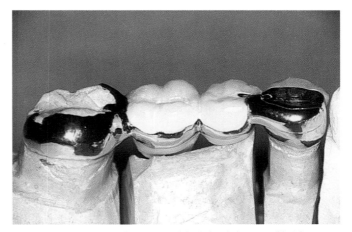

Fig. 12.20 Long-span fixed-movable hybrid design of bridge. Note the bracing arm milled palatally on the premolar crown in addition to the non-rigid connector distally.

Fig. 12.19 Minor retainer of fixed-movable design of resin-bonded bridge. The rest seat preparation has been waxed into the retainer at LR5 for a non-rigid connector.

bridges may be employed successfully even in long spans (Fig. 12.20).

Hybrid bridges

These are ideal where a heavily restored or previously crowned tooth exists at one end of an edentulous span and there is a sound abutment tooth at the other end. Resin-bonded retainers may be used in combination with conventional bridge retainers when a fixed-movable connector is employed. If a fixed-fixed design was used, cementation would be complicated by the need for mixing and using different cements simultaneously. In addition, if there is cementation failure of the resin-bonded retainer, caries of the abutment is invited because the bridge is still retained by the more retentive conventional unit. For hybrid bridges the resin-bonded retainer should be made as the major retainer (Fig. 12.21). Debonding will therefore not require replacement of the original retainer. It is also easier to create room for a removable joint within the confines of a conventional retainer. Placing the joint extra-coronally in the pontic section is not recommended as the lever arm created invites failure. Alternatively, a telescopic or sleeve crown may be permanently cemented to the carious or restored tooth and a fixed-fixed design employed whereby a chemically active resin cement is used to retain the resin-bonded unit and a temporary conventional cement is used to cement the conventional crown over-

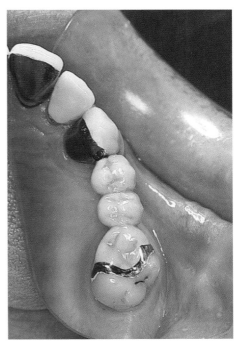

Fig. 12.21 Hybrid fixed-movable bridge with resin-bonded onlay major retainer on molar.

casting to the telescopic crown. If the resin-bonded unit becomes uncemented, it is an easy matter to remove the bridge, and if the overcasting becomes uncemented, the telescopic crown protects the conventional unit from caries.

Resin-bonded versus conventional bridges

Resin-bonded bridges should always be considered first and rejected as a possible option before a conventional bridge design is considered. This is because they are highly conservative, involving minimal tooth preparation. No anaesthesia is required unless there is dentine involvement. Modern dentine-bonding agents have expanded the indications and versatility of resin-bonded bridges. Whilst the tooth preparation is quick, it is also exacting because of the 'white on white' effect of confining preparations to enamel during development of retention and resistance form. There is no risk of soft tissue trauma because of the supragingival finish lines for these impressions and this simplifies preparation. There is usually no need for any provisional restoration. Occlusal clearance can be maintained by spot-etching and placement of a small amount of composite on the opposing tooth to act as a centric stop (Fig. 12.22).

Where dentine is involved at the base of a groove or occlusal offset, this can be covered temporarily with a polycarboxylate cement. An air scaler is useful to remove the cement without further damage to the preparation at the time of cementation. Whilst modern designs of resin-bonded bridge usually incorporate retention and resistance form together with a precise path of seating, it is frequently not possible to assess the need for occlusal adjustment until the bridge has been seated. Cementation or 'bonding' is more technique-sensitive than for a conventional bridge and requires considerably more time; hence the time that is gained during tooth preparation and provisional prosthesis is offset during cementation. *Resin-bonded bridges must not be seen as a quick-fix solution.*

Metal/resin retention techniques

Reliable retention of resin cements to prepared enamel surfaces may be obtained with the acid-etch technique. This bond is micromechanical in nature. The retention techniques for resin to metal are based on mechanical, micromechanical or microchemical techniques with or without the use of chemically active resin cements. The Rochette design has limited retention and the framework

is weakened by the perforations and the fact that the composite lute is exposed to the oral environment (Fig. 12.23). However, Rochette bridges still have a role as immediate or interim replacements or as part of a complex treatment plan. Where the prognosis for a bridge is in doubt because of questionable support, a Rochette bridge may be constructed as a diagnostic measure with no tooth preparation. Once it has been established that the periodontal support is sufficient, then it is a relatively easy matter to remove this type of bridge by simply drilling out the resin composite from the retention holes and tapping the bridge off.

Other types of mechanical retention such as mesh and particle roughened retention have fallen out of favour because they add bulk to the casting and are not as retentive as alternative designs. The most popular type of micromechanical retention involves grit-blasting with 50 µm aluminium oxide, followed by silicon oxide coating (the Silicoater technique) or use of a chemically active resin cement. In this situation, retention is both mechanical and chemical (microchemical). Electrolytic and chemical etching techniques have fallen out of favour because the laboratory technique was highly sensitive to error and special apparatus was required. In addition, beryllium-containing nickel chrome alloys, which were most amenable to etching, are now not considered safe for routine laboratory use. Chemically active resin composite cements form bonds to the oxidised surfaces of non-precious alloys. Two effective materials are Panavia 21 (Kuraray) and Metabond (Parkell). The former contains an active phosphate ester and the latter 4-META as the active chemical agents.

Contamination of the grit-blasted non-precious alloy surface must be avoided as this seriously impairs the bond. Even momentary contamination with saliva will reduce the bond by 50% and contaminated surfaces are very difficult to clean effectively. This can involve 30-minute ultrasonic treatment in a suitable surfactant solution at high temperature. Chairside grit-blasting units allow metal

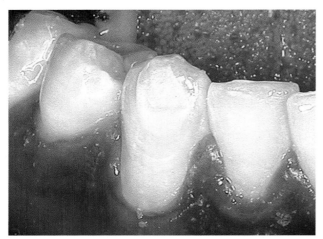

Fig. 12.22 Spot-etch resin to stabilise occlusal relationships between preparation and bonding of resin-retained bridge.

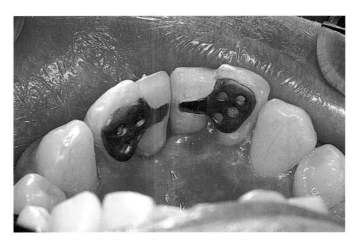

Fig. 12.23 Two simple cantilever Rochette bridges.

surface treatment between try-in and cementation. In the case of precious metals, effective adhesion of resin to metal may be obtained either by tin plating (Fig. 12.24) or by heat treatment of hard gold alloys which contain more than 8% copper (Fig. 12.25).

An alternative technique for chemical bonding is based on the adhesion of a resin to silane-bonding agents. The Silicoater technique allows a very thin glass-like layer to be built up on the roughened metal fit surface of the bridge. This surface has to be protected with an opaque layer or a layer of resin if the bridge is not to be cemented within 30 minutes of treatment. This has limited the widespread application of this technique.

Non-precious alloys (Ni/Cr or Co/Cr) are preferred for resin-bonded bridge frameworks because they are more rigid in thin section. Their modulus of elasticity is twice that of a type 4 gold. In addition, they are more amenable to bonding with chemically active resins and simply require grit-blasting of the surface after try-in. Precious metal alloys for metal ceramic frameworks (Au/Pd) are best tin-plated or silicoated after try-in and then cemented with

a chemically active resin. Type 3 or type 4 gold alloys (containing more than 8% copper) can be heat-treated for 4 minutes at 400°C after try-in and grit-blasting to make them amenable to bonding with a chemically-active resin cement.

Guidelines for resin-bonded bridges (assuming metal framework used)

Abutment tooth preparations

Appropriate preparation improves the retention of resin-bonded bridges by increasing the available area of enamel for bonding and by reducing functional stresses on the resin composite lute. Preparation also provides increased occlusal clearance and creates a positive path of insertion and seat for the restoration during try-in and bonding. The removal of the outer enamel surface layer, which is frequently aprismatic and rich in fluoride, allows for more predictable etching. By removing axial undercuts and developing guide plane retention, the effective preparation length is increased.

The aim of tooth preparation should be to cover the maximum enamel area consistent with (i) aesthetic considerations, (ii) occlusal constraints, and (iii) the need to fit a rubber dam. A precise path of insertion and seating should be developed by the preparation for the metal framework. A retentive framework design limits the stresses placed on the cement lute and dramatically increases the success rate. Preparation features and sufficient alloy thickness should be allowed to reduce stresses on the bonded joint.

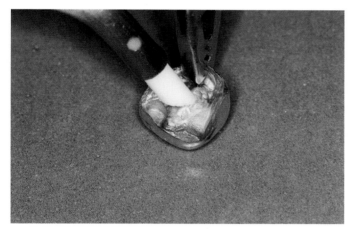

Fig. 12.24 Chairside tin-plating of fit surface of full veneer gold crown.

Anterior preparations

* Reduce palatal enamel to allow 0.5 mm interocclusal clearance in all functional mandibular excursions. Less reduction is required/indicated for mandibular teeth. Allow 1 mm clearance for regions of heavy occlusal load.
* Extend cervically to 1 mm from gum margin.
* Extend within 1–2 mm of incisal edge depending on functional and aesthetic considerations.
* Extend proximally (adjacent to the edentulous space) as far as appearance permits.
* Extend proximally (opposite to the edentulous space) to within 1 mm of the contact area.
* Provide a cingulum rest to aid resistance form.
* Use proximal grooves and/or cingulum pinholes as substitutes for labial wrap circumferential retention. Stabilise the framework on each abutment in the plane perpendicular to the path of insertion with these features.

Posterior preparations

* Replace any small proximal amalgam restorations with composite and/or glass ionomer cement or use a dentine adhesive.

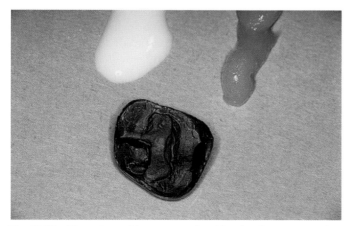

Fig. 12.25 Fit surface of heat-treated gold onlay for upper molar with luting resin composite.

- Reduce proximal and lingual/palatal axial surfaces to provide a >180° 'wrap-around' effect. When crown height is limited, a 360° sleeve coverage can be used whilst maintaining occlusal stability. Obtain a minimum of >3 mm guide plane retention axially.
- If necessary, accept knife-edge finish proximally and/or lingually to avoid dentine exposure.
- Use occlusal onlay coverage to supplement bonding area on short teeth.
- Make occlusal rest seat preparations.
- Use shallow proximal grooves and occlusal inlays to assist retention and compensate for lack of circumferential retention.
- Join intracoronal retention features to the extracoronal part of the preparation with offsets and isthmuses to maximise retention and resistance (Fig. 12.26).

Try-in and cementation or bonding

- Try-in the bridge to check for fit, contour and path of insertion.
- Assess occlusion at this stage if the bridge is sufficiently stable.
- Place a rubber dam, allowing slack in pontic region for passive seating of the bridge.
- Clean the prepared teeth with a pumice/water slurry, rinse and dry.
- Protect adjacent teeth with matrix strips and acid-etch enamel, rinse and dry.
- Check for characteristic frosted appearance of correctly etched enamel.
- Apply enamel-dentine (ED) primer to exposed enamel and dentine surfaces for 60 seconds.
- Evaporate solvent with air.
- Apply mixed Panavia 21 to retainer fit surfaces.
- Seat bridge promptly and remove gross excess with a brush or suitable instrument.
- Maintain seating pressure. Apply barrier agent (Oxyguard 2) to the bridge retainer margins after removal of excess cement.
- Remove excess cement after set from margins with suitable hand and/or rotary instruments.
- Remove rubber dam. Check and adjust occlusion.
- Final finishing of resin/metal margins (using water-cooled burs) is best delayed until 1 week after cementation.

Longevity of resin-bonded bridges

Whilst there is currently little consensus on what is optimal design for resin-bonded bridgework, there is good evidence from clinical investigations that rigid framework designs coupled with retentive abutment tooth preparations dramatically increase longevity. The preparation and retainer design must protect the resin/enamel bond from high stresses to avoid fatigue failure. Non-perforated metal frameworks make removal and re-cementation of partially debonded fixed-fixed resin-bonded bridges difficult and less successful. Single retainer simple cantilever designs are the first choice wherever possible; if circumstances do not permit then fixed-movable or hybrid designs are the next best.

There is a higher failure rate for perforated retainers, multiple abutments and/or pontics, mobile teeth and young patients. Common reasons for failure include:

- poor case selection
- inadequate bridge design
- inadequate tooth preparation
- faulty bonding procedure
- occlusal factors.

Whilst some authors advocate the re-cementation of a debonded resin-bonded bridge, such a procedure frequently leads to repeated failure. The risk increases with each rebond. Frequent debonding and replacement of restorations is clinically frustrating and economically unsound. Rebonding a resin-bonded bridge involves much more time and effort than merely re-cementing a loose crown or conventional fixed prosthesis. It is necessary to remove contaminants from both adherent (bridge fit surface and tooth) surfaces and to re-prepare them for rebonding. This procedure inevitably reduces the precision of fit and increases the luting resin film thickness. Indications for rebonding are given in Box 12.9.

The main cause of debonding must be remedied, provided this does not compromise restoration design.

REMOVABLE PROSTHESES (REMOVABLE PARTIAL DENTURES)

If the decision has been made to undertake a removable partial denture (RPD) then a provisional design is completed at the initial treatment planning stage on the articulated casts before undertaking any other restorative treatment. This must be drawn up on a design sheet. Whilst undertaking a design, the following decisions are made when assessing whether mouth preparation is required:

- *Rest seat preparation.* This is undertaken to provide both sufficient space and a horizontal surface for any support component of a cast metal partial denture. It also aims to prevent any interference with the occlusion.

Box 12.9 Indications for rebonding

Rebonding is indicated where there is an identifiable fault with:
- Abutment surface treatments
- Framework fit surface treatments
- Nature of the bonding agents
- Handling errors
- Correctable occlusal errors
- Any combination of the above

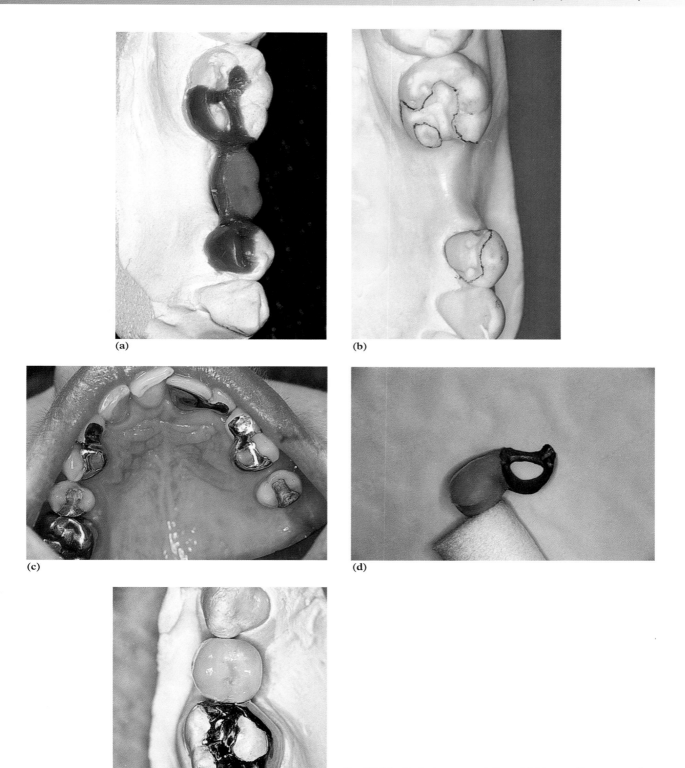

(a)

(b)

(c)

(d)

(e)

Fig. 12.26 Posterior presentation. (**a**) Diagnostic wax-up of resin-bonded bridge to replace lost deciduous molar. (**b**) Cast of tooth preparations. (**c**) Occlusal view of three simple cantilever design resin-bonded bridges. Note the rigid design for premolar preparations created by circumferential wrap-around with joining of palatal and occlusal components of retainers. (**d, e**) Fit surface and occlusal view of simple cantilever resin-bonded bridges showing proximal slots and wrap-around retainer designs.

- *The tooth contour may require modification.* This may necessitate grinding of the tooth or the addition of light-cured composite resin, to improve the placing of clasp arms. The occlusal relationship may require adjusting by removing prominent cusps or reducing over-erupted teeth. In some cases this may involve the placement of crowns with guide surfaces incorporated in the restoration (Fig. 12.27).

The design is then transferred to the study cast and this is combined with a design diagram, which is clear, neat and labelled where necessary. These study casts are kept throughout the treatment for future reference and the definitive design is produced when other restorative treatment has been completed. A *definitive design* must also be clear, neat and adequately labelled, which allows the technician to complete the requested task correctly (Fig. 12.28). The design should include details of the path of insertion, any mouth preparation such as rest seats and guide surfaces. The components are labelled where this is needed for clarity. To assist the technician, the approved definitive design is also drawn up on the diagnostic cast. This should be all completed before the master impression is obtained.

Surveying

The initial step in producing any design is a survey of the casts; a dental surveyor is used for this purpose. This instrument is used to determine the relative parallelism of two or more surfaces of the teeth or other parts of the cast of a dental arch (Fig. 12.29). Several tools are used with the surveyor, including an analysing rod, undercut gauges, a graphite marker and wax/plaster trimmer. It is the clinician's responsibility to survey the casts and use this information to design the denture. The surveyor is used to *identify*, *mark*, *measure* and *eliminate* undercuts on the teeth.

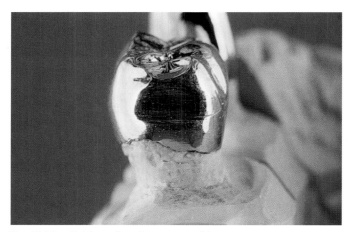

Fig. 12.27 Guide surface incorporated into crown.

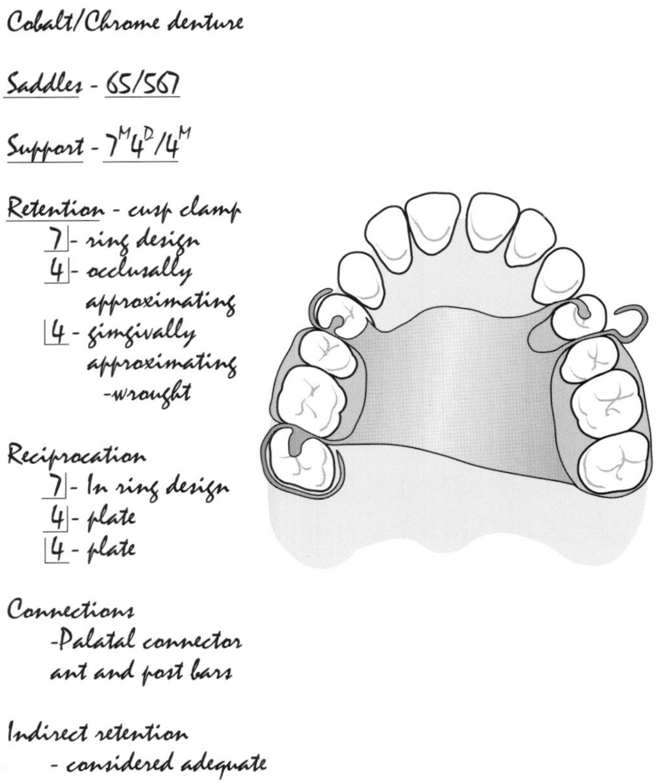

Cobalt/Chrome denture

Saddles - 65/567

Support - 7^{M}4^D/4^M

Retention - cusp clamp
  7⌋- ring design
  4⌋- occlusally
      approximating
  ⌊4 - gingivally
      approximating
      -wrought

Reciprocation
  7⌋- In ring design
  4⌋- plate
  ⌊4 - plate

Connections
  -Palatal connector
  ant and post bars

Indirect retention
  - considered adequate

Fig. 12.28 Design sheet correctly and neatly drawn up.

Identify

When examining the casts, movement of the RPD away from the cast is identified. Any denture will have a path of displacement away from the cast/mouth. It is possible to introduce a path of insertion and removal which is different from the path of displacement (Fig. 12.30). Usually the two are coincident and the clinician will rely on clasps and guide surfaces for retention of the RPD. However, a path of insertion and removal different from the path of displacement will lead to a more retentive denture.

In this identification process, guide surfaces are sought. They consist of two or more parallel surfaces on the abutment teeth which are used to define the path of insertion. They also help to aid in stabilising the denture. These surfaces can be either natural or artificially prepared. This latter procedure involves either altering the shape of the tooth with a dental bur or the use of a restoration, which may range from the simple addition of composite material to the use of a cast restoration. Retentive surfaces receive the same identification process. Undercuts around the teeth are examined and the depth measured. If a clasp is to be placed, the last third (the retentive part) must rest in the undercut. This is the elastic element of the clasp which sits within the undercut. It is the elastic recoil of the clasp that needs to be overcome as the denture is removed. A

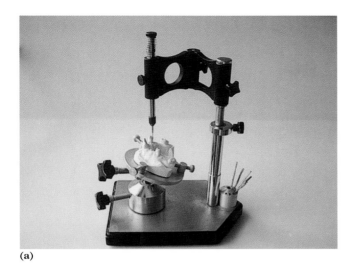

(a)

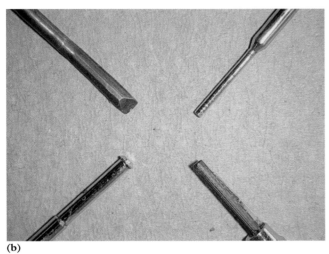

(b)

Fig. 12.29 (a) Dental surveyor. (b) Surveying tools used (clockwise from bottom left): analysing rod, undercut gauges, graphite marker, wax trimmer.

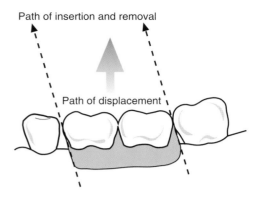

Fig. 12.30 Diagram showing insertion and removal different from path of displacement.

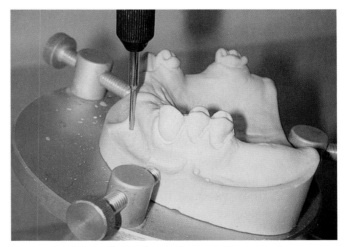

Fig. 12.31 The cast is tilted with the heels down to take advantage of the labial undercut.

cast cobalt chrome (Co/Cr) clasp requires a 0.25 mm undercut and a wrought clasp requires a 0.5 mm undercut to be effective.

If the undercut were 0.75 mm or greater, it would cause permanent deformation of the clasp. An inverted depth gauge is used to measure such undercuts on the tooth, and if required the use of a bur or composite material will either reduce or create potential undercuts. If natural surfaces are favourable then tilting of the cast will allow the RPD to utilise them. This additional surveying is carried out with both anterior and posterior tilts. This is sometimes referred to as 'heels down' or 'heels up' (Fig. 12.31). This will result in two survey lines, which may help with clasp position, especially in cases with difficult tooth angulations. Good aesthetics may be important, especially at the front of the mouth, and the insertion of the denture may lead to unsightly gaps between it and the natural teeth. If these occur, they should be eliminated. Other problems that may be identified include the presence

of bony undercuts, prominences or inclined teeth, which can be avoided by the use of an anterior or posterior tilt.

Mark

Once the cast has been thoroughly examined and the areas of interest or concern identified, it is necessary to mark on the survey lines with the black graphite marker. An alternative colour, such as red, is used to mark any tilting that is needed.

Measure

Any undercuts that are present are then measured with the undercut gauge (0.25–0.75 mm), which will enable decisions to be taken on the type of clasp material (wrought stainless steel vs. cast Co/Cr) and its subsequent design (gingival/occlusal approaching). A decision is made as to the best orientation of the cast for the final survey, which gives the best path of insertion together with optimal retention.

165

Eliminate

The clinician can then prepare to eliminate the problems and assess the need for mouth preparation. Undercuts can be blocked out using plaster of Paris, which is done on the master cast.

The information from the surveyor needs to be recorded to enable the survey to be interpreted correctly in the laboratory. The best method for achieving this is by the process of tripoding, which involves the placement of three marks on the palatal surface of the cast by the graphite marker, with the vertical arm of the surveyor locked at a fixed height (Fig. 12.32).

Design stages

After surveying the cast, the design is drawn up and this can conveniently be seen as comprising six stages: saddles, support, retention, reciprocation and bracing, connection and finally indirect retention (Fig. 12.33).

Saddles

Saddles rest on and cover the alveolar ridge and include the artificial teeth and gum work. It is this component of the denture that carries the replacement teeth (Fig. 12.34).

When reviewing the design of the saddle area, the extension of the base is considered and should follow complete denture principles. It should extend to the depth of the functional sulcus, unless there are aesthetic considerations such as at the front of the mouth, posteriorly onto the buccal shelf and halfway up the retromolar pad. The positioning of the teeth may dictate the saddle position. Where a tooth is missing, it does not necessarily mean that a replacement is required, especially when replacing posterior teeth at the end of the arch. The saddle material

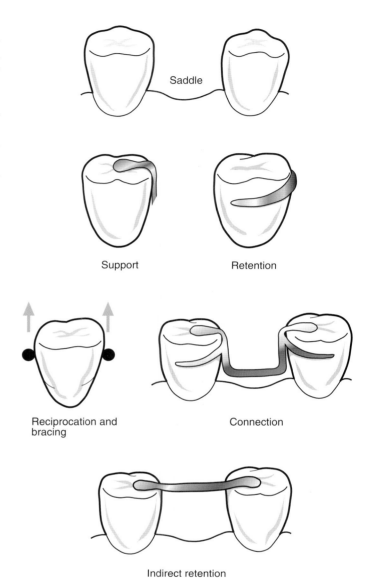

Fig. 12.33 Useful images to remember the design stages for removable partial dentures.

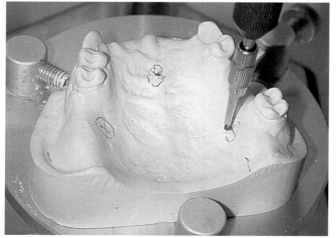

Fig. 12.32 An illustration of the tripoding technique to record the angle of tilt of the cast.

is either all acrylic or a Co/Cr substructure supporting the acrylic teeth and gumwork. The saddle cannot enter the undercut around the tooth and therefore, although a wax trial denture may be satisfactory, if the undercuts have not been blocked out it will be impossible to seat the partial denture at the insertion stage. This situation is prevented by giving instructions to the technician to process the denture on a duplicate cast where such undercuts have been previously blocked out.

The occurrence of edentulous areas lends itself to a simplistic classification. The Kennedy classification identifies the number and positioning of the saddles (see Fig. 12.35a). It has the disadvantage that it only indicates the missing teeth and does not provide information on the nature of the support that is present.

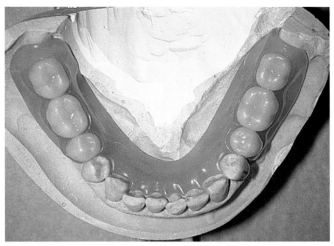

Fig. 12.34 Two unbounded saddles are shown on this wax trial denture saddle.

Support

Support is the resistance to vertical force (i.e. masticatory forces) directed towards the teeth and mucosa. The partial denture should dissipate these forces and resist downward pressure. Resistance to masticatory forces is provided by either the mucosa or the teeth, or by a combination of the two. The way in which this resistance is provided determines the classification of the support (Fig. 12.35b).

Quality of the support. The type of support available may vary and assessment of its quality is made during design procedures. Tooth support will be dependent upon the root area of the abutment teeth, their periodontal status, conservation status and whether they are able to withstand occlusal forces. The root area of the abutment teeth will vary and both molars and canines are the best suited for this purpose as they have the greatest root surface area. The saddles will also influence this support. Large saddle areas (three to four teeth) will exert a large

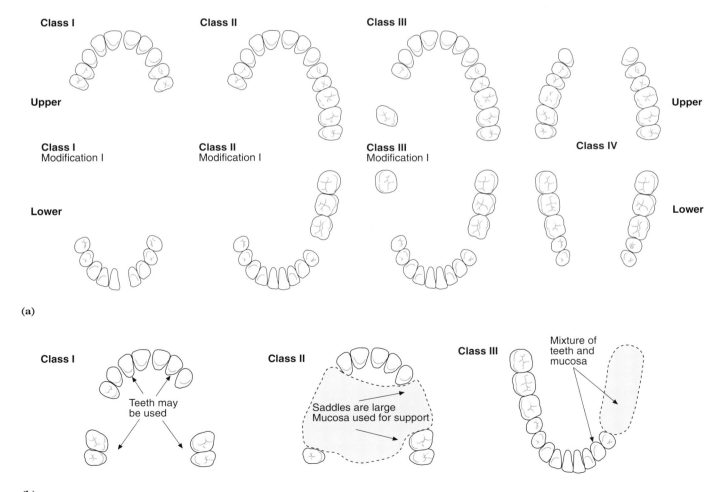

Fig. 12.35 (a) Diagram of Kennedy classification. Note that the Kennedy IV has no modifications. (b) Support classification.

force on the adjacent teeth. If large masticatory forces from opposing natural teeth are expected, this will increase the loading on the saddle areas and therefore onto the supporting elements.

Mucosal-borne dentures may work well in upper arches, especially if the palatal area is used for support. An area of approximately 5 cm^2 in the centre of the palate does not resorb and it is this which assists in the retention and stability of upper dentures. Lower acrylic dentures are often provided but they can cause problems by 'sinking' into the tissues under occlusal loading. This will lead to gum stripping and other periodontal problems. Therefore lower mucosal-borne dentures should be avoided unless they are seen as transitional in nature (i.e. ready for future immediate additions).

The 'Every' type acrylic partial denture is a special design which attempts to minimise periodontal damage and maximise retention (Fig. 12.36). There are six principles involved in its construction:

- Point contact between adjacent standing and artificial teeth – intact upper dental arch with contact points which are buccally placed. Point contacts between natural and artificial teeth are distributed mesiodistally along the arch.
- Wide embrasures between contiguous standing and artificial teeth.
- 'Free occlusion' – a free occlusion with no tendency for the upper and lower cusps to interlock or hinder movement.
- Uncovered gingivae – no contact with the gingival tissue. Palatally the acrylic should be at least 3 mm from the gingival margins.
- Contact of the denture with the distal surface of the last standing tooth – distal stabilisers contact posterior teeth and maintain point contact by preventing drifting.
- Maximum retention following the principles used in full denture construction – the denture base covers as large an area as possible; the fit of the denture is accurate and polished surfaces should be shaped to assist muscular forces.

The open design allows a hygienic denture to be constructed which is retentive and stable and minimises damage to the supporting and surrounding tissues. It does require the presence of bounded saddles so that point contact can be maintained throughout the arch form. Even where the most distal tooth is missing, however, 'Every principles' can still be incorporated into the denture design.

Decisions on the nature of the support are based on the teeth and the mucosa. A tooth-supported denture will require rest seat design and tooth preparation. A rest enables the forces to be directed down the long axis of the tooth (Fig. 12.37). During the design stages, teeth are identified which can support the denture, usually with a rest. Clinical decisions are made on how the tooth should receive the supporting element. The tooth may naturally have a depression within the occlusal surface within which the rest can sit. If this is not present then the tooth is shaped with a diamond bur. The rest is saucer-shaped with a deeper portion towards the centre of the tooth (Fig. 12.37).

A natural tooth may not allow the operator to cut a rest too deeply due to problems of breaching the enamel. However, the presence of a restoration or the prescription of a crown will allow the operator to make a more distinct shape to the rest design. A mucosa-supported denture will rely on maximum saddle extension and on the quality of the mucosa and underlying bone. An area that requires special consideration is the combined support from the teeth and the mucosa. This clinical situation is better known as the free end saddle.

Management of the free end saddle

The clinical situation. The unbounded free end saddle is commonly seen following posterior tooth loss. It presents

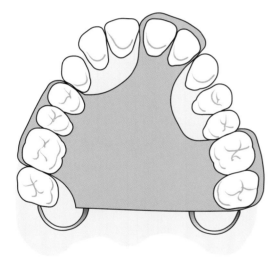

(a)

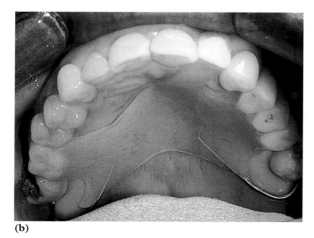

(b)

Fig. 12.36 An Every denture.

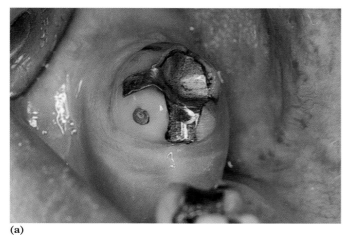

(a)

Fig. 12.37a A mesial rest prepared in the tooth with guide surface.

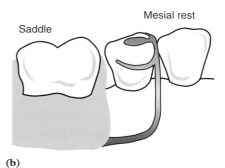

(b)

Fig. 12.37b Diagram of mesial rest.

a difficult clinical situation with its characteristic mixture of tooth and mucosa support. Near to the abutment tooth there is a predominance of tooth support, but further away there is more mucosal support (Fig. 12.38). This differential support is the problem during loading of the saddle area. The upper free end saddle is often easier to treat, as support is gained from the palate. Generally it is the lower free end saddle that presents the greatest difficulty due to the reduced anatomical area.

Clinical procedure. A good history of the presenting problem is taken and the saddle area is assessed during the clinical examination. A past history is also taken to see what previous treatment has been carried out and whether it was successful. Both the periodontal and conservative status of the abutment teeth will also influence the clinical

decision. Where possible, a purely mucosal-borne lower denture in acrylic should be avoided due to the lack of support available. However, if the teeth have poor periodontal support then an acrylic denture is provided which is transitional in nature. Where there are teeth present which have a poor prognosis and will require eventual extractions, it is easier to make additions to an all-acrylic denture than to a metallic one. After examination of the free end saddle problem, a diagnosis of the situation is made and a treatment plan is drawn up to resolve it.

Initially a preliminary impression in alginate is obtained and this should record the abutment teeth together with detail of the free end saddle area. Support of the alginate impression is assisted by the use of impression compound in the edentulous areas of the tray. Following pouring of the casts, if it is not possible to hand articulate them, an assessment of the occlusion is required and the patient is brought back for a preliminary registration.

Design considerations

A simple rigid design. A well-designed but rigid Co/Cr framework is a simple method of treatment. Modifications may be indicated if the abutment tooth does not possess an ideal crown shape with suitable undercuts. The tooth may be modified using composite or guide surfaces created by grinding with a diamond drill. In the case of heavily restored teeth, crowning may be indicated. Where the abutment tooth has poor bone support, the design should spread the loading away to other adjacent teeth. In order to dissipate the loading, clasping of the tooth is made with wrought clasps as distinct to cast clasps. In theory, the more elastic wrought material will act as a shock-absorber, reducing loading on the tooth.

Modifications. Where there is a free end saddle present, conventional designs should incorporate a mesial placement of the rest. This will reduce anterior posterior forces acting on the tooth. As mentioned previously, potentially

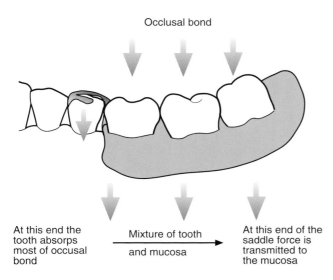

Occlusal bond

At this end the tooth absorps most of occusal bond

Mixture of tooth and mucosa

At this end of the saddle force is transmitted to the mucosa

Fig. 12.38 Diagram showing differential support.

damaging lateral forces on the tooth can be reduced by the use of more flexible wrought clasps and gingivally approaching clasps.

Use of the altered cast technique. This technique is a selective impression technique, which imparts a functional load to the denture. A Co/Cr denture constructed for a free end saddle will need the differential support offered by the abutment tooth which is relatively rigid in its socket, supported by the periodontal ligament and the more displaceable denture-bearing mucosa. This impression technique takes into account the differential support provided by both the oral mucosa and the teeth. The treatment follows the use of both preliminary and master impressions. The Co/Cr casting is constructed ready for trial fitting in the mouth (Fig. 12.39).

A close-fitting acrylic special tray is constructed on the free end saddle of the casting. An impression is taken of the free end saddle using either zinc oxide/eugenol impression paste or a medium-viscosity silicone. When the framework is placed in the mouth, the impression is taken with loading on the support elements of the framework only. No finger pressure is applied on the saddle area as this would lead to over-displacement of the mucosa. Border moulding is carried out as the impression material is setting. In the laboratory, the free end saddle areas on the master cast are sectioned and removed. The denture is positioned on the cast and the new saddle areas are poured. The resulting cast represents the free end saddle areas under conditions which attempt to mimic functional load. The original technique used functional waxes and was described as the Applegate technique. The altered cast technique improves the distribution of loading on the free end saddle and the denture is more stable. However, the technique requires good cooperation with the laboratory and may lead to disruption of the occlusion, especially if it is undertaken as a rebasing of the finished denture. This can lead to considerable adjustment at the chairside.

The Co/Cr casting over the free end saddle may either contact or sit 1–2 mm above the ridge. The latter is preferable as it allows relining at a later date. Generally, the saddle area is a mesh design which allows the acrylic to be processed underneath. To help with seating, a 'foot' (small part of Co/Cr which contacts the posterior region) is incorporated into the casting. This acts as a valuable reference point when the fit of the framework is checked, both on the cast and in the mouth. Any lack of contact may be eliminated by the altered cast technique. There is debate on whether this technique is useful but it does provide an improved impression of the saddle area.

RPI system. Studies on the differential loading of free end saddles suggested that the mesial placement of occlusal rests and the use of wrought clasping on the abutment tooth led to more favourable distribution of loading. This concept is further modified in the RPI system (R = *r*est; P = distal *p*late; I = gingivally approaching *I*-bar). The mesial rest contacts the mesiolingual surface of the abutment tooth and, with the distal plate, reciprocates the action of the retentive I-bar clasp. The abutment tooth is held in a mesial–distal direction (Fig. 12.40).

Under functional load the denture will tend to rotate around the mesial rest. Both the plate and I-bar will move downwards and forwards and disengage from the tooth. This will limit the stresses placed on the tooth during function. Although often well understood theoretically, the RPI is not always drawn on designs correctly.

Balance of forces. This can be considered as a further refinement of the RPI system. It consists of a mesial rest and guide surface with a lingual clasp arm extending into the distal undercut from the rest. The aim is to ensure that the loads during function are directed vertically along the long axis of the tooth in order to avoid torque and leverage (Fig. 12.41).

The tooth is held in a similar fashion (i.e. mesial–distal) to the RPI system, but both a mesial rest and guide surface are prepared in the tooth. The guide surface may be

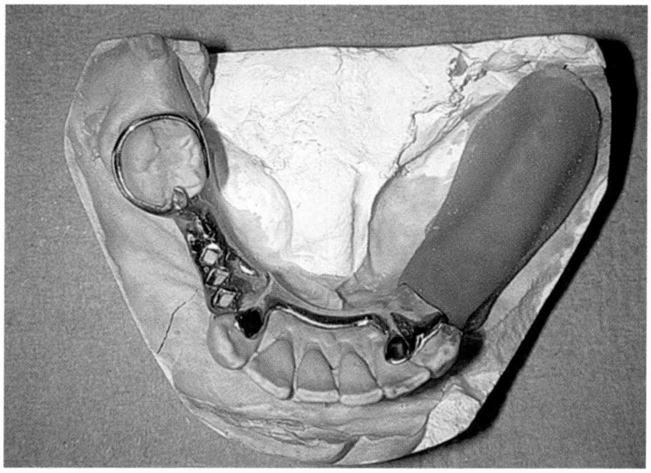

Fig. 12.39 The use of the altered cast technique – a special tray is made over the free end saddle area.

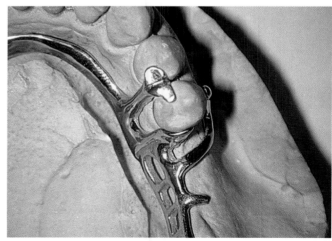

Fig. 12.40 The RPI system.

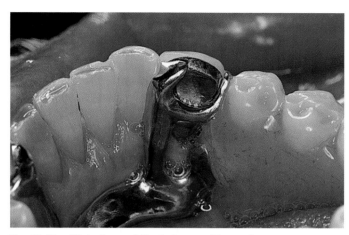

Fig. 12.41 Clinical use of the balance of force clasp.

unsightly and will often require preparation of the natural tooth. This will not be a problem if the treatment plan involves the placement of a full veneer crown as the mesial guide surface can be designed into the crown. The clasp is designed so that the retentive tip of the clasp arm is positioned on the interproximal surface of the abutment tooth adjacent to the edentulous saddle.

Retention is achieved mesiodistally as opposed to buccolingually. During function there is similar rotational movement to the RPI system and the clasp will disengage. In the UK and the USA, dentures using the balance of force system are constructed under licence (Equipoise designs).

Use of stress breakers. These designs attempt to provide some degree of flexibility between the clasp unit and the free end saddle. They can have either a movable joint or a flexible connection between the direct retainer and the saddle. Precision attachments may be used to provide the movable joint. An example of the flexible design is where the Co/Cr casting is split to enable the differential loading between the saddle and tooth-supported elements. Although such designs can be useful, they can be complicated and involve excessive coverage of teeth leading to periodontal problems.

Design of saddle and occlusal table. The design of a free end saddle should also follow traditional guidelines for denture construction. Such measures should include maximal extension of the saddle (halfway up the retromolar pad, extension into the buccal shelf). This will reduce the load per unit area being placed on the saddles during function. Narrow posterior teeth will reduce the degree of lateral force applied by the musculature during function. Omitting the most distal tooth will reduce the amount of loading on the abutment tooth by reducing leverage. The use of narrow teeth will assist in tooth position and improve the occlusal loading by allowing the patient to penetrate food more effectively without increasing the load to the saddle area.

Relining of free end saddle. This can prove to be a frustrating clinical experience. If a saddle is not seating

correctly then application of an autopolymerising acrylic to define the saddle area at the chairside is indicated. The setting of the material should be made under functional occlusal load, taking care not to allow material to set into undercuts. (This will be embarrassing clinically as it will prove impossible to remove the denture unless acrylic is removed – the *true* prosthetic emergency!) Laboratory relining of impressions may also be technique-sensitive and can lead to disruption of the occlusion.

Retention

Retention of a RPD is achieved by the following means:

* mechanical – clasps engaging undercuts on tooth
* neuromuscular – muscles acting on the polished surfaces
* physical forces – arising from maximal coverage of mucosa
* other means – guide surfaces, precision attachments.

Clasping of the tooth by thin flexible metal remains the conventional method of achieving retention. A clasp is a metal arm, which retains or stabilises a denture by contacting a tooth. It can be described as either occlusally approaching or gingivally approaching (Fig. 12.42).

The material, length and cross-sectional shape influence the flexibility of a clasp. The metal clasps may be either cast Co/Cr or wrought stainles steel, with the latter having greater flexibility. Typically occlusally approaching cast Co/Cr clasp needs to be 15 mm long in order to enter into an undercut of 0.25 mm. This is feasible on a molar tooth but would not be possible on a premolar tooth. A wrought clasp can enter the 0.25 mm undercut with a length of 8 mm and still retain its flexibility. Alternatively, the cast clasp can maintain a length of 15 mm if it is designed as a gingivally approaching clasp.

An additional feature of the gingivally approaching clasp is that it has a trip action on removal that assists with retention. Finally, if the cross-sectional shape of the clasp is changed from a round section to a half-round one then it is more resistant to movement in the vertical plane and will maintain its position relative to the undercut. These are the physical properties of the clasp arm but there are other factors which influence the choice.

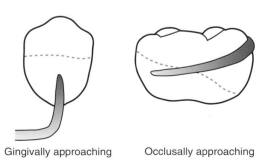

Gingivally approaching   Occlusally approaching

Fig. 12.42 Occlusally and gingivally approaching clasps.

The depth of undercut on the tooth has a direct influence on the retentive force of the clasp but its position is also important. Typically an occlusally approaching clasp is placed on molar teeth, and gingivally approaching clasps are placed on the premolar being influenced by both flexibility and aesthetics. There are two designs of occlusally approaching clasp: the three-arm clasp and the ring clasp. The use of either design depends on the relative position of the undercut on the tooth. For instance, a mesial lingual undercut may be best clasped using a ring clasp, whilst a distal lingual undercut may require a three-arm clasp.

Extra forces on insertion and removal will be placed on a tooth when it is clasped. Teeth which have reduced periodontal attachment may require a more flexible clasp such as wrought stainless steel.

The sulcus shape will influence decisions on the choice of clasp design. A gingivally approaching clasp may interfere with bony prominences, prominent frenal attachments and shallow sulci. Taking it away from the tissue undercut may make it more noticeable to the buccal tissues.

The length of the clasp may be reduced if only premolar teeth are available for clasping. In order to maintain a flexible clasp for the appropriate undercut on the premolar tooth either a short, occlusally approaching wrought clasp or a longer, cast Co/Cr gingivally approaching clasp may be selected.

Finally, aesthetics will dictate the positioning of the clasps. Metal is unsightly and an occlusally approaching clasp anterior to the premolar teeth should be avoided where possible; the gingivally approaching clasp is to be preferred. However, there are special tooth-coloured porcelain clasps which can overcome this problem (Fig. 12.43)

Reciprocation and bracing

When a tooth is clasped, the arm exerts a lateral force onto the tooth during insertion and removal of the RPD. If this lateral force is not resisted, the tooth will be moved orthodontically during placement and removal, eventually leading to non-function of the clasp arm. A reciprocating arm is used to prevent this lateral movement during denture displacement (Fig. 12.44).

The reciprocating element is rigid and therefore forces the retentive element to flex as it moves out of the undercut over the bulbosity of the tooth. This leads to effective use of the clasp forces on the tooth. Reciprocating elements may be contained within the arm of the clasp, as in a ring clasp, or in an extra arm which is positioned on the opposite side of the clasp arm on the tooth. Other reciprocating elements may be the minor connectors, occlusal rests or guide surfaces which are designed to keep the rest in its correct position and prevent tooth escape when the clasp is activated during displacement.

Bracing provides resistance of the whole partial denture to forces to which it may be subjected during mastication. These forces attempt to dislodge the denture in both anteroposterior and lateral directions. The lateral forces may inflict damage on the periodontal and alveolar tissues. Bracing elements may include rests, reciprocating elements and clasps, or other parts of the denture including the saddles (Fig. 12.45).

Connection

The saddles, clasps and reciprocating elements need to be connected in order to function as a complete unit. Minor connectors include parts of the Co/Cr framework which hold these local elements together, while major connectors connect the main saddles of the denture.

In the upper metal partial denture, these will cross the palate and there are many variations on the design. The main consideration is that all the parts are connected together. The simplest connector design is a full metal plate that covers the palate (Fig. 12.46). This has the advantage of rigidity and ease of design; however, the full coverage may not be comfortable for every patient and

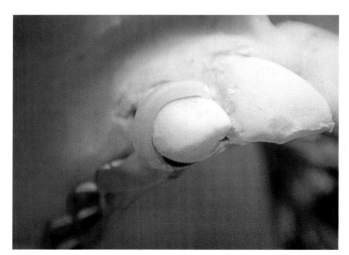

Fig. 12.43 Tooth-coloured clasps.

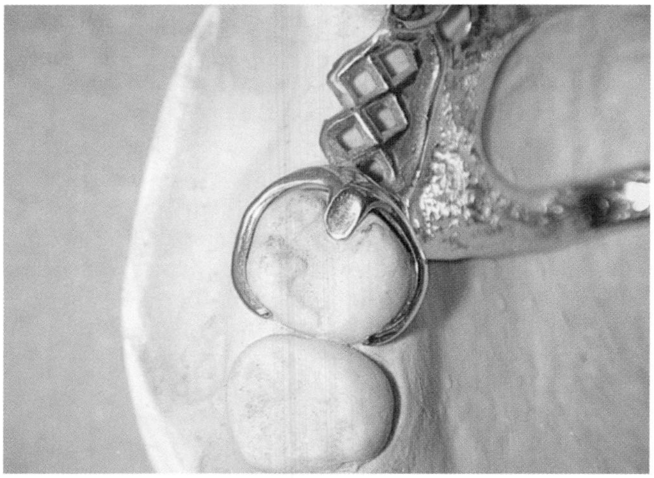

Fig. 12.44 The buccal clasp is reciprocated by the palatal arm.

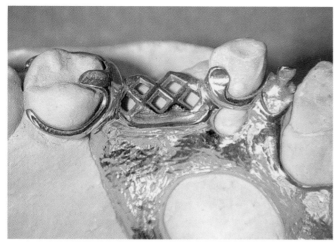

Fig. 12.45 The palatal components act as bracing by preventing lateral movement of the denture.

does increase the weight of the denture. An alternative approach is to use anterior and palatal bars where the central portion of the palate is left uncovered. This may be necessary if there are palatal tori present which need to be left uncovered. Other designs are a variation on the theme and include anterior only, posterior only and mid-palatal bars. The choice of design may relate to patient preference or problems with tolerance.

The lower major connector will be influenced by both the space available and periodontal considerations (Fig. 12.47). A lingual bar is the best choice where there is clearance of approximately 1 cm from the lingual sulcus to the gingival contour of the lower incisors. This allows a rigid bar to be constructed which does not interfere with either the sulcus or the gingivae of the teeth. Where space is limited, a sublingual bar may be made which lies in the lingual sulcus and is pear-shaped in cross-section. A good impression of the sulcus area, recording its depth and

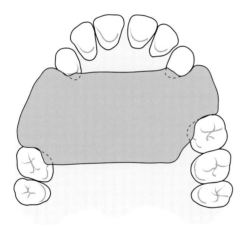

(a) Full coverage

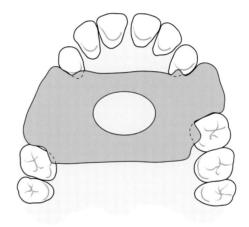

(b) Anterior and posterior palatal bars

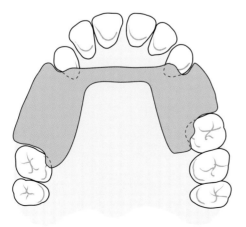

(c) Anterior palatal bar

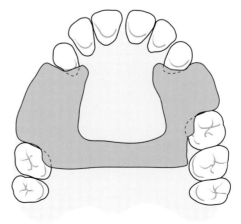

(d) Posterior palatal bar

Fig. 12.46 Examples of upper connectors.

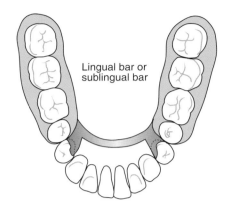 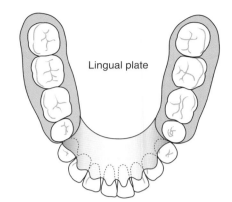

Fig. 12.47 Examples of lower connectors.

width under function, is required. The quality of the impression of the sulcus directly influences the design of the bar. The bar should sit in the lingual sulcus with minimal discomfort to the patient. An alternative solution is to use a lingual plate, which lies on the tooth surface above the cingulum. This is surprisingly comfortable to the patient but also results in total coverage of the periodontal tissues. This design should be selected with care and should not be constructed if there are problems with oral hygiene. Other designs such as the lingual bar combined with a continuous clasp or the use of a dental bar resting on the cingulum surfaces of the teeth are complicated castings and often prove to be poorly tolerated by the patient.

Indirect retention

The RPD unit will have a tendency to rotate around an axis formed by the tips of the clasps. The eating of sticky foods will cause the saddle to move occlusally around this clasp axis. It is analogous to a see-saw: if the saddle moves upwards then the components anterior to the clasp will rotate downwards. If there is no resistance to this movement, damage to the underlying soft tissues may result. A support unit, an indirect retainer, is placed anterior to the clasp axis to prevent this movement (Fig. 12.48).

Indirect retainers do not prevent displacement towards the ridge. This movement is resisted by the occlusal rest on the abutment teeth and by the maximal extension of the saddle. Decisions on indirect retention are made at the end of the sequence of design stages. However, there are two common design situations where it proves to be a problem. In the lower bilateral free end saddle situation, support units need to be positioned anterior to this clasp axis and the example of a design with such indirect retainers is shown in Figure 12.48.

The upper RPD replacing anterior teeth (Kennedy class IV) is problematical. The forward position of the saddle makes indirect retention of the denture a problem. The design uses support from the posterior teeth and retentive

clasps are placed on the molar teeth. The clasp axis will be posteriorly placed and allow rotation of the anterior saddle during function. To prevent this, indirect retainers are placed on the most posterior teeth or the palatal connector is extended towards the soft palate (Fig. 12.49). If this is not possible, the lack of indirect retention will be a problem. A path of insertion may also be considered to utilise any anterior buccal undercut that is present.

Final considerations

The overall design is checked and the occlusal relationship is reviewed to ensure that there are no interferences present. The design should be correctly drawn on an accompanying piece of paper which should include details of all the components and the teeth involved. Clarity is essential for the technician to understand the correct design and any problems are resolved with direct communication. The design is also drawn on the cast to assist the technician.

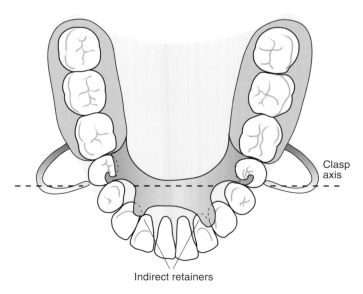

Fig. 12.48 Example of an indirect retainer.

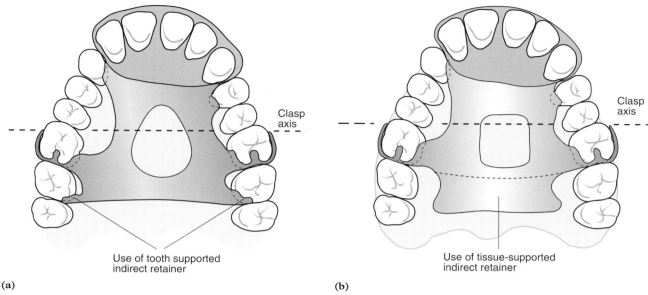

Fig. 12.49 Kennedy class IV and solutions. **(a)** Tooth-supported indirect retainer. **(b)** Tissue-supported indirect retainer.

There has been much progress in the use of computer-aided design programs, of which RaPiD is the most advanced. RaPiD stands for removable partial denture design, artificial intelligence, and contains rules based upon a wide range of specialist prosthetic opinion. The designs produced are drawn on the screen and the program verifies each design before it is sent via an internet connection to the local laboratory (Fig. 12.50).

A summary of the visits required in the process of producing a partial denture is given in Box 12.10.

OVERDENTURES

Introduction

Edentulous spaces may be replaced by more advanced prostheses such as an overdenture. Such dentures may prove useful where there is loss of tooth structure due to tooth wear or difficulty in placing a conventional RPD. An overdenture is a prosthesis that derives support from one or more abutment teeth which may have been reduced in

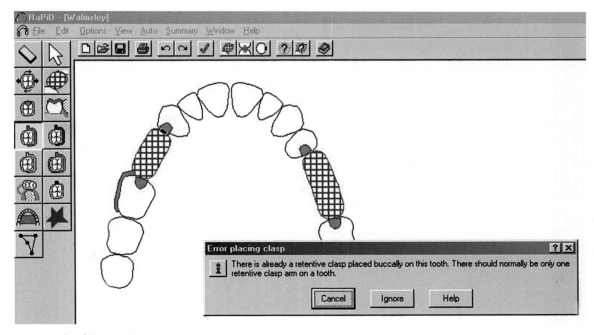

Fig. 12.50 An example of the RaPiD computer-aided design program.

Box 12.10 Summary of the visits required to produce a partial denture	
Clinical	**Laboratory**
1. History and examination Preliminary impressions	
2. Registration of jaw relations	Surveying Mounting of casts on articulator Preliminary design Proposed tooth alteration Draw out partial design on: <ul><li>design sheet</li><li>study cast</li></ul>
3. Tooth modifications Master impressions	
4. Try-in of frame work	
5. Try-in of frame work/wax denture	
6. Delivery of denture	

height and which encloses them beneath its impression surface. Figure 12.51 shows a typical situation where an overdenture is indicated. The canines have a high root surface area and are often the only teeth remaining in the arch. In this situation the provision of a partial denture may prove difficult and the crown/root ratio of the teeth is not favourable. Following root canal therapy, the teeth are reduced in height. Finally, complete upper and lower dentures have been provided. The lower prosthesis is an overdenture.

Overdentures can range from this simple example to more complex forms of overlay on the teeth. The procedure brings together many different components of restorative dentistry, such as periodontal, preventative care and endodontics. It is also a demanding form of treatment and requires great care in the selection of suitably motivated patients. Overdentures offer several advantages:

- alveolar bone is maintained
- sensory feedback is provided
- psychological trauma is reduced.

Alveolar bone maintained

The retention of teeth maintains the alveolar bone around the root. Over a 5-year period, Crum & Rooney (1978) observed the bone changes that occurred in two groups of patients who still had their natural teeth prior to prosthetic treatment. The two groups can be summarised as follows: in group 1 the lower canine teeth were retained and the patients were provided with a lower overdenture; in group 2 all the remaining lower teeth were extracted and a lower complete denture provided. Cephalometric radiographs

were taken over a 5-year period to assess the resulting bone levels. The amount of bone loss in the two groups is shown in Figure 12.52.

Findings from this study showed that, in the lower jaw, where roots had been retained there was a reduction in the bone resorption over the edentulous group. Furthermore, it was found that the retention of roots helped to maintain bone not only in the immediate vicinity of the teeth but also in adjacent areas such as along the edentulous ridges. The study also observed the bone loss that occurred in the maxilla. There were no observable differences between the resorption ridges whether the roots had been retained or the maxilla was edentulous. The retention of roots in the maxilla offers other advantages, by absorbing increased loads that may be delivered by an opposing natural dentition.

Sensory feedback

It is recognised that the teeth are rich in proprioceptive fibres. These confer several advantages to the patient:

- control of the amount of masticatory force
- recognition of the size and texture of objects
- help with spatial positioning of the mandible during masticatory function.

Where there are teeth present, there is increased tactile discrimination which allows a dentate patient to exert high occlusal loads during mastication with more precision. In contrast, a complete denture-wearer is six times less efficient at detecting small objects.

Teeth with large surface areas, such as canine teeth, are rich in mechanoreceptors and therefore able to help with location. Natural teeth are more sensitive to lateral than to axial forces. Such sensory perception is not as readily detected by the edentulous patient. Therefore it can be argued that the patient with overdentures will retain the advantages of sensory feedback associated with the retained roots. However, the wearing of an acrylic prosthesis may also reduce this sensitivity but it will still be superior to a complete denture.

Reduction of psychological trauma

The retention of roots will often help the patient to come to terms with the need for restoration of the remaining dentition. This can help in transitional situations where a patient is eventually going to lose teeth due to past neglect.

Overdenture cases

Overdentures are a useful treatment option in many clinical situations. A simple complete lower overdenture which encloses the roots of two root-treated canines has been shown above (Fig. 12.51). Cases can be more complicated

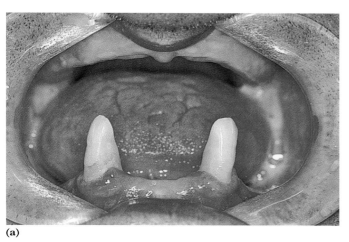

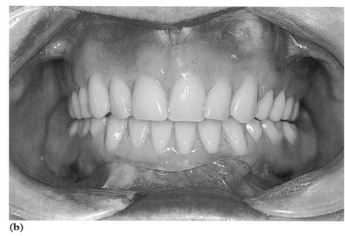

(a)

(b)

Fig. 12.51 (a) The canines are the last teeth remaining but have an unfavourable crown/root ratio. (b) Overdentures have been constructed which completely enclose the remaining roots.

than this. The reduction in the crowns of the teeth may have occurred due to tooth wear from a combination of erosion and attrition. In the elderly, where such tooth reduction has occurred, root canal treatment may not be necessary. The removal of the roots will not benefit the patient and the overdenture is the best form of treatment.

Less common situations, such as partial anodontia, cleft palate or loss of tooth crown substance in dentinogenesis imperfecta, may also require restoration using overdentures. The distinction between an onlay and an overdenture is not clear-cut and a potentially difficult partial denture treatment, such as the restoration of a free end saddle, may be helped by the coverage of a canine or molar tooth with a reduced crown rather than a more involved crown restoration.

In the case illustrated in Figure 12.53, an elderly patient has severe tooth surface loss. The aetiology of this wear must be diagnosed before treatment is commenced. For instance, is this wear a result of parafunction or erosion

from the consumption of acidic drinks? The remaining dentition has been restored and a definitive overdenture placed.

Clinical synopsis

Successful overdenture treatment involves careful patient selection and treatment planning. Similar criteria to those used in selecting bridge or partial denture abutments are employed.

Selection of abutments

When selecting the appropriate teeth for overdenture abutments, there are many factors which influence the clinician's choice. The abutment teeth should exhibit good periodontal health with adequate bone support. There should be minimal attachment loss and ideally they should be surrounded by attached gingivae with no bleeding and

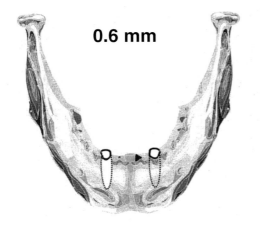

0.6 mm

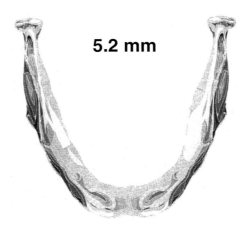

5.2 mm

Fig. 12.52 The resulting bone loss over the 5-year period of the Crum & Rooney (1978) study (see text).

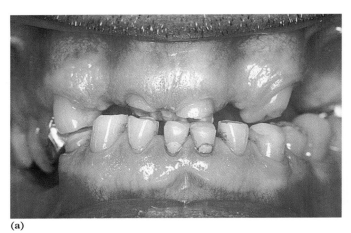

(a)

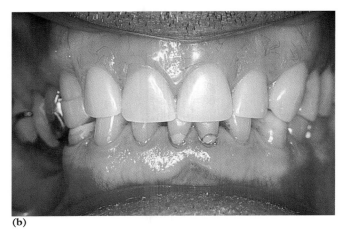

(b)

Fig. 12.53 (a) This elderly patient has lost tooth structure over many years in the upper arch. (b) The remaining dentition has been restored and a final overdenture placed. (Courtesy of Mrs E.A. McLaughlin.)

minimal plaque deposits present. The potentially damaging lateral loads are reduced with a more favourable crown/root ratio. This can be achieved by reducing the height of the abutment tooth following root canal treatment.

Ideally, the abutments must be located on both sides of the arch and evenly distributed. The best teeth for overdenture abutments are those with the largest root surface area such as canines and molars. If less favourable teeth, i.e. lower incisors, are to be used for overdenture abutments there should be a number of them together in order to spread the loads. The teeth should be restorable and have enough supragingival tooth structure to allow them to be used as abutments. If root canal treatment is required then the tooth should have canals that are readily negotiable and the long-term prognosis of the tooth should be good.

Although a tooth may be in a suitable position for use as an abutment, there may be a large bony prominence that would preclude the use of a flange for the final prosthesis. Such a situation may occur with the retention of upper canines as overdenture abutments, where a large bony eminence will often prevent the placement of a flange and/or detract from aesthetics. It may be necessary to incorporate a precision attachment and this will require a tooth that has sufficient strength and root surface area to support the increased loading.

Overdenture treatment is sophisticated and may require many clinical visits and there will be a high cost element. All of this will influence the patient's suitability for such treatment and should be dicussed with the patient at the planning stage.

Sequence of treatment

Following the drawing up of the treatment plan, preliminary preparation may be started. Such treatment should include any periodontal work and conservation and/or root canal treatment of the abutments. If advanced work is required, such as copings or attachments, this should be completed

prior to manufacture of the overdenture. The prosthesis is completed towards the end of the treatment unless there is a need for a provisional denture to stabilise the occlusion during treatment. Finally, the importance of follow-up, careful maintenance of the overdenture and regular review of the state of the oral tissues must be stressed to the patient (see Box 12.11).

Types of overdenture

There are three methods of providing overdentures:

- They may be placed immediately on reduction of the teeth.
- If the patient wears a removable partial denture, this may be converted to an overdenture.
- Existing overdentures may require replacement.

A patient may already have an existing prosthesis, in which case it is possible to convert the existing partial denture into an overdenture at the time of reducing the abutment teeth. Such dentures may be constructed at the chairside or in the laboratory.

Box 12.11   Typical stages involved in overdenture provision

1. Examination
2. Diagnosis, treatment plan
3. Preparatory treatment:
   - periodontal
   - abutments
   - conservation
   - root canal treatment
4. Other treatment
5. Denture construction
6. Follow-up and maintenance

After a period of time, overdentures may require replacing due to occlusal wear or fracture of the acrylic baseplate. Other problems that may occur include damage to the underlying abutments either by parafunctional forces or due to caries. Poor oral hygiene may have led to increased periodontal breakdown leading to tooth loss.

The clinician may wish to replace the overdenture if this has served well using a duplicate denture technique. This may prove to be a more successful method than a conventional technique. If there has been fracture of the baseplate due to excessive occlusal loads, a metal base of Co/Cr may be required.

Copings and attachments

Copings

In some cases, the root face of an abutment tooth may have been damaged by caries or there may be a need to protect the root face. A coping consists of either a gold thimble over the tooth or a post-retained dome and is constructed in a similar fashion to a post crown (Fig. 12.54). Copings are used to protect a weakened tooth from fracture and wear but they do not prevent caries.

Attachments

Precision attachments can be used to aid retention from the root. However, they are expensive items and their maintenance is difficult. If required, they should only be placed in the more motivated patient. The increased retention brings about higher loading of the teeth, particularly in the lateral direction, and such forces are potentially damaging to teeth. If precision attachments are not maintained properly, failure due to caries around the attachment or periodontal breakdown is a potential hazard.

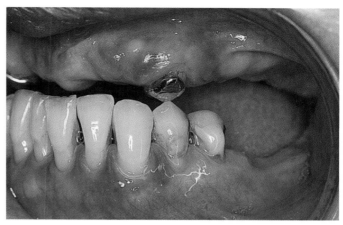

Fig. 12.54 A coping used to protect the root surface.

There are generally three different types of precision attachments available: studs, bars and magnets. Studs are generally placed in the root face and the attachment, in the form of a press clip, is retained in the denture (Fig. 12.55a). Bars have the advantage of spreading the loading between the abutment teeth. However, they impart high loading to those teeth, are difficult to clean and relining is complicated. The bar is attached to the root face via a post system and the clip or sleeve is held in the denture (Fig. 12.55b). Magnets used in dentistry are made from either cobalt–samarium or iron–neodymium–boron. They have the advantage that they are less likely to cause lateral stresses to the abutment tooth and are clinically easy to use. Their disadvantage is that they are liable to corrode in oral fluids over time. Special base metal is supplied for use with magnets, which is cast into copings and cemented into the root face. The magnets are positioned in the mouth and retained in the denture using a self-cure acrylic (Fig. 12.56).

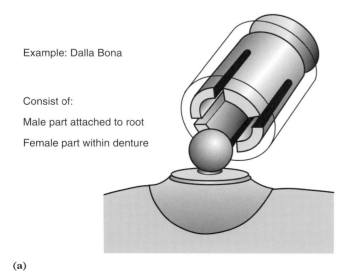

Example: Dalla Bona

Consist of:

Male part attached to root

Female part within denture

(a)

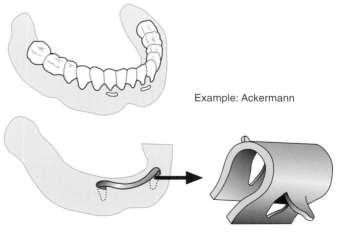

Example: Ackermann

Other systems – Dolder, Kurer

(b)

Fig. 12.55 Examples of (a) studs and (b) bars used to retain dentures.

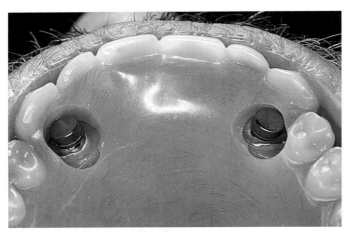

Fig. 12.56 Dental magnets placed on abutment keepers ready to be cured to the denture.

When planning treatment for overdentures, the clinician should consider whether the support will come from the teeth, the mucosa or a combination of the two. Increasing the support provided by the tooth root may lead to increased lateral stresses which may be detrimental in the long term. A mucosal-supported denture receives increased retention and support from the greater amount of alveolar bone that is present.

Maintenance

The continual after-care of the prepared teeth underlying the overdenture is aimed at preventing both carious attack and periodontal destruction, which would lead to root extraction. This would then require modification or construction of a new overdenture. The prevention of such problems should form part of the management in this restorative procedure.

Caries

Root caries may take place on an unprotected root face. Patients should be given correct dietary advice together with advice on measures aimed at protecting the roots. It has been shown that, in those patients who used a fluoride gel daily, only 5% of teeth developed caries. This is in contrast to those patients who did not use such a gel, in whom 20% of the teeth developed caries.

Periodontal disease

Studies show that 35% of patients wearing overdentures experience some loss of attachment. Furthermore, when examining patients' dentures, only 50% of their prostheses were plaque-free. All these findings were related to poor oral hygiene status of the patient.

Maintenance regime

It is imperative that the patient receives regular maintenance with plaque control of the abutments and care of the root face. A fluoride gel, which can be placed in the recess of the denture where it contacts the abutments, should be prescribed. Regular oral hygiene appointments with the hygienist must be mandatory.

Within 1 month of preparing the abutment teeth for the patient in Figure 12.57, the UR3 had developed recurrent caries. The caries was removed and a new restoration was placed. A strict regime of regular recalls was commenced, including application of a fluoride gel containing 0.05% fluoride. Four years later, the abutment UR3 had an extended amalgam present but both root faces had been stable for this period of time. The darkening of the root dentine is a result of the high levels of fluoride. In contrast, the patient shown in Figure 12.57(b) was not well controlled and after placement of the overdentures did not

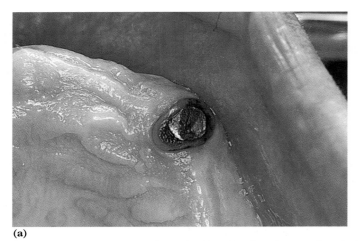

(a)

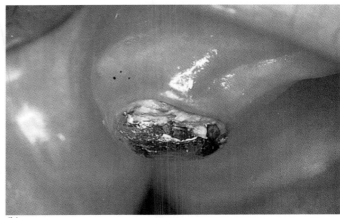

(b)

Fig. 12.57 Both these root faces developed caries. The root face in (a) has been restored and a strict regime of oral hygiene and topical fluoride instigated. In (b) the root required extraction.

return for review. Three years later the root face had recurrent caries and the root required extraction.

Summary

Overdentures are a useful form of restorative treatment when replacing teeth. They are indicated where teeth are to be covered or where there is crown loss which is not restorable by other methods. The procedure requires the careful interaction of periodontal treatment, good operative procedures and root canal treatment, thus allowing the final placement of the removable prosthesis to be successful. This success is built on appropriate treatment planning and a high quality of clinical care. As with any advanced procedure, it is important to maintain a careful review of the ongoing function of such treatment.

IMMEDIATE DENTURES

Introduction

An immediate denture is a denture that is made prior to the extraction of the natural teeth, which is inserted into the mouth immediately after the extraction of those teeth. It is seen as a provisional prosthesis (Figs 12.58–12.61).

The provision of an immediate denture has may advantages for a patient including maintaining the soft tissue contour of the face and helping the patient at a time when losing a tooth or teeth may be a traumatic and difficult emotional process. An immediate denture has the big advantage in that it aids in the process of adaptation to dentures. As patients' dental health has improved, the provision of immediate dentures has changed from extensive removal of all the teeth to simple additions to existing dentures. Once again such dentures are seen as transitional in nature (Figs 12.62–12.64).

They are used to assist in aesthetics or mastication over a period of time (6 to 12 months) prior to provision of a

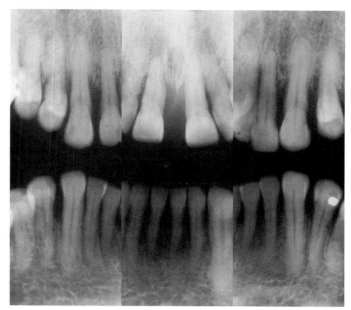

Fig. 12.59 Radiograph shows poor bone support for the anterior teeth.

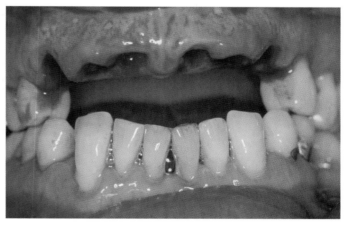

Fig. 12.60 The teeth have been removed.

more permanent restoration. They are also used to help a patient gradually acclimatise to dentures, as the teeth are lost over a period of time. Advantages and disadvantages are outlined in Boxes 12.12 and 12.13.

Treatment planning

The treatment planning of the patient will dictate which of the existing teeth require extraction (Box 12.14). For instance, it may not be necessary to extract the teeth as they may be used for overdenture abutments or if they have a poor prognosis they may be temporarily kept for the transition to denture wearing. Other options include extracting teeth of poor prognosis and not fitting the denture for approximately 6 months. This is only done for posterior teeth, which allows resorption to take place and

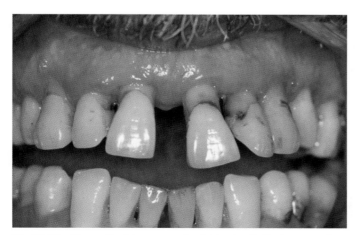

Fig. 12.58 The patient has several anterior teeth that are causing problems.

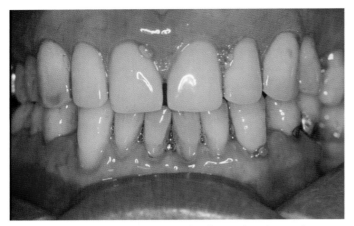

Fig. 12.61 The immediate denture has been placed over the extraction sockets.

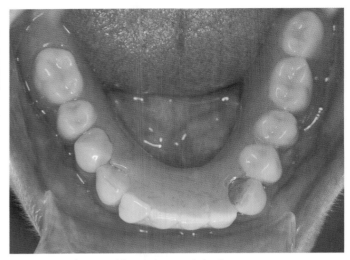

Fig. 12.64 The transitional denture is in situ.

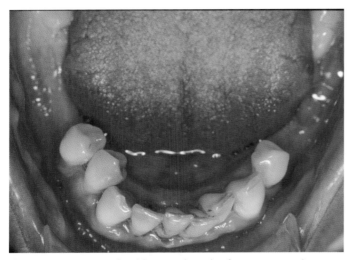

Fig. 12.62 Lower arch with several teeth of poor prognosis.

then provides a stable base for subsequent partial denture treatment. Anterior teeth will always be extracted and wherever possible immediately replaced with a restoration such as an immediate denture.

When immediate dentures are proposed, it is important that patients are advised of the necessity for early relining and/or remaking with associated additional visits and extra costs. Communication and understanding of such involved treatment and potential difficulties will prevent any mis-

---

Box 12.12 Advantages and disadvantages of immediate dentures to clinicians

Advantages
- Potential to use the existing occlusion of the natural teeth for jaw registration procedures
- Presence of the teeth to be extracted allows the clinician to make a suitable assessment of the aesthetics

Disadvantages
- There is no trial denture stage possible and therefore there is the potential for the final result not to be exactly what the patient was expecting
- Gross irregularities of the teeth including broken-down teeth, which require surgical extraction, may result in an uneven ridge or ill-fitting dentures

---

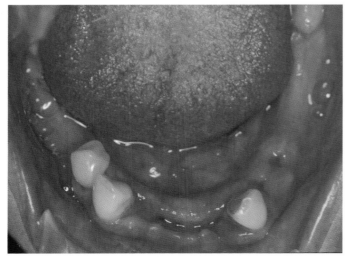

Fig. 12.63 Following extraction, three teeth have been retained which will assist in the transition to a complete denture.

Box 12.13 Disadvantages to undertaking immediate dentures from the patient's viewpoint

- There will be many visits required and as the bone resorption sets in following the loss of teeth, there will be progressive loss of fit of the dentures. The patient should be ready to expect this and appreciate that it will also result in an increased cost. Therefore good cooperation is necessary

understanding or potential future disagreements. It is useful to provide the patient with written instructions of what is involved in the immediate denture process.

Design of immediate dentures

When providing immediate dentures the replacement teeth on the denture should be supported by a flange. This provides strength and stability to the dentures and allows the area that is healing to be protected. Subsequent relining of the denture is straightforward as the flange acts as a template allowing further addition of acrylic in place. Dentists may come across dentures where the teeth sit into sockets of the extracted teeth. These are termed socketed immediate dentures and will lead to long-term problems. Whilst this technique is favoured by technicians as it will provide good initial aesthetics, over time this is lost. Typically the appearance is only satisfactory for a couple of weeks, after which the resorption of bone leads to a poor aesthetic result. Furthermore, the denture will become unretentive and difficult to reline.

Additions of teeth to partial dentures

When providing additions an alginate impression in a stock tray is used. The impression is taken over the correctly seated denture *in situ*. The full functional width and depth of the sulcus is recorded in the area of the tooth to be extracted. It is useful to mark teeth to be added to the denture with indelible pencil to avoid confusion and mistakes. It may be necessary to use a wax or silicone interocclusal record if there are several teeth to be replaced. An opposing alginate impression is taken. This is sent to the laboratory with correct patient and clinical information after appropriate cross-infection precautions. An appointment is arranged for both tooth extraction and insertion of denture at the same visit.

Provision of new immediate denture

If there are substantially more teeth to be removed then the treatment is spread over several appointments. Preliminary alginate impressions for study casts are taken and once customised special trays are constructed the working impressions are taken at the second clinical visit. The teeth are cleansed of debris, plaque and calculus and the impressions are taken in alginate. There is then a clinical decision:

* If sufficient tooth contact is present for jaw relationship, then an interocclusal record is taken with shade and mould of teeth.
* If there is insufficient tooth contact, then occlusal rims will be required and the registration will have to take place at an extra clinical visit.

Instructions are given to the laboratory and the teeth for extraction indicated on working casts. If the immediate restoration is a partial denture, those undercuts to be blocked out are specified. The technician will set up the artificial teeth in the edentulous spaces for trial insertion in the mouth.

At the trial insertion stage the occlusion and aesthetics are checked but it will not be possible to see the finished result, as the teeth to be extracted are still present. At this visit arrangements for the tooth extraction are made.

Before the trial denture and cast is sent in for processing, it is the responsibility of the clinician to prepare the cast ready for placement of the artificial teeth by the technician. The clinician will then determine bone levels around teeth using a periodontal probe and assessing radiographs of the teeth. This provides an estimation of the amount of soft tissue collapse that will take place immediately following tooth extraction. Therefore the clinician will trim the cast appropriately.

At the next visit the teeth are extracted and the immediate dentures inserted. In order to avoid trauma to the anaesthetised tissues, any acrylic pearls, spicules and undercuts are removed from the fitting surface of the denture. This will help with the insertion of the denture. Any obvious occlusal discrepancies and overextension are corrected. It is best to leave any finer adjustments of the dentures including the occlusion to a later appointment because of subsequent swelling that occurs.

Instructions are given to the patient that the dentures should not be removed for 24 hours and post-extraction instructions are given as for routine tooth removal.

The patient is reviewed at 24 hours, when the dentures are removed from the mouth and cleaned with brush, soap and water, and the mouth is examined for areas of soreness. The dentures are adjusted to relieve any overextensions, excessive pressure from denture base or obvious occlusal discrepancies. Instruction on oral and denture hygiene is given together with a patient handout.

At the next review, which should be at one week, all factors at 24-hour review are checked again with evaluation and adjustment of occlusion. Regular review appointments are then arranged for the patient at suitable periods as follows: 1 month, 3 months, 6 months and then annually thereafter (Box 12.15). It is also good practice to remind the patient that temporary relining will be necessary at a review in the near future and that permanent relining or the construction of new dentures will be necessary at a later stage.

Box 12.15	Review timetable
24 hours	Simple check on patient status – adjustments geared to make patient comfortable
1 week	More involved check of patient status – thorough examination followed by adjustments of impression and occlusal surfaces
1 month	Review for further adjustments. Any placement of temporary or permanent linings should be delayed until 3 to 6 months unless absolutely necessary
6 months	Review the need for reline of denture as much of the resorption will have taken place
12 months	Provision of new dentures

COMPLETE DENTURES

Although patients are keeping their teeth longer and the demands for fixed prosthodontic solutions in restorative dentistry are growing, there will still remain a sizable number of patients who are edentulous. This group of patients will generally be elderly and with current life expectation increasing will live without teeth for a substantial number of years. This will pose several problems including the ability of the patient to adapt. Also the skill base of clinicians who are capable of providing such treatment will slowly decrease as the demands for other types of treatment increase. In short complete denture cases will become more clinically challenging. This text can only serve as an introduction to the provision of complete dentures and the reader is advised to further such knowledge by the use of postgraduate courses following graduation.

A simplistic way to consider complete dentures is to look at how they are designed in a similar manner to partial dentures. This concept of designing then assists during the diagnosis of the patient's problem and subsequent treatment planning. Complete dentures may be considered in four different ways (Box 12.16).

Mechanistic approach

In this approach the artificial teeth will be set up on the crest of the remaining alveolar ridges. The concept here is that the underlying ridges will take the occlusal stresses during function. This is simple and straightforward to understand. Unfortunately it does not consider the biological consequences of adopting such an approach in the longer term. The edentulous ridge will resorb over time and therefore their position will change. The associated soft tissues will also be compromised. For instance in the lower arch, the mechanical positioning of the teeth on the ridge will often produce an occlusal form that takes no account of the positioning of the tongue. This may lead to soreness of the tongue and instability of the lower denture.

Copy dentures

Many patients present with dentures that they have been wearing for several years and are generally comfortable with them. Their presenting problems are often related to looseness or difficulty with eating. The patient has developed good neuromuscular control over the years. Therefore the polished surfaces of the dentures (i.e. the general denture form) are correct. The problem is either related to the artificial teeth that have worn leading to a poor occlusion or the impression surface no longer corresponds to the ridge shape that has resorped over the years. It may be sufficient in such cases to undertake a copy denture technique (Fig. 12.65).

Biometric

Watt and MacGregor demonstrated in the early 1960s that there is a remnant of the palatal gingival vestige that remains as a stable anatomical structure. This may be identified on the upper edentulous denture-bearing area even after many years of bone resorption. This vestige may then be used to assist in the placement of the artificial teeth. The subsequent guidelines can prove to be very useful in knowing where the teeth should be placed. Further reading on this technique may be found in the further reading section at the end of this book (Fig. 12.66).

Box 12.16	Designing complete dentures	
Mechanistic	Artificial teeth placed on the ridge	Simple to understand Does not take account of biological changes
Copy dentures	Use of a template of old dentures which is modified	Builds on previous success May be more expensive to produce from laboratory
Biometric	Uses guidelines of previous position of natural teeth	Useful guidelines Not always applicable as a rule to every case
Neutral zone	Places teeth in context of muscular structures such as the lip, cheeks and tongue	Assists where lower denture stability is a problem Not always a success

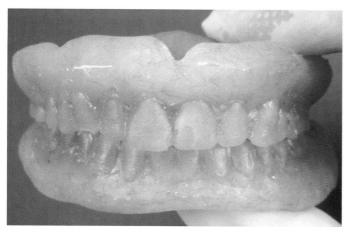

Fig. 12.65 This is a copy denture template which has been produced from impressions of a patient's old dentures.

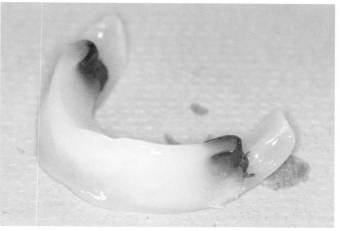

Fig. 12.67 A typical neutral zone impression where a rim of a tissue conditioning material has been moulded into the neutral zone.

Functional approach

The neutral zone technique is an alternative approach for the construction of lower complete dentures. It is defined as the area between the tongue on one side and the cheeks and lips on the other where soft tissue displacing forces are least. It is most effective for dentures where there is a highly atrophic ridge and a history of denture instability. The technique aims to construct a denture that is shaped by muscle function and is in harmony with the surrounding oral structures. The technique is by no means new but is a valuable one to use in difficult cases (Fig.12.67).

Conventional approach to complete dentures

The following description of examination and subsequent treatment follows a traditional outline of treatment.

Assessment of the patient

As in any patient consultation, a careful history is essential and leading questions will often open up a more detailed assessment that will have consequences for the subsequent treatment of the patient. Asking the patient a few leading open questions assists in drawing up the picture of the patient's problems. For instance: how many dentures have been made for you? When did you become edentulous? Which denture has been the most successful? The scenarios can be many and varied but the following are examples. A patient who has been edentulous for many years where each denture has lasted well over 5 years may be considered to be a relatively successful denture wearer. However, a history of a couple of years of edentulousness with a series of dentures that have not functioned well will

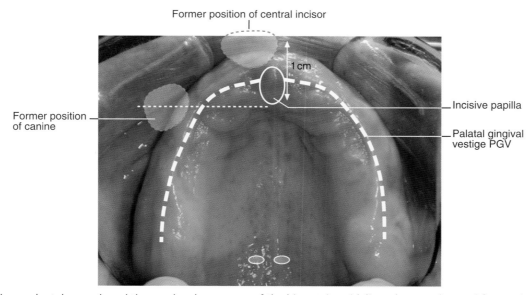

Former position of central incisor

1 cm

Former position of canine

Incisive papilla

Palatal gingival vestige PGV

Fig.12.66 This is an edentulous arch and the overlay shows some of the biometric guidelines that may be used for tooth positioning.

send warning signs. These typical examples will immediately give a clinical impression to the operator to what has gone before and how it will influence the subsequent success. The provision of complete dentures is an area of dentistry where the psychological profiling of the patient is an important component of the diagnosis and treatment planning. Figure 12.68 shows examples of upper and lower edentulous arches.

The previous medical history is taken as outlined in Chapter 3 (p. 15). However, many of these patients will be elderly and will be taking a complex cocktail of medications. One of the common problems with many of these patients is that the variety of drugs they are taking may lead to a reduced salivary flow. The consequences of this include a dry mouth which may lead to poor denture retention.

Social history may reveal more details of their personality and other non-dental considerations which may have a direct impact on the treatment. As such patients are elderly there may be pressures such as transport arrangements, care of elderly relatives, etc., all of which may have an impact on treatment.

The first visit with a patient requiring complete dentures is an opportunity to find out why the patient wishes new dentures and to diagnose any problems. At the end of the visit, as a clinician, you should be in a position to draw up a treatment plan. The subsequent examination allows you to bring in the patient's presenting complaint with the clinical presentation.

Examination

The examination of the edentulous patient will include visual inspection of the soft tissues. This will be followed by examination of the denture-bearing tissues which will include the upper ridge, where the shape of the ridges is observed and noted (i.e. 'u' or 'v' shaped, high or low palate), and any soft tissue that is present. The health of the tissues should also be noted. Any inflammation over the area that the denture fits indicating the presence of *Candida albicans* in the denture is recorded.

The lower edentulous ridge is examined and an estimation of its shape, health and the bone quality is made.

The previous dentures, if present, are then examined and placed in the mouth. These will provide important clues to both the clinical problem and methods of how to possibly resolve the situation. The denture may be examined in the following manner.

Impression/fitting surface – the extensions of the border of the denture are examined to determine if it is adequately extended. Overextension may reveal pain and soreness whilst underextensions may relate to the complaint of looseness and lack of retention.

Occlusal surface – when the patient closes the teeth together, the maximum number of teeth should meet. If the patient is then asked to move the teeth over one another this should occur in an even gliding movement without any cuspal interference. If this is present then the teeth are in occlusal balance. The lack of such balance will often present as either pain underneath the denture or looseness during function. Often clinicians will look to the fitting surface of a denture as to the source of such discomfort or denture instability without considering occlusal discrepancies as the potential source of the problem.

Polished surfaces – the tongue, lips and cheeks contact the denture whilst in function and may be major factors in retaining and stabilising it during function. If the surfaces are not in balance with such soft tissues then this will present as denture looseness. An assessment of the lower denture in the neutral zone is made.

An estimation of the vertical dimension of occlusion is made. Typically patients require approximately 2 to 3 mm space between the teeth at rest. This interocclusal clearance

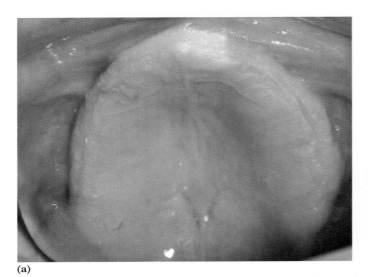

(a)

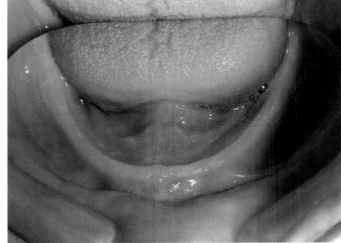

(b)

Fig. 12.68 **(a)** and **(b)** Examples of upper and lower edentulous arches.

(freeway space) may be measured with a Willis bite gauge (Fig. 12.69). If there is excessive freeway space then this will lead to instability and looseness with the patient appearing overclosed. Too little or no freeway space will not allow the patient to rest and the underlying tissues will be under constant stress. This will lead to discomfort and may also interfere with speech.

Finally the most difficult assessment to make is the psychological profile of the patient and their ability to cope or adapt to the wearing of dentures. Sometimes the complaint is out of proportion to the clinical results found following clinical examination of the dentures. Alternatively the remaining hard and soft tissues do not lend themselves to the provision of dentures. It is useful to explain at this stage to the patient what complete dentures are 'A replacement of no teeth'. Patients' expectations run high and simple communication of why there may be difficulties with the wearing of dentures following the loss of natural teeth is an important factor in the overall care of the patient.

The clinician will by now have made an assessment of the patient and a diagnosis is made of the clinical problem. From this diagnosis a treatment plan is drawn up as to the overall clinical techniques that will be used.

An example of provision of a set of complete dentures

History-taking, examination and treatment planning

The following patient presented edentulous following the removal of all his teeth for medical reasons. He had been edentulous for over a year and the intraoral presentation immediately shows the problem that may be faced in the treatment of this patient (Fig. 12.68).

The period of edentulousness has allowed the tongue to spread laterally and this will compromise the position of the teeth. It is possible to identify several structures on the upper denture-bearing area including the incisive papilla and the palatal gingival vestige. These may be useful as a potential guide to positioning the teeth. For instance, in general the central incisors should be placed approximately 1 cm in front of the posterior border of the incisive papilla. This has been determined to be close to the previous position of the natural incisors.

The lower denture-bearing area reveals a narrow ridge and the tongue spread may make the positioning of the posterior teeth very difficult. The subsequent determination of the neutral zone for tooth placement may well be difficult.

The *diagnosis* was an edentulous situation where complete dentures were required. However, care and attention to the placement of the artificial teeth in relation to the soft tissues is important.

The treatment plan was to construct the complete dentures using a conventional approach but using biometric guidelines to assist in the provision of the complete dentures. A decision on the placement of the lower teeth would be made at the registration stage (Box 12.17).

Preliminary impressions

Preliminary impressions were taken using impression compound (Fig. 12.70). The stock trays were selected for both the upper and the lower arches. The material was warmed in a water bath at 37° and both upper and lower impressions were taken. Impression compound is a thermoplastic material made up of a mixture of resins, shellac and powder. It is a high viscosity material that is able to support itself and thus compensate for any deficiencies of the stock trays. A high viscosity alginate may also perform the same task.

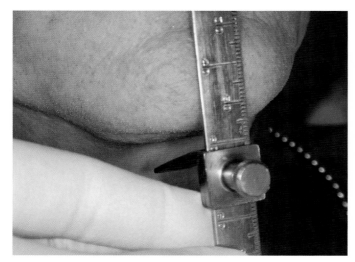

Fig. 12.69 The free space is being measured with a Willis bite gauge. Typically the difference from resting position and occlusal contact position is 2–3 mm.

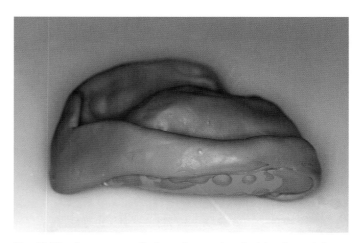

Fig. 12.70 An upper preliminary impression that has been taken in impression compound.

Master Impressions

A laboratory request for the provision of upper and lower light-cured special trays is made. The upper is spaced (2 mm) and the lower is close fitting. The upper tray is tried into the patient's mouth and checked that the extensions relate to the functional depth of the sulcus. Corrections may be made to the tray with a suitable autopolymersing acrylic resin. A portion of 'carding' wax is placed on the impression surface of the tray to maintain the necessary spacer present for the alginate impression material.

The upper impression is taken with a low viscosity alginate (Fig. 12.71). This is a mucostatic material, which gives detailed reproduction of the upper denture-bearing area. It is dimensionally accurate but not dimensionally stable and therefore the subsequent cast should be poured straight away.

The lower special tray is constructed as a close fitting for a wash impression with zinc oxide eugenol (Fig. 12.72). The close fitting special tray provides a mucodisplacive force on the lower ridge. Zinc oxide-eugenol is a mucostatic impression material that provides an accurate representation of the fine detail of the mucosa. Other materials that may be used include medium-bodied silicone. The additional benefit of using a close fitting tray is that there

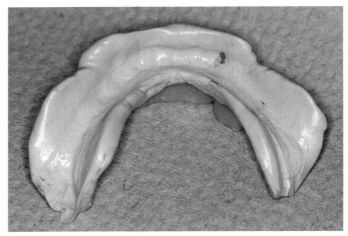

Fig. 12.72 The lower impression shown has been taken with zinc oxide/eugenol.

is minimal saliva contamination during the taking of the impression.

In order to protect the representation of the sulcus on the dental cast, red carding wax is added to the lower impression; this creates a land area when the impression is poured. The process is called beading.

Registration

This is the most involved stage of the construction of complete dentures. There are several important objectives to be achieved at this clinical stage (Box 12.18).

The laboratory will have been asked to provide wax occlusal record rims. The upper is strengthened by the use of a shellac or polystyrene base and the lower will have a wire strengthener. Do not be tempted to use all wax bases as they distort. Occasionally heat-cured (i.e. processed) bases may be made from the casts. These are useful if you want to know at an early stage how your denture will fit. However, the cast will no longer be with you and if excessive trimming is required then you will quickly learn that wax is much easier to adjust than acrylic.

It is useful to consider the registration stage in three separate stages.

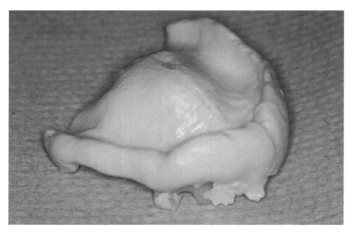

Fig. 12.71   An upper impression that has been taken in alginate.

Stage 1. If previous dentures are present then it is wise to ask the patient whether they liked the look of the dentures or have a preference on how their previous teeth looked as this can then be incorporated into the new denture.

The upper rim is tried into the mouth and it is adjusted to an ideal vertical level, which is generally accepted to be 1 to 2 mm below the upper lip to give a pleasing appearance. To ensure that the rim is trimmed to the correct level, a Fox's occlusal record plane is used.

Once the rim is correctly trimmed, then the centre line and the canine lines are added. Furthermore, ask the patient to smile and mark the extent the lip rises up the record rim. All this information helps the technician, who has not seen the patient.

Stage 2. The aim is to establish the occlusal vertical dimension and register this at the ideal horizontal dimension. This can be a difficult procedure. The Willis bite gauge is used to measure the free space. The lower record rim (only) in the mouth is placed in the mouth, and with the patient in a relaxed position the distance between two fixed points (i.e. under the chin and nose) is measured. The upper record rim is placed in the mouth and the patient is asked to close together and the distance is remeasured. You may need to adjust the lower record rim but do not alter your correctly trimmed upper rim. The difference between the two measurements should typically be around 2–3 mm.

As discussed earlier, if dentures are provided with no freeway space then this will affect speech and comfort as the patient will always be clenching on them. If there is too much (i.e. 12 mm) freeway space then this will lead to overclosure and unretentive dentures. There are different ways of approaching the correction of such a large freeway space and this includes incremental additions to the denture or assessment on closing the free way space to a smaller value such as 6 mm. During measurement of the resting face height the lower record rim is placed in the mouth, which allows the tongue to adopt a correct position. If there are difficulties with the measurement of the resting face height using the Willis bite gauge, such as no chin (i.e. the chinless wonder) or the patient with a beard, it may be prudent to use marks or stickers on the face.

The important stage is reached when the lower record rim is trimmed so that it is contacting the upper rim evenly and at the suitable freeway space for the patient (Fig. 12.73). The rims are then sealed together in the 'retruded jaw position'. The retruded jaw position is the most posterior position of the condyles on the retruded arc of closure. Studies have found that it is a reproducible position.

The rims may be sealed together with a variety of materials including wax or zinc oxide/eugenol. The material should have good flow properties and not distort when set. Always cut the notches on the upper rim as this will assist the technician in the setting up of the upper rim on the articulator.

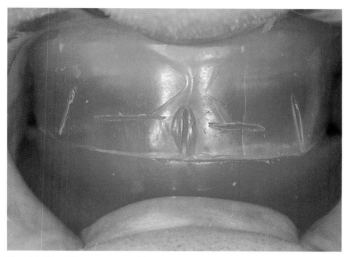

Fig. 12.73 The upper and lower record rims are shown correctly trimmed and ready for sealing.

Stage 3. Finally the selection of teeth is made. This procedure is very much an art form and is subjective. In its simplest form the shape and size of the teeth are selected to harmonise with the rest of the face and more importantly with the patient's wishes. The shade of the teeth is selected with similar considerations.

The laboratory is asked to set up trial dentures in wax on preferably an average movement articulator (Fig. 12.74).

Trial dentures

The trial dentures are presented with the artificial teeth in wax. The clinical work undertaken at the last stage is checked. Check the stability of the dentures, the vertical dimension with a Willis bite gauge, that the occlusion meets evenly on both sides and there are no interferences

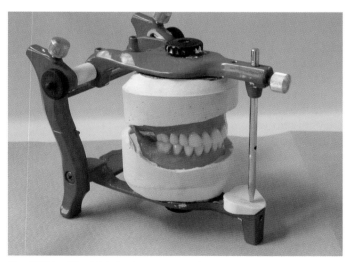

Fig. 12.74 The trial dentures are made on an average movement articulator.

between the opposing teeth. Retention is not a major issue at this stage as the trial dentures are primarily composed of a wax base that will distort and does not provide a good border seal. Reassure patients that it will be better at the finished stage and that this looseness is not an indication of what is to come. The patients are also asked to check on the appearance of the teeth and whether the shade and mould is to their liking.

If all is satisfactory then it is a simple matter of asking the technician to flask, process and finish the dentures in pink acrylic.

However, try-in may not be accurate, with a common problem being that the registration is incorrect. If the teeth are not meeting correctly then certain decisions need to be made. If the aesthetics of the upper rim are satisfactory then the lower premolars and molar teeth are removed and the posterior segment will with placement of extra waxwork revert to a lower record rim. Then it is a matter of re-registering the trial dentures. The dentures are then sent back to the laboratory to be reset for a further trial denture visit.

Delivery of complete denture

The processed dentures will arrive wrapped up in moist gauze to prevent the acrylic from drying out. The fitting surface of the dentures is first checked for any spicules or acrylic pearls which will irritate the mucosa and if present these are smoothed away with an acrylic bur. The dentures are placed in the mouth and the retention and stability checked. The vertical and horizontal dimension is also checked and the aesthetics. The placement of the lower denture is inspected and the neuromuscular control reviewed as the patient is trying out the dentures.

Always check the occlusion as there may be processing faults that can occur during the processing of the complete dentures. The occlusion may be checked with articulating paper and any prematurities removed. Unfortunately the mouth is not a good vehicle for assessing such interferences as the patient will adapt to any problems and therefore avoid them. If there is a larger discrepancy present then a 'check record procedure' is required. In this a layer of wax is placed on the occlusal surfaces of the teeth, softened and then the patient is asked to close in the retruded arc of closure. However, he is prevented from making tooth contact as if this occurs his adaptive processes will then 'kick in' and you will record an incorrect registration. The dentures are sent into the laboratory and lightly 'tacked' into position on an articulator (Fig. 12.75). The wax is removed, the incisal pin removed and the artificial teeth are allowed to contact. The technician will then adjust the occlusion accordingly.

Instructions to the patient

The patient is provided with instructions on what to expect with wearing his denture and what to do if he

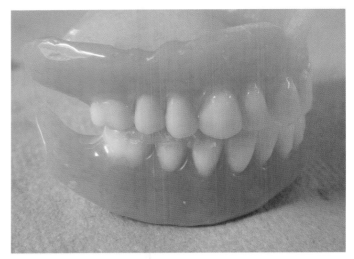

Fig. 12.75 The finished dentures have been registered with some wax to enable them to be transferred to an articulator for adjustment.

experiences any problems. The advice includes not to wear the dentures at night and to soak them in an appropriate hypochlorite cleaner overnight. Further brushing with a scrubbing brush and soap and water is more than sufficient to maintain cleanliness and prevent the colonisation of the dentures with *Candida albicans*. If the patient experiences any pain or discomfort during the wearing of the dentures then he should leave them out of the mouth. They should only be worn for 24 hours before the review appointment in order for the clinician to identify where the dentures are causing problems.

Review appointment

At the review appointment the patient may have experienced several problems from the dentures. Problems may be related to the patient such as undercuts, poor amount of bone, or poor adaptation to dentures. There may be faults with the denture and these will be related to the three surfaces of the denture. Generally, looseness may be attributed to faults with all three surfaces of the denture (impression, occlusal and polished) whilst pain and discomfort may be attributed to problems originating from the impression and occlusal surfaces. At the review appointment a detailed history is taken of the problems and an examination is made of both the denture bearing areas and the dentures themselves.

Other techniques

Both copy dentures and the use of a neutral zone technique provide an alternative technique or approach to the construction of complete dentures. Space does not allow a full detailed description of their use. The copy denture technique involves duplicating the patient's previous dentures and then adding modifications to the resulting templates. Registration follows similar principles as those described in this text. Impression taking is relatively straightforward as the duplicate dentures will act as a special tray allowing wash impressions to be taken. The neutral zone technique is introduced at the registration stage of denture construction. Once the upper rim is trimmed the lower rim is built up in a suitable mouldable material such as the tissue conditioner Viscogel. This is allowed to mould to the neutral zone as the patient is asked to speak, sip some water, thus allowing the tissues to influence the shape of the rim. The teeth are subsequently set up within the space created by this rim.

Final considerations

If there are some teeth left then these may be root filled and overdentures provided. If the present techniques do not provide satisfactory retention and stability of the dentures then an implant-supported overdenture may be considered for the patient.

INTRODUCTION TO IMPLANTS

The use of implants in the field of dentistry has grown rapidly since its introduction in the early 1980s. This specialised area is generally considered a postgraduate subject and the majority of the work takes place in the private sector. However, a small percentage of dental implants are placed within the NHS, mainly for priority cases and for the purposes of clinical trials. This section serves as an introduction to the subject and aims to encourage further reading.

Osseointegration

A successful dental implant must be biologically accepted in the bone and is termed osseointegration. There is direct apposition of the bone to the implant material and there is no intervening fibrous tissue present. Osseointegration is a misnomer because there is no actual integration occurring between implant and bone, only close apposition of the bone to the implant material. There are many materials which are biologically acceptable and can serve as dental materials. However, titanium metal is the material of choice owing to its high compatibility and the ability to machine the material into the required shapes. The titanium oxide surface layer makes the material relatively inert and also provides a degree of bonding with the bone.

The main advantage of an implant is that it replaces lost teeth with a non-removable restoration. In doing so, it helps to restore function, aesthetics and speech. Although successful, there are some disadvantages associated with the treatment. The provision of an implant-borne restoration requires long-term care and this requires high patient cooperation. This also makes such treatment costly for the patient in comparison to more conventional forms of tooth replacement, such as dentures or bridges. Furthermore, patient exceptions may be high and it is often not possible to restore every mouth using implants. Often situations where an implant is suitable can be resolved with the use of a bridge or RPD. The clinician must prevent a denture/bridge problem becoming an implant problem through incorrect treatment planning.

The success of such treatment is assessed by the following four clinical parameters:

- implants are clinically immobile
- no peri-implant radiolucency
- vertical bone loss less than 0.2 mm/year
- no pain or infection.

Modern implantology is very successful but there were many other methods used by clinicians in an attempt either to improve denture-wearing or to provide support for a crown and bridgework. Initially, surgeons used pre-prosthetic surgery to improve the denture-bearing area. These were mainly soft tissue operations and included vestibuloplasties which aimed to improve the buccal sulcus. Such operations had mixed success rates.

Early techniques focused on subperiosteal implants. First the mucosa was reflected and an impression of the bone made. A framework was constructed and placed under the periosteum. These failed as the body attempted to encapsulate the metal framework with epithelium, and inevitably they were lost due to infection. An early forerunner of the modern implant was the blade implant. These were hammered into the bone, which was allowed to grow around the design, thus providing anchorage. The metal used was stainless steel and these implants had a poor success rate, with infection being the usual reason for failure.

Blocks or crystals of hydroxyapatite were used in an attempt to augment the resorbed ridge and met with limited success. These blocks were of limited value, as they tended to be unstable and migrate under the periosteum. This resulted in a flabby rather than a firm denture-bearing area.

It was the studies undertaken by Professor Brånemark and his team in the early 1980s that introduced the concept of osseointegration into implantology. Their work showed that implants constructed from titanium and placed under a certain clinical protocol brought about high success. The following is a brief description of these techniques.

Clinical procedure

Most modern implant treatment consists of a two-stage procedure. After treatment planning, the bone is surgically exposed and a pure titanium metal implant is placed therein. This is left buried in the bone and unloaded, usually for 3 months in the mandible and 6 months in the maxilla. After this healing period, the implant is uncovered and the final prosthesis is placed. There is an exception with one system (Straumann/Bonefit) which allows the implants to communicate with the mouth during the healing phase and this enjoys similar rates of success. Professor Brånemark based his clinical protocol on experience gained over a 10+ year period of implant treatment in over 700 patients between 1965 and 1982 and demonstrated a high success rate. It paved the way for extensive research and clinical reports which demonstrated the success of the implant technique. It is now known that the success of osseointegration in well controlled clinical trials is > 95% in the mandible and > 90% in the maxilla. The lower success in the maxilla appears to be related to the bone density and structure.

Present implant systems

Although the implant is made of commercially pure titanium, many of the systems that are available attempt to improve osseointegration by increasing the surface area (Fig. 12.76). This is done by:

- providing a hollow screw
- spraying implant surface with titanium plasma hydroxyapatite
- surface roughening by titanium blasting
- providing external threads on the implant.

The final restoration may be either a fixed or a removable prosthesis, and fixed restorations are all implant-supported designs. There are also specialised single tooth restorations. The removable implant designs are based on traditional overdenture procedures and may be retained by the use of studs, bars and magnets in a similar fashion to conventional overdentures.

Treatment planning

The best planning is via a team approach. This should ideally involve the oral surgeon and restorative dentist (specialities generally involved are fixed and removable prosthetics and periodontology). The dental technician should be involved in the planning process and the hygienist during the maintenance phase.

Treatment planning is very important, as is a good history. The clinician can quickly select on the psychological profile and personality of the patient. The patient's attitude to dentistry and motivation towards a long and intense form of treatment are also important. A clinical examination is undertaken followed by radiographs such as sectional CT scanning to assess the bone levels. An acrylic stent may be used to assist this process, and can be converted to a surgical stent to assist the oral surgeon (Fig. 12.77).

All surgical/prosthetic implant kits come with a selection of burs and various instruments for use with fixture and abutment placement. The burs supplied have a marking system to allow the clinician to determine the depth of hole cut in the bone. Ideally a fresh bur should be used for each patient.

Surgical procedure

A mucoperiosteal flap is raised and the tissues are reflected to reveal the underlying bone. The holes are cut using a saline-cooled bur driven by a torque reduction handpiece. The cutting temperature must not exceed 60°C, otherwise the bone cells will be destroyed leading to implant failure. Depending on the system used, the hole may either be tapped for placement of a threaded implant or receive a self-threaded implant. A depth gauge is used to verify the correct length of implant to be placed. The implant is handled by instruments and delivered to the surgical site. The mucoperiosteal flap is then closed and the area left to heal. The implants should not be loaded, thus enabling osseointegration to take place.

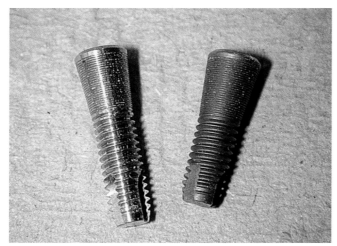

Fig. 12.76 Examples of a commercially available implant with screw thread. One surface is machined titanium (left) and the other has been titanium-blasted (right).

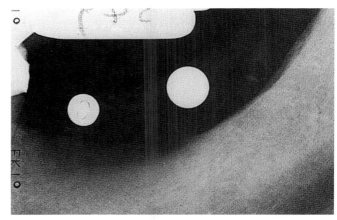

Fig. 12.77 An acrylic stent with metal markers to assist in the planning of where to place the implants.

The implants are left buried and unloaded for 3 months in the mandible and 6 months in the maxilla. During this time, dentures, if present, are lined with a tissue conditioner. If sufficient natural teeth are present then a temporary bridge may be placed. Wherever possible, any loading of the site which may prevent osseointegration taking place is avoided.

During the surgical procedure, if there is a bone deficiency, a non-resorbable membrane such as Gortex may be used to promote bone infill during implant placement.

After the healing phase, a small incision is made and the implant is uncovered. An abutment connector or a healing cap is placed and a period of time allowed for the peri-implant mucosa to heal within a controlled environment (Fig. 12.78). Following healing, the bridge is constructed as shown in Figure 12.79.

Single tooth implant

Single tooth implants follow similar procedures. After radiographic analysis and ridge mapping (depth gauging

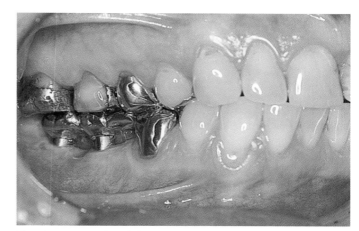

Fig. 12.79 Completed clinical case of a free end saddle replaced with implants.

with a graduated probe under local) to determine the presence of adequate bone, an implant is placed and allowed to osseointegrate (Fig. 12.80). After the second surgical phase, the abutments are placed and the crowns constructed

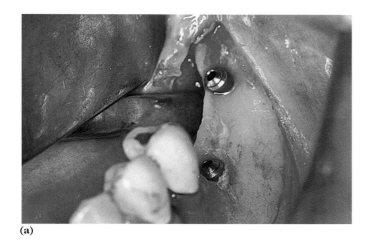

(a)

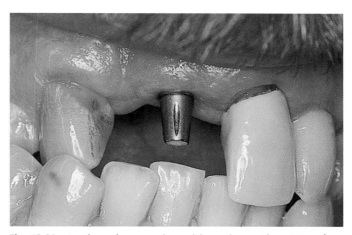

Fig. 12.80 Implant abutment in position prior to placement of a cantilever bridge.

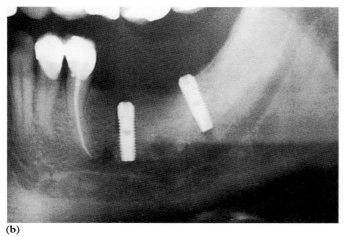

(b)

Fig. 12.78 (a) Implants correctly placed with cover screws prior to closure. (b) Radiographs of the implants in situ.

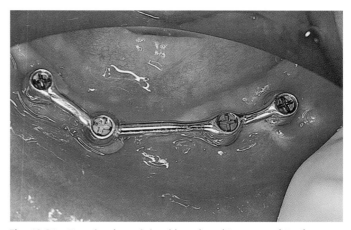

Fig. 12.81 Four implants joined by a bar. (Courtesy of Professor W.R.E. Laird.)

following conventional clinical and laboratory procedures. A transfer coping at the impression stage is passed to the laboratory to assist in the crown manufacture.

Overdentures

Implant-borne overdentures offer a simple and effective method of retaining dentures. This is done using a bar, studs or magnets. A bar prosthesis provides positive retention and stability to the complete lower overdenture. The clip is retained in the denture and the bar is linked to between two and four implants in the lower jaw (Fig. 12.81). The retentive clips are held in the denture. The bar is attached to caps which are retained by screws on the abutments. It is important that good oral hygiene is maintained around the abutments, especially at the join of the bar.

The ball-and-socket attachment relies on the frictional attachment of the gold housing over the stainless steel ball. The grip of the housing may be adjusted by opening or closing the gold wings. Sufficient retention may be gained by the use of two implants. A clinical picture showing the

housing situated in the denture and the stud attached to the abutment is illustrated in Figure 12.82.

Magnets provide a simple and effective method of retaining overdentures. They are made from iron–neodymium–boron encapsulated in a steel housing and are retained in the denture. They attach to a ferrous keeper which is attached to the implant abutment (Fig. 12.83). Up to two to four implants may be used for magnetic retention of the denture in the lower jaw.

Failure of implants

Plaque and calculus will attach to titanium implants, which will lead to inflammation of the tissues (Fig. 12.84). All these situations respond to increased awareness of oral hygiene procedures. An early complication of the implant placement is infection. This occurs within a few days of placement and will often lead to non-integration of the implant. Other common failures are related to the attachments. Single tooth crowns and bridges may fail due to

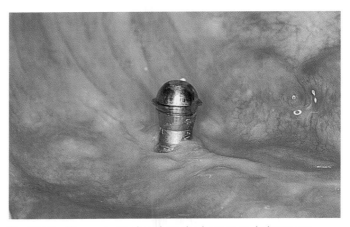

Fig. 12.83 The magnet placed on the keeper and abutment which will be processed into the denture.

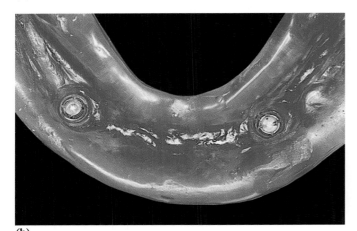

(a)

(b)

Fig. 12.82 (a) Two implant abutments with stud attachments. (b) The associated clips are cured into the denture.

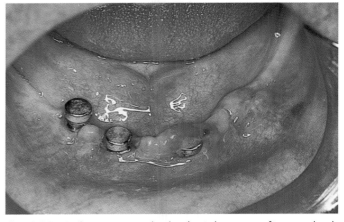

Fig. 12.84 Patients may receive implants but poor after-care leads to failure.

Table 12.3 Advantages and disadvantages of treatment options

Type of treatment	Advantages	Disadvantages
Fixed restoration 1. Conventional bridgework	Fixed	Involves tooth preparation which can result in pulp death
	Good aesthetics	Failure due to decementation and caries of abutment teeth may lead to further tooth loss
	Medium-term predictability is good for short-span bridges	Moderately expensive
	Good control of occlusion possible	Highly operator-dependent, requiring exacting techniques both clinically and technically
	Minimal compromise of oral hygiene	Requires lengthy clinical time and temporary restorations
		Irreversible
2. Resin-bonded bridgework	Minimal or no preparation	Lack of predictability Average life span 5–7 years
	Good aesthetics if ideal spacing exists	Requires high operator technique and enamel surface area for bonding
	Less expensive than conventional bridges	Change in colour/translucency of abutment teeth due to presence of retainer
	Consequences of failure are relatively small	May interfere with occlusion, particularly incisal guidance
		Debonding of retainer may lead to reduction in life span
Removable partial denture	Replaces multiple teeth in multiple sites	Patient acceptance may be poor
	Mucosa and/or teeth support	Connectors cover soft tissue such as palate and gingiva
	Generally do not require extensive preparation of abutment teeth	Coverage of gingival margins will lead to plaque retention and increase periodontal disease and caries
	May be designed to accommodate future tooth loss	Aesthetics compromised by retentive elements such as clasps
	Replaces missing soft tissue and provides soft tissue support	Moderate maintenance requirements and durability
	Aesthetics may be very good	
	Low cost	
Implant-retained prostheses	Fixed or removable	Requires the presence of adequate bone quantity and quality
	Independent of natural teeth for retention of crowns, etc.	Involves surgical procedures
	No dental caries, reduced or altered response to dental plaque	High operator technique/technique-dependent
	High level of predictability	High initial expense and lengthy treatment time
	Good maintenance of supporting bone	Moderate maintenance requirements especially for removable or extensive fixed prostheses

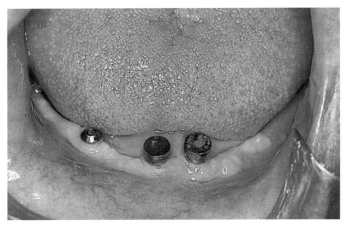

Fig. 12.85 Failure of attachments. One of the attachments (LR3) has fractured, leaving a screw thread in place.

incorrect assessment of the occlusion, leading to excessive forces being placed on them; consequences include loss of crowns and breakage of the attachments. Overdenture attachments are prone to wear and tear in the clinical environment. Clips used for either studs or bars may wear with use and require replacement (Fig. 12.85). If the steel casing is broken around a magnet, it will quickly corrode.

SUMMARY

This chapter has covered many different methods of restoring the edentulous space. Each has advantages and disadvantages and these are summarised in Table 12.3. The restorative care, as has been seen, can be complex and there are different indications for each treatment.

13 Integrated treatment planning

Restorative dentistry covers many different disciplines. It is relatively easy to consider undertaking treatment such as root canal therapy, restorations involving occlusal or proximal surfaces, or the provision of a removable partial denture. However, bringing all these events together in a logical clinical sequence is the decision process involved in a restorative treatment plan. There may be many different approaches to similar problems and these can vary from simple monitoring to more elaborate restoration of an occlusion. When considering a treatment plan, the skills and experience of the treating clinician are applied to the problem, at the same time taking account of the patient's wishes and demands.

SIMPLE RESTORATIVE TREATMENT PLANS

Simple restorative plans often arise when a patient is a regular attender and there are no presenting complaints. Such treatment planning will often contain the following items of treatment. In the first instance, the patient will require oral hygiene instruction. The teeth are disclosed and the patient is shown an appropriate toothbrushing technique. If there are concerns about the level of oral hygiene, it will be necessary to monitor the patient over subsequent visits. The most useful clinical tools in this case are simple plaque and bleeding indices. The patient may require a scaling with the removal of both supra- and subgingival calculus followed by polishing of the teeth. Simple plastic restorations may be undertaken and usually the patient is discharged with a recall being set for 6–12 months. Such treatment planning is simple and undemanding and the majority of regular attenders fall into this category.

Complications

This simple approach will change if the patient presents in pain or has other problems such as lost fillings or fractured teeth. The emphasis of any treatment planning must include aims to eliminate the immediate cause of this pain. Once this is solved, the routine treatment can be carried out. Elimination of the pain may well require temporisation. Decisions are made to resolve the situation and then the clinician can move back to the simple plan. An example of such emergency treatment is the construction of an immediate denture prior to the removal of a tooth. This may involve the addition of an artificial tooth to the patient's denture. Once resolved, it is then possible to return to simple treatment planning, eventually remaking the denture. Emergency treatment planning can involve different parts of restorative dentistry. Teeth marked down for extraction are removed. Simple root canal therapy is started and the patient is made comfortable. It may be possible to complete the root filling quickly, but usually the root canal is dressed with calcium hydroxide and stabilised. Gross caries is removed from the teeth, which are then stabilised.

The majority of treatment plans will include an initial phase of periodontal treatment. Such clinical work can give the clinician an idea of the patient's motivation and this may influence subsequent treatment. This phase will enable the clinician to motivate the patient and work at establishing a baseline from which further complicated procedures can be done.

OVERVIEW OF THE SPECIALITIES AND THEIR INFLUENCE ON THE TREATMENT PLAN

Periodontal procedures

As discussed in Chapter 3, the basic periodontal examination (BPE) provides an indication of the treatment needs of the patient (Box 13.1). This initial screening can be expanded to involve plaque and bleeding scores, recording of probing depths where indicated and the use of radiographs. Following this treatment the patient will be reviewed, and where a BPE score of 3 or 4 has been recorded, there may be a further series of appointments for root planing of the teeth in these areas. A need for periodontal surgery may become evident on subsequent review appointments.

Finally, a maintenance phase is put into place to see the patient regularly and check on the condition of the periodontium. This maintenance phase is important, as the patient needs to be monitored so that there are no lapses in home care. This periodontal treatment may then indicate the need for further treatment or, if there is poor patient compliance, the patient may only require simple restorative treatment. This is not the end of the periodontal considerations in the treatment planning process. Assessment of the conservation work may reveal overhanging ledges or poor crown margins that need attention. The design of any removable partial denture must take account of any detrimental effect it may have on the associated periodontal tissues. Finally, there is always the need to monitor and maintain periodontal health.

This approach to integrated planning involves the use of periodontal treatment and its subsequent influence as the first phase of therapy. This would then be followed by any operative or endodontic procedures. Fixed bridgework or removable partial denture options are undertaken towards the end of the treatment. Unfortunately, in many patients treatment is not straightforward and, as previously discussed, some patients may well require several visits to help draw up a provisional treatment plan, which may change during treatment.

Simple operative procedures

Many operative procedures involve the placement of plastic restorations. These are done in sequence either by quadrant or by complexity. Their placement follows any emergency treatment and the periodontal phase of therapy and any treatment plan may be modified as such (Box 13.2).

Anterior restorations may need to be completed first where aesthetics is important to the patient. Treatment of root caries or abrasion cavities will be completed at this stage as well. This is followed by the placement of posterior restorations. This may be all that is required and the patient can be discharged and recalled at an appropriate time in 6–12 months. This recall will be dependent upon the previous caries exposure and periodontal problems but many patients may generally be seen on a 12-monthly basis. More advanced operative procedures such as inlays, crowns, adhesive bridgework, and the placement of veneers would be left towards the end of the treatment plan and may require articulated casts and diagnostic wax-ups to assess the situation. A single crown may be incorporated into the plan comfortably; however, multiple crown work would necessitate articulation of casts and the use of radiographs to assist in the treatment planning process.

Endodontic therapy

Simple endodontic procedures are positioned early in the treatment plan in a similar manner to operative work. Single-rooted teeth such as the anterior incisors or canines may only require one to two visits to complete treatment. However, other teeth may exhibit variations in root canal morphology, and if complications occur during treatment it may be wise to stabilise the tooth with a dressing and leave further intervention until later on in the treatment plan. Any root canal treatment must take into account the subsequent restorative procedure, such as a pinned retained amalgam core and placement of an extracoronal restoration.

If there are anticipated problems with the final restoration, such as insufficient tooth substance remaining to support a crown or compromised periodontal health, then an early decision should be made as to whether the tooth is viable as a functional unit. Options such as hemi-

Box 13.1 Periodontal procedures
1. Basic periodontal examination (BPE)
2. Plaque and bleeding scores
3. Recording probing depths where indicated
4. Use of radiographs
5. Root planing
6. Reassess for surgery
7. Maintenance phase

Box 13.2 Modified treatment plan for simple operative procedures
1. Plaque and bleeding scores. Probing depths recorded
2. Scale and polish
3. Root planing where indicated
4. Placement of anterior and posterior plastic restorations

sectioning or crown root lengthening may appear to be solutions but are advanced procedures about which the patient must be fully informed, including the likely prognosis. It is often easy to overlook alternative options such as tooth removal and bridge provision in favour of a more complicated and potentially less successful procedure if the tooth has a poor prognosis. Molar root canal procedures are best left to the latter stages of a plan and may require specialist intervention. The overdenture procedure will require early endodontics prior to the provision of the removable prosthesis. The use of overdentures brings together many restorative procedures and a typical plan is as follows:

1. Extraction of non-viable teeth
2. Root canal treatment (RCT) of canines
3. Reduction in height of teeth
4. Fitting of overdenture.

Apical surgery is an important part of endodontic procedures and if a conventional approach is not successful then on reassessment an apicectomy is performed and retrograde root filling may be indicated.

Fixed and removable prosthetics

The placement of bridges or removable partial dentures will often require the production of casts and their articulation. This will allow the clinician to assess the problem prior to the subsequent appointment with the patient.

Casts production and articulation

Casts are important aids in treatment planning. They may require two visits in order to obtain secondary impressions which are made from special trays constructed on the preliminary casts. The master casts need to be articulated on a semi-adjustable articulator and this information is obtained from a registration and the use of a face bow recording. Such a diagnostic procedure will assist the clinician in the formation of a treatment plan for a complex case. As the case proceeds, the original treatment plan may need to be revisited using the articulated casts to assess the need for fixed and removable designs. It is at this stage that it will be possible to draw up the definitive denture design. Following this, the advanced crowns can be undertaken followed by the provision of the removable partial denture.

MAINTENANCE

Once advanced work is complete, the patient should be kept on a review regime. If advanced fixed prosthetic work has been undertaken, this should be protected by the use of an occlusal guard to prevent damage from parafunctional activities such as the grinding of teeth during sleep.

MODIFICATIONS TO INITIAL TREATMENT PLANNING

If a patient presents with a high caries rate (Box 13.3) then one of the first considerations is the implementation of a diet sheet. This will be undertaken over three visits. First, the sheet is given to the patient to take away and record food consumed over three separate days, one of which should be during the weekend when eating habits are often different. The times at which food is eaten are required together with the time that the patient retires to bed. At the second visit the diet sheet is collected, and it is analysed prior to the third visit (Fig. 13.1).

Sugar, fizzy and acidic drink consumption is identified together with any other caries or erosive foodstuffs. The time at which the last meal/snack is taken prior to bedtime is also identified. The simple rules are that sugar/erosive drinks should be consumed immediately after main meals and any snacks should be non-carious. No food or drink other than water should be taken within 30 minutes of going to sleep. All this is aimed at reducing the frequency of the sugar intake. This advice should be given to patients early in the treatment and reinforced periodically during subsequent clinical visits.

Tooth surface loss is becoming more commonplace. The causes of this condition are multifactorial and a diagnosis is required before advanced restorations are commenced. Compliance with dietary advice will quickly

---

Box 13.3 Treatment plan in patients with a high caries rate

1. Dietary advice (usually over three visits)
2. Temporise/stabilise gross caries
3. Reassess after a short recall (3 months)

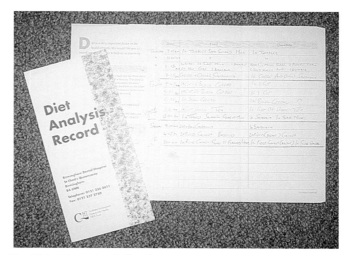

Fig. 13.1 Example of diet sheet.

become apparent during treatment. Examples of ongoing tooth surface loss include amalgams becoming proud of the surrounding tooth substance and obvious carious cavities that do not show signs of arresting (Fig. 13.2). A simple way of assessing tooth loss is by the production of casts, which are given to the patient to take away. At recall these casts are brought along to be re-examined and changes can be quickly detected.

CASE STUDIES

The discussion above gave some guidelines to approaching the integration of the different specialities that are involved in restorative dentistry. However, each patient is very different and it is difficult to cover all scenarios the clinician may come across. The following pages present a series of cases which involve different approaches to restorative treatment planning together with their eventual outcome. These cases should serve as an example of how to integrate the different specialities into a logical treatment plan. Each case is discussed using a layout that follows the sub-headings (and their abbreviations) for examining a patient that were introduced in Chapter 3 (Box 13.4).

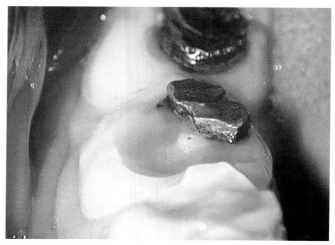
Fig. 13.2 Erosion occurring on a tooth which has left the amalgam proud.

Case 1

Mrs PS (25 years old)

RFA. This female patient was referred by her local dentist for replacement of her upper anterior crowns. They had been replaced 1 year earlier due to the poor gingival condition, which was thought to be due to poor crown margins. The new crowns had not improved the situation.

CO. The patient complained of gums that bled on brushing around the upper anterior crowns. The rest of the mouth did not have any symptoms (Fig. 13.3).

HPC. The original crowns had been provided 5 years ago as the teeth were heavily restored. The problem had occurred shortly after the original crowns were fitted.

MH. There was no relevant medical history.

DH. She attended regularly for treatment. She received routine care from her dentist, including scaling and polishing every 6 months.

Box 13.4 Aide-memoire

Referred by:	Reason for referral:
Date of referral:	Date seen:

1. Reason for attendance — RFA
2. Complains of — CO
3. History of present complaint — HPC
4. Medical history — MH
5. Dental history — DH
6. Personal/social history — PH/SH
7. Examination
   (a) *Extraoral* — EO
   (b) *Intraoral* — IO
     Soft tissue exam
     Hard tissue exam
     Periodontal assessment
     BPE screen
     Assessment of edentulous areas
     Assessment of removeable/fixed appliances
     Static/dynamic occlusion of teeth/prosthesis
8. Special investigations
9. Diagnosis
10. Treatment plan
11. Signature

*An 11-point structure to history-taking, examination, diagnosis and treatment planning with appropriate abbreviations (these may differ between teaching institutions but the general approach will be similar)

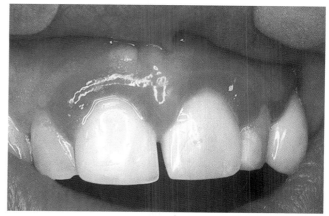
Fig. 13.3 Bleeding gums.

PH/SH. The patient brushed her teeth three times a day and occasionally used floss. Her diet was normal.

Extraoral. There were no problems with the temporomandibular joints (TMJs) and no other extraoral abnormality was diagnosed.

Intraoral. The oral soft tissues were healthy except in the upper anterior region adjacent to the porcelain crowns.

Teeth present:

7654321	1234567
7654321	1234567

Periodontal assessment

BPE:

4	3	4
4	2	4

There were very low plaque accumulations around the teeth.

Conservative assessment

The patient had few restorations present and these were in a satisfactory state.

Static/dynamic occlusion of teeth

The occlusion was normal with no significant deviations.

Special investigations – radiographic examination

Full-mouth, long cone periapicals were taken. There was no generalised bone loss except early loss noted around the anterior crowns.

Diagnosis

A diagnosis of early adult periodontitis was made, associated with the subgingival crown margins.

Treatment plan

The main objective of treatment was to provide an excisional flap to move the gingival margins apically away from the edges of the crowns. This would permit healing of the grossly inflamed gingival tissues.

Therefore, the following treatment plan was drawn up:

1. Check on home care measures
2. Scale and polishing
3. Periodontal excisional flap to reduce the gingival height to the level of the crowns (Figs 13.4 a, b, c).
4. Follow-up and maintenance (Fig. 13.5).

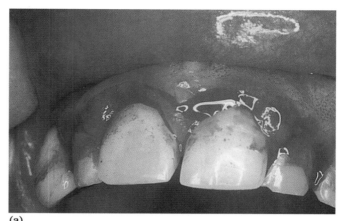
(a)

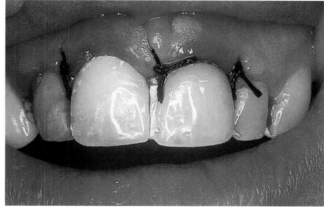
(b)

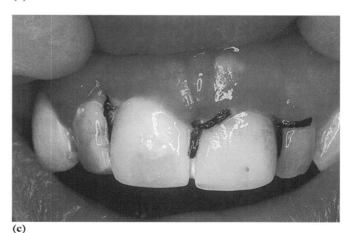
(c)

Fig. 13.4 Periodontal excisional flap to reduce gingival height to the level of the crowns.

5. Replace the crown if the revealed margins are seen to be deficient.

Discussion

Another possible treatment would be to remove the crowns and replace them with ones with excellent margins. This, combined with good subgingival plaque removal, will result

201

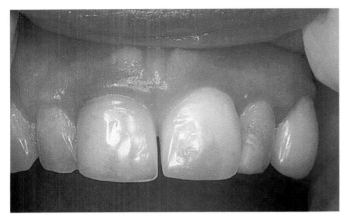

Fig. 13.5 Follow-up and maintenance.

in resolution of the inflammation. However, in this case this had already been attempted and the hoped for improvement had not occurred, perhaps due to the subgingival location of the crown margins in this periodontally susceptible patient. In this case an excisional flap may be undertaken to move the gingival margins apically away from the edges of the crowns. Ideally the crown margins should be left at the gingival margin as shown in this example.

Outcome

The patient's gingival health around the crowns improved dramatically and the periodontal condition was stabilised during the review period, which was for 2 years. The patient was then returned to her general dental practitioner who keeps her under regular review. She receives a hygiene appointment every 6 months.

Case 2

Mr KG (23 years old)

RFA. The patient attended the emergency department of his own accord.

CO. Pain from the lower jaw.

HPC. He had several broken teeth but had neglected visiting a dentist due to apprehension of having dental treatment. He had general pain on eating, especially on the right side of the mouth, but it had not been keeping him awake at night.

MH. There was no relevant medical history.

DH. Irregular attender.

PH/SH. He used to drink 10 cans of sugared cola a day but was trying to cut down and was now at three per day. He worked as a telephone engineer.

Extraoral There were no problems with the TMJs and no other extraoral abnormality was diagnosed.

Intraoral The soft tissues were healthy.

Teeth present:

8765321	1235678
8765321	123567

Clinical photographs of the case are shown in Figures 13.6a, b, c.

Periodontal assessment

BPE:

2	2	2
3	2	3

The level of oral hygiene was adequate but there was chronic marginal gingivitis present.

Conservative assessment

The patient had one restoration present. Frank caries was observed in the LR56 and the UL7. There was evidence of erosive tooth wear which was most evident on the lower anteriors.

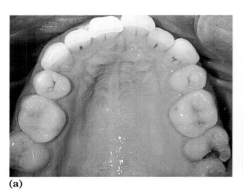
(a)

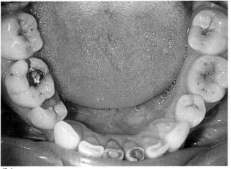
(b)

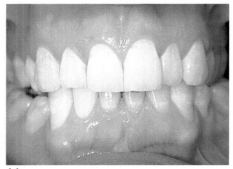
(c)

Fig. 13.6 Clinical photographs of Case 2 pre-treatment.

Static/dynamic occlusion of teeth

The patient came together in an intercuspal relationship and was canine guided on lateral excursions.

Special investigations – radiographic examination

Left and right bite wings and selected long cone periapicals were taken (Figs 13.7a–f). These show caries in several teeth and a periapical area associated with the LR1. Radiolucencies are present where the caries has involved the dentine in the following teeth:

$$\frac{\quad|\quad 78}{65\quad|\quad 5}$$

The LR1 has a radiolucency, which involves the apices of the LL12 teeth. The root filling in the tooth is not well condensed. Following the radiographs the lower incisors were subjected to electronic pulp testing and it was found that all were responsive except LR1.

Diagnosis

The following was diagnosed:

- caries
- chronic marginal gingivitis (some evidence of historical bone loss)
- periapical infection related to the non-vital LR1
- tooth wear.

Treatment plan

The main objective of treatment in this situation was to relieve the patient's pain and then encourage him to become a regular attender at the dentist. The treatment plan should include a regime to prevent further tooth loss by caries and erosion and to improve the patient's oral hygiene. Early on in the treatment plan those teeth that were not considered restorable should be extracted. The following visits should be aimed at improving the periodontal care, removing caries and giving dietary advice. Once the active disease was stabilised, the restorations, including the root canal treatment (RCT), could be undertaken. Finally the patient should be recalled on a regular basis to ensure that the preventative regime is being followed.

Therefore the following treatment plan was drawn up:

1. Relieve pain by temporary dressing to LR5
2. Extraction of non-restorable teeth:

$$\frac{\quad|\quad 78}{5\quad|}$$

3. Instigate oral hygiene procedures with scale and polish, oral hygiene instruction. Issue diet sheet
4. Remove caries and stabilise LR6 and LL5. Collect and advise on diet sheet
5. Restorations:

$$\frac{\quad|}{7\quad|\quad 5}$$

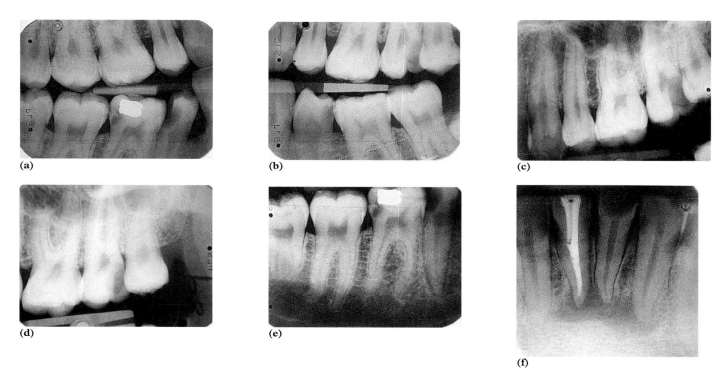

(a) (b) (c)

(d) (e)

(f)

Fig. 13.7 Radiographic examination of Case 2.

6. RCT LR1
7. Assess RCT LR6 or extraction
8. Aesthetic restorations on lower incisors
9. Study models for patient and reassess for possible advanced restorations
10. Recall.

Discussion

The clinical pictures show that the acid erosion (from cola) had affected many teeth, as seen by their glassy appearance, and ridging of the incisal tips. There is little staining on the smooth surfaces, in spite of inadequate oral hygiene. This suggests that regular 'acid washing' was present, preventing stain from forming. The treatment plan includes both dietary advice and the use of study models, which are a record of the tooth surfaces and can be examined at subsequent appointments.

Outcome

The patient had the teeth removed and is undergoing treatment successfully. The RCT of the LR1 showed that there was an extra canal present that had not been treated (45% of lower central incisors have an extra canal). The patient has complied with dietary advice but the real evidence will be the observation of no change with silicone index impressions taken at review appointments and compared with the patient's study models.

Attendance and motivation were high and eventually the molar RCT was undertaken towards the end of the treatment plan. If compliance had been low, the option of extraction would have been considered. This plan shows the need to stabilise dentitions, instigate preventative regimes and undertake more complicated procedures such as molar RCT later in the treatment plan.

Case 3

Mr NS (26 years old)

Endodontic problems may arise in association with periodontal disease. Examples include sensitivity due to exposed cervical dentine or an abscess. In such situations it is important to analyse the situation in a systematic manner as the abscess may be periodontal or endodontic in origin.

RFA. This man was referred to the periodontal department for management of his periodontal disease.

CO. One year previously the patient had been advised by his own dentist that he had gum disease. He was aware of an abscess in his lower jaw near the front of his mouth and this was troubling him.

HPC. There was a 2-year history of bleeding gums and his own dentist had prescribed a course of antibiotics for an intraoral swelling.

MH. There was no relevant medical history.

DH. The patient was a regular attender every 6 months.

PH/SH. He brushed twice a day and for interdental cleaning used a bottle brush and floss. He smoked three cigarettes per day.

Extraoral. No problems with TMJs and no lymphadenopathy.

Intraoral. Subgingival calculus present, swelling LL2 region.

Teeth present:

87654321	12345678
87654321	12345678

Periodontal assessment

BPE:

4	4	4
4	4	4

Conservation assessment

Some small amalgam restorations were present. No active caries was noted.

Occlusal relations

The patient had a class I relationship. On right lateral excursion there was contact on LR2 and on left lateral excursions on LL2. Both the LL2 and LR2 were over-erupted by 1 mm.

Special investigations

Pulp test. LL2 positive, LL3 negative, LL4 positive.

Radiographic examination. Bone loss 60–70% generally, 50% on LL3. There was a periradicular radiolucency on LL3.

Diagnosis

1. Rapidly progressive periodontitis with secondary occlusal trauma
2. Perio-endodontic lesion LL3.

Treatment plan

The objectives of the treatment plan were to stabilise the periodontal condition and provide endodontic treatment LL3:

1. Reinforce oral hygiene with attention to interproximal cleaning
2. Full-mouth fine scaling
3. Endodontic treatment LL3
4. Review oral hygiene with view to further periodontal therapy.

Discussion

The radiographs of this patient show an example of complex root canal anatomy (Figs 13.8–13.10). The LL3 had two root canals, which merge apically. One lateral canal can be seen in the coronal third, two in the middle third and there is an apical delta. The periradicular lesion lay on the mesial aspect of the root, reflecting the position of the portals of exit/entry. The LL3 was not carious but the degree of bone loss could have exposed the more coronally placed portals of exit/entry. This, together with the previous periodontal instrumentation, may have resulted in pulp necrosis.

The obturation film shows sealant overfill through the portals of exit. The coronal and middle third communications lie adjacent to the periodontal pocket. The follow-up radiograph shows bone infill with an absence of sealer laterally (Fig. 13.11). The infill has occurred as a result of managing the microbiological problem in the root canal.

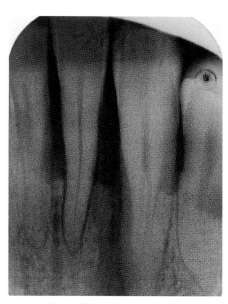

Fig. 13.8 Preoperative radiograph showing periradicular lesion and periodontal bone loss associated with LL3.

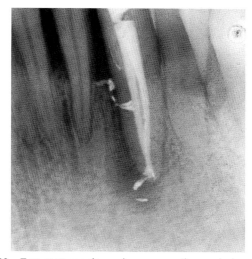

Fig. 13.10 Two root canals can be seen on the angled postoperative radiograph.

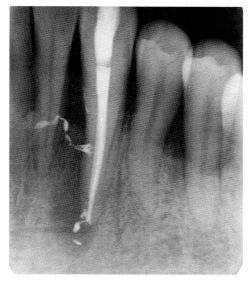

Fig. 13.9 Postoperative radiograph showing complex root canal anatomy (straight on view).

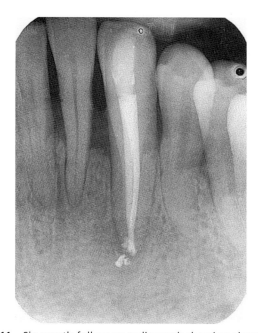

Fig. 13.11 Six-month follow-up radiograph showing absence of sealer and bony infill laterally. Apical healing is also progressing satisfactorily.

The sealer excess may have been washed out by gingivo-crevicular fluid or removed during subsequent scaling procedures. Apical healing is progressing well despite the sealer, although it may be slightly delayed.

Outcome

This case illustrates that healing will occur in the presence of excess filling material, provided treatment is directed at microbiological management. It also highlights the importance of a systematic approach and the use of appropriate special tests to reach a diagnosis.

Case 4

Mr RC (23 years old)

RFA. Referred by general practitioner following a fall.

CO. The patient complained of broken teeth which were sensitive.

HPC. The patient fainted in the heat and fell down on the pavement after finishing his degree examination! He fell on his chin, which led to shearing of several teeth and cuts to his tongue. There was a midline fracture of the mandible. Emergency treatment consisted of dressing the broken teeth and monitoring the fracture, which was stable. He was anxious to get treatment underway as he was having job interviews outside the area.

MH. There was no relevant medical history.

DH. He was a regular attender and had undergone little dental treatment previously.

PH/SH. The patient cleaned his teeth twice a day and was a non-smoker.

Extraoral. Initially following the accident there had been problems with pain on opening over the left TMJ and limited opening. Now there was no pain and he had normal opening. Mouth opening at time of examination was approximately three fingers.

Intraoral. The soft tissues were healthy.

Teeth present:

87654321	12345678
87654321	12345678

Clinical photographs of the case at the time of presentation are shown in Figures 13.12 a, b, c.

Periodontal assessment

BPE:

2	2	2
2	2	2

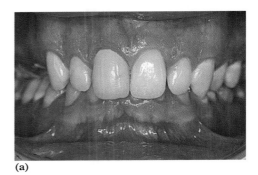
(a)

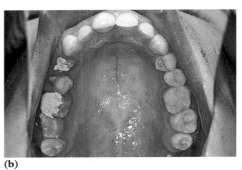
(b)

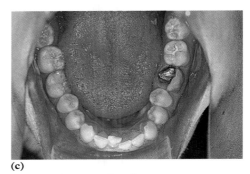
(c)

Fig. 13.12 Clinical photographs of Case 4 pre-treatment.

The mouth was well cared for but gingival inflammation was present around those teeth that were fractured.

Conservative assessment

The following teeth were fractured:

654	4
6 1	6

The UR456 were badly fractured whilst the others were less severe. The UL1 had a porcelain jacket crown although this had an overhanging margin. The other amalgams were simple surface restorations in apparent good order.

Static/dynamic occlusion of teeth

The patient was able to achieve an intercuspal position.

Special investigations

Radiographic examination. Anterior long cone periapicals and a panoramic radiograph were taken and these are shown in Figure 13.13. A hairline fracture is associated with the lower incisors. UR4, 5 and 6 have fractures, which are at or below the bone level with evidence of pulpal involvement. LR6 and LL6 crowns are fractured with no pulpal involvement. LL7 has occlusal caries.

Thermal and electrical pulp testing. This revealed that all teeth with the exception of the severely fractured teeth were responsive to testing.

Diagnosis

Fracture of mandible and several teeth due to fall after fainting. Gingivitis is also present.

Treatment plan

The main objective of treatment was to remove those teeth which were severely fractured and restore function and aesthetics of the other teeth in the arches. Therefore the following treatment plan was drawn up:

1. Investigate UR 4, 5 and 6 with a view to their immediate extraction
2. Instigate oral hygiene procedures with a scale and polish
3. Restore UL6, LR6, LL6 and UR7 with amalgam
4. Articulated study casts for upper partial denture
5. LR6, LL6 and UR7 full veneer gold crowns
6. UL1 replace porcelain jacket crown
7. Upper cobalt/chromium removable partial denture (RPD).

Discussion

The patient received the initial emergency treatment at a local casualty department. Radiographs were taken to assess for any facial fractures and the midline fracture was considered to be stable so that dental treatment could be carried out. The impact on the chin resulted in shearing of

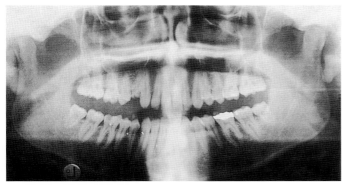

Fig. 13.13 Radiographic examination of Case 4.

the teeth as they met violently in occlusal contact at the time of the fall. A decision was made early on to assess which teeth were not restorable and this was immediately apparent: UR4, 5 and 6 were removed by a minor oral surgery procedure. Fortunately aesthetics was not a problem and there was not a need to provide an immediate replacement.

Following healing the patient can receive hygiene treatment after which the teeth can be restored. Before advanced restorations are carried out, impressions are taken and the resulting casts are articulated. The provisional RPD design is made and then the crowns can be commenced. Finally the RPD is constructed. In this case it was not possible to fill the space with a fixed bridge as the span was too large. Furthermore, the UR3 was intact and the UR7 had been fractured in the fall and therefore there was a question-mark over its ability to support such a bridge design.

Outcome

Although a well-thought-out treatment plan was drawn up, there were complications during treatment. This was related to the LL6 and LR6. A few months after the accident both teeth became sensitive and caused pain and discomfort. The LL6 started to give pain of a throbbing nature. This was worse on biting and on presentation had interrupted sleep. A diagnosis of acute apical abscess was made. Root canal treatment was commenced but over four visits it was not possible to achieve a dry and symptom-free mesiolingual canal. It was concluded that the root might be fractured and the tooth was extracted. A month later the LR6 gave similar symptoms and this time the patient requested extraction in preference to the RCT option. All other restorative treatment was completed and the RPD was provided. The final result is shown in Figures 13.14 a, b, c.

Case 5

Mr IE (50 years old)

RFA. Practitioner referral requesting a periodontal assessment of the patient and a request for treatment.

CO. The patient complained of loose teeth and poor aesthetics.

HPC. The problem of loose teeth had become apparent over the last few months. However he had had several gum infections which had been treated with antibiotics.

MH. There was no relevant medical history.

DH. Not a regular attender but has started to visit the dentist due to concerns about his teeth. He needed to have his upper posterior teeth removed in the last few weeks due to looseness and infection.

PH/SH. The patient brushed occasionally but tended to rely on mouthwashes. He smoked 20 cigarettes per day.

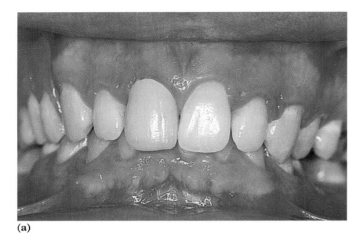

(a)

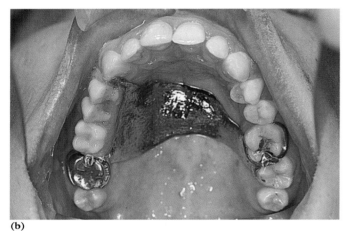

(b)

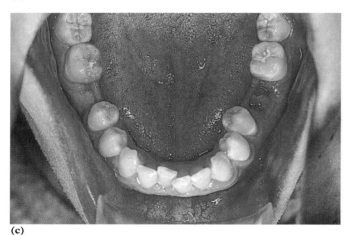

(c)

Fig. 13.14 Case 4 after restorative treatment.

Extraoral. There were no abnormalities detected.

Intraoral. The soft tissues were healthy.

Teeth present on examination:

54321	2345
654321	123456

Clinical photographs of the case are shown in Figure 13.15 a–d.

Periodontal assessment

BPE:

4	4	4
4	4	4

There were large deposits of plaque and calculus on the teeth. Mobility of several teeth was present and this was most pronounced in the upper arch. The lower teeth did not show excessive mobility.

Conservative assessment

The patient had few restorations present and these were in a satisfactory state, although the lower restorations were poorly contoured.

Static/dynamic occlusion of teeth

The patient closed together in intercuspal position which was not fully stable due to mobility of upper teeth.

Special investigations – radiographic examination

Full-mouth, long cone periapicals were taken prior to removal of the upper posterior teeth (Fig. 13.16). This shows generalised bone loss which is most pronounced in the posterior sextants. The upper canines show better bone support than the other teeth in the upper arch.

Removable prosthodontic assessment

The patient was wearing an ill-fitting upper acrylic partial denture to replace the UL1. This was unstable and unretentive with poor aesthetics.

Diagnosis

A diagnosis of chronic adult periodontitis was made.

Treatment plan

The main objective of treatment was to improve the periodontal status of the patient which had led to considerable loss of bone around the teeth. The prognosis for the majority of the teeth was poor and the patient faced the prospect of wearing an upper and lower complete denture. However, it was considered possible to conserve the lower arch and, with the potential use of the upper canines as abutments, an overdenture could be provided.

Therefore the following treatment plan was drawn up:

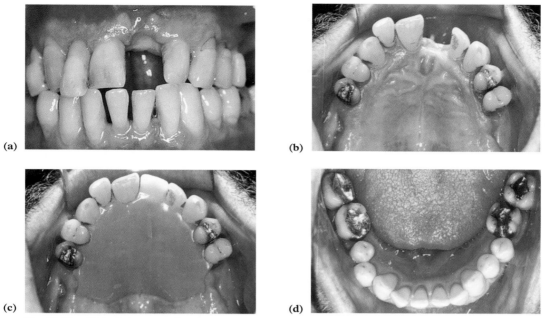

(a) (b)

(c) (d)

Fig. 13.15 Clinical photographs of Case 5 pre-treatment.

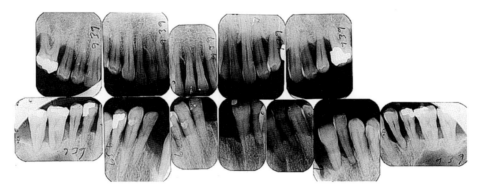

Fig. 13.16 Radiographic examination of Case 5.

1. Oral hygiene instruction and improve motivation towards dental treatment
2. Probing depth measurements in sextants scoring 4
3. Scale and polish followed by root planing
4. Removal of all upper teeth with the exception of the canines and the construction of an immediate replacement denture
5. RCT on upper canines
6. Removal of crowns, convert canines to overdenture abutments and addition of artificial teeth to present denture
7. Review and monitor situation until new complete denture made in 12 months' time.

Discussion

The periodontal condition of this patient was poor and there was a strong possibility that the majority of the teeth

would be extracted. A decision was made to keep those teeth that had a reasonable prognosis. The lower arch had reasonable bone support and the periodontal treatment focused on this area. The teeth in the upper arch had a poor prognosis. However, the canines could be saved and they would prevent bone resorption from the loads applied by the lower natural teeth. This would prevent the formation of a flabby ridge where the tissue remained but where there was resorption of the underlying bone. The abutment teeth would also help with retention and stability of the upper denture.

Outcome

The periodontal treatment was carried out and the patient made exceptional progress. The teeth were cleaned and this was followed by root planing of the lower quadrants. The removal of the upper teeth was undertaken as planned and at the time of extraction an immediate denture was placed. Root canal therapy was undertaken after which the crowns were removed and replacement teeth added to the denture. After 12 months a final complete upper overdenture was made. In order to assist with retention, the new denture incorporated magnets within its fitting surface. The keepers were made from ferromagnetic metal and fashioned into overdenture abutments. This magnet retention was successful and the patient has been stable for over 5 years, only requiring the re-cementation of one of the copings (Figs 13.17 a, b, c).

Case 6

Mr AG (60 years old)

RFA. An opinion from the patient's local general dental practitioner was requested.

CO. The main complaint was a loose upper denture.

HPC. The patient had been losing teeth progressively over a number of years and now the dentures were causing problems. This was mainly due to the difficulty of wearing a denture that covered his palate which was causing him to gag due to the looseness. The lower denture was also loose and was causing similar problems.

MH. There was nothing relevant.

DH. The patient was a regular attender at his own dentist and had worn his present dentures for about 5 years.

PH/SH. The patient brushed twice a day and occasionally suffered from bleeding gums.

Extraoral. On talking it was noticed that the occlusal plane of the teeth sloped downwards on one side but no other abnormalities were observed.

Intraoral. The soft tissues were healthy.

Teeth present:

$$\frac{3^x \quad 2^x \quad 1}{7 \quad\quad 321} \bigg| \frac{12 \quad\quad\quad 7}{123 \quad 4_x}$$

Clinical pictures of the case are shown in Figures 13.18a–d.

Periodontal assessment

BPE:

–	2	3
3	2	–

The standard of oral hygiene was poor, with deposits of plaque and calculus.

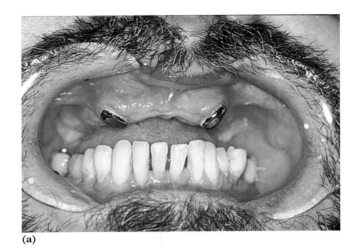

(a)

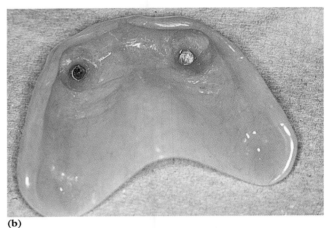

(b)

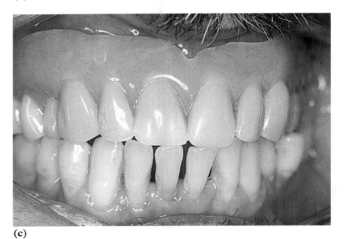

(c)

Fig. 13.17 Case 5 post-treatment. The keepers (**a**) are cemented with the magnets processed in the denture. The completed case is showned in (**c**).

Conservative assessment

UR23 were overdenture abutments and required restoration due to root caries. LL4 was grossly carious. Other problems included UL12 crowns that had deficient crown margins and evidence of tooth wear on the lower anterior teeth.

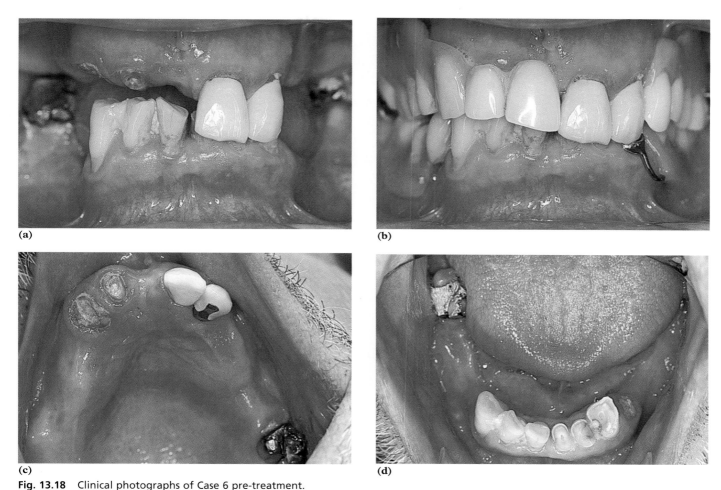

Fig. 13.18 Clinical photographs of Case 6 pre-treatment.

Removable prosthodontic assessment

The upper denture-bearing area was well formed but denture-induced stomatitis was present across the hard palate. The lower denture-bearing area was well formed in the edentulous areas. The present dentures were mucosal-borne. The upper denture was constructed from cobalt/chromium but there was minimal palatal coverage with no attempt at support from the teeth. The lower denture was acrylic but its stability and retention were poor and appeared to contribute to the high level of plaque formation and gingival trauma that occurred around the teeth.

Static/dynamic occlusion of teeth

The face height was decreased and there was an occlusal stop on the UL12 without the dentures placed in the mouth. The present dentures had worn occlusal surfaces and had led to a sloping occlusal plane and this resulted in an adaptive muscular position where the patient protruded forward onto the anterior teeth. There was minimal contact on the left side of the teeth.

Special investigations – radiographic examination

Long cone periapicals are shown in Figure 13.19. These show fracture of the UR3 overdenture abutment, deficient crown margins and radiolucent areas associated with the LL4 root and the LL2.

Diagnosis

Chronic adult periodontitis, root caries and unstable dentures.

Treatment plan

The main objective of treatment was to prevent further tooth surface loss from both parafunctional activity and poor diet. The patient had received restorative work previously which had included an overdenture option. However, neglect and poor diet had resulted in root caries. Once the preventative treatment was seen to be working, further restorative work could be commenced. This would be aimed at restoring the patient's occlusion with upper and lower removable dentures but designed so as not to

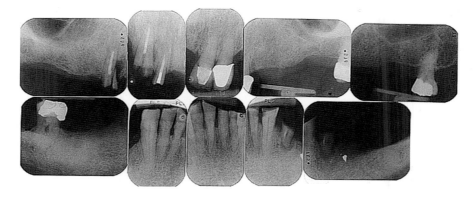

Fig. 13.19 Radiographic examination of Case 6.

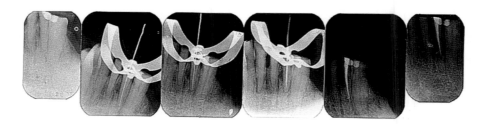

Fig. 13.20 Endodontic treatment of LL2 in Case 6.

compromise gingival health. Some of the teeth were not restorable and would require extraction, to be carried out early in the treatment plan.

Therefore, the following treatment plan was made:

1. Scale and polish and intensive oral hygiene instruction – this to be undertaken by a hygienist. The instructions to the hygienist should include particular emphasis on denture hygiene
2. Extraction of UR3 and LL4
3. RCT LL2 (Fig. 13.20)
4. Restore LL23
5. Draw up provisional removable partial denture design
6. Provisional occlusal splint to increase the occlusal vertical dimension
7. Gold coping UR2
8. Replace porcelain-bonded crowns UL12, incorporating rest seats in the cingulum area
9. Construction of upper and lower removable partial dentures
10. Maintenance.

Discussion

This plan brought together all the specialities involved within restorative dentistry. The patient had worn his present denture for 5 years but had not been on regular maintenance visits. Consequently, his dentition had been neglected. There was fracture of an overdenture abutment, periapical pathology and deficient crown margins related to root caries. The treatment plan aimed to remove those teeth that were not restorable and then to provide preventative treatment. Very early on in the treatment, a provisional denture design should be drawn up and this would help with the subsequent restorative treatment. A provisional appliance should be placed to correct the increased occlusal vertical dimension and to protect the replacement crowns prior to the construction of the final denture. Then it will be possible to undertake the root canal treatment and the replacement of the crowns. Finally the dentures should be made and the patient placed on a strict maintenance regime.

Outcome

In this case the treatment progressed without complication according to the original plan that was made. Maintenance has been ongoing for 2 years and at the 24-month stage it was noticed that wear of the occlusal surfaces of the acrylic teeth had occurred and a new denture was constructed. The periodontal condition and other restorative work has remained stable and there has not been any new root caries diagnosed (Figs 13.21a–e).

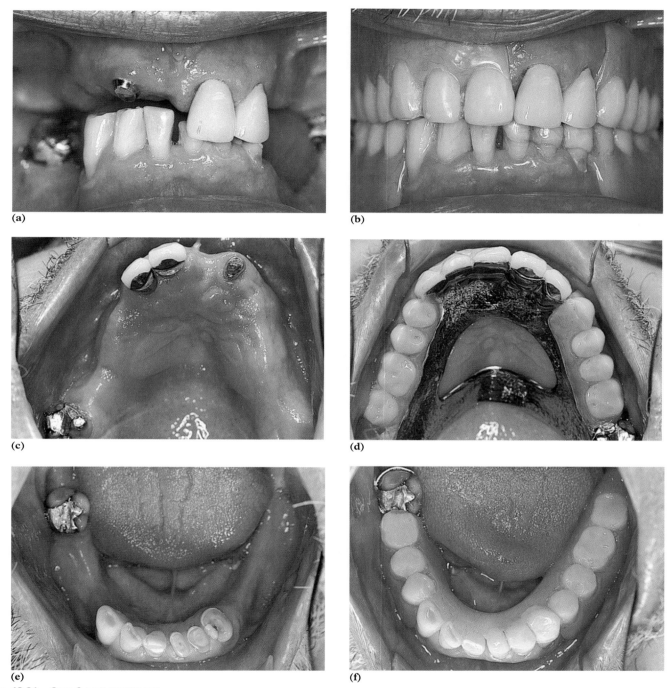

(a)

(b)

(c)

(d)

(e)

(f)

Fig. 13.21 Case 6 post-treatment.

Case 7

Miss MM (27 years old)

RFA. The patient attended, having complained that her teeth were sensitive to hot and cold drinks at a meeting with a psychologist at an eating disorders self-help group. The psychologist subsequently arranged a dental appointment.

CO. The patient complained of sensitivity to cold drinks on several posterior teeth and additionally stated that she was aware that her anterior teeth were 'chipping' and becoming shorter.

HPC. The patient had experienced similar problems for approximately 3 years but stated that the problem was worsening on the right side of her mouth.

MH. The patient stated that she had been bulimic for 4 years and that she had previously vomited up to 15 times per day. She also said that, now that she was attending the self-help group, she was getting the habit under control and that she now wished to have the appearance of her teeth improved and the sensitivity treated.

DH. She had been a regular attender in the past, when she had received a number of amalgam restorations, but had only received one course of treatment since she started suffering from bulimia. That treatment had involved the placement of three crowns in the upper left quadrant for the treatment of sensitivity.

PH/SH. The patient brushed her teeth many times per day, usually after vomiting. She rarely used floss. Her diet history was vague.

Extraoral. There were no problems with the TMJs, no facial asymmetry and no cervical lymphadenopathy.

Intraoral. The soft tissues were generally healthy. Plaque deposits were noted on the buccal aspects of some upper posterior teeth.

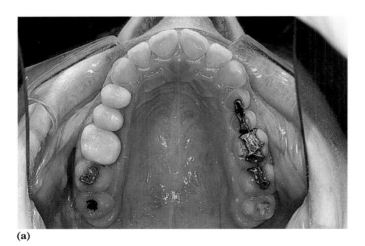

(a)

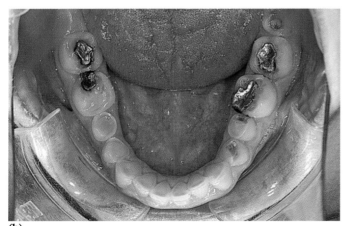

(b)

Fig. 13.22 Mirror view of upper arch (a) and lower arch (b) at presentation in Case 7.

Teeth present (Fig. 13.22):

87654321	12345678
7654321	1234567

BPE:

1	1	1
1	2	1

The standard of oral hygiene was fair with some plaque and calculus deposits.

Conservative assessment

Full crown restorations were present at UL 654. Restorations of amalgam were present in many posterior teeth. In many of these teeth, dentine was exposed occlusally and amalgam restorations which were present stood proud of the tooth surface (Fig. 13.23). Such features are typical of the patient suffering from bulimia. Dentine was exposed on the palatal aspects of the upper anterior teeth, with the incisors being particularly affected. The incisal edges of the upper anterior teeth were chipped, and in UL12 they were translucent due to the loss of support for the incisal enamel (Fig. 13.24). The mandibular incisor teeth also exhibited tooth substance loss (TSL), with dentine being exposed at the incisal edges of these teeth.

Many teeth contained restorations in amalgam. Many required replacement because of tooth substance loss around the restorations and because of the patient's complaint of sensitivity. The full crown restorations in the maxillary left quadrant were of good fit. Caries was noted in a number of mandibular posterior teeth.

Static/dynamic occlusion of teeth

This was class I and was canine-guided on both sides.

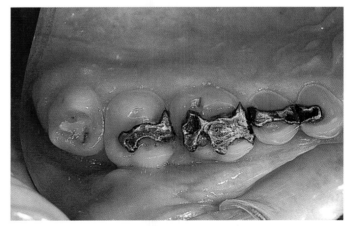

Fig. 13.23 In teeth affected by erosive tooth substance loss, amalgam restorations may stand proud of the remaining tooth surface.

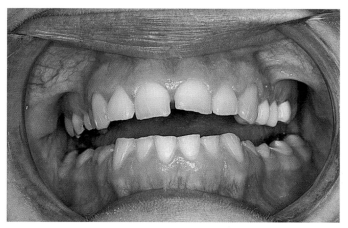

Fig. 13.24 View of anterior teeth with teeth apart.

Special investigations – radiographic examination

Full-mouth, long cone periapical radiographs were taken. These showed no loss of bony support, that there was some secondary dentine formation in the maxillary anterior teeth, and confirmed the presence of caries in a number of mandibular posterior teeth. No teeth were found to have areas of periapical radiolucency.

Diagnosis

Diagnoses of erosive tooth substance loss and caries were made.

Treatment plan

Treatment objectives were to counsel the patient in respect of the causes of the erosive TSL, to cover the areas of exposed dentine which were causing sensitivity, to treat the caries, to improve oral hygiene and to improve the appearance of the upper anterior teeth.

It was decided that the caries would be treated by placement of amalgam restorations. The TSL, which was particularly severe at UR456 and LL54, would be treated by placement of full coverage restorations, except at UR6 in which it was considered that an onlay-type restoration would be satisfactory. Because of the erosive TSL, the teeth to be crowned were of reduced crown height. It was therefore considered that conventional crowns would be likely to be poorly retained, so adhesive restorations were indicated, i.e. dentine-bonded crowns.

The anterior teeth should also be crowned. Palatal veneers in ceramic or composite could be provided. These would effectively cover exposed areas of dentine but would have no impact on the poor aesthetics about which the patient had expressed concern. It was therefore decided that minimal preparation full crown restorations should be placed, i.e. dentine-bonded crowns. In these restorations, there is no metal framework, so the preparation is less than

necessary for a metal-ceramic restoration. The crowns are luted with a dual-cure resin cement, with the dentine being treated by a dentine-bonding agent.

Other teeth suffering from TSL, but for which restoration was not considered necessary at this stage, would be kept under review and treated if TSL was thought to be continuing.

The treatment plan was therefore as follows:

1. Counsel patient with regard to her bulimic habit. The patient was advised not to brush her teeth after vomiting, as this will lead to excessive loss of dentine from the surfaces which have been affected by acid. Instead, the patient was advised to rinse her mouth with a sodium bicarbonate mouth rinse, and to brush her teeth 30 minutes later. In view of the presence of caries, a fluoride mouth rinse was also prescribed.
2. Reinforce home care, provide dietary advice, scaling and polishing.
3. Treat caries in mandibular posterior teeth with amalgam restorations.

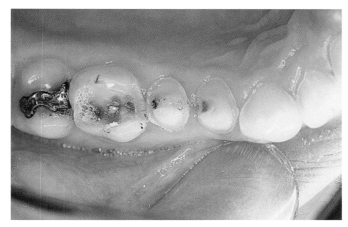

Fig. 13.25 Preparation for full-coverage dentine-bonded crowns on UR45 and onlay at UR6.

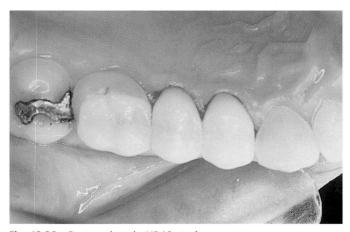

Fig. 13.26 Restorations in UR46 at placement.

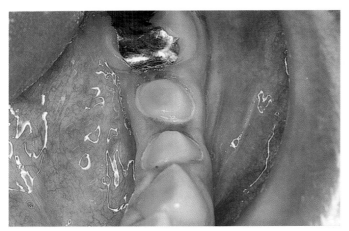

Fig. 13.27 Preparations for full-coverage dentine-bonded crowns at LL45.

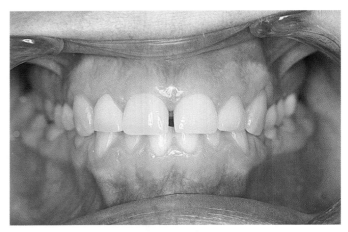

Fig. 13.30 Crowns at UR12UL12 at placement.

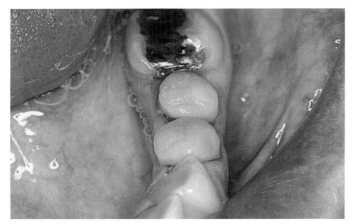

Fig. 13.28 Restorations at LL45 at placement.

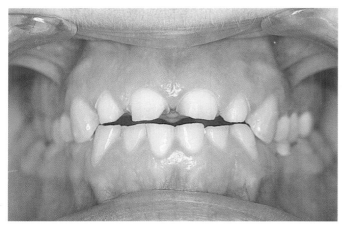

Fig. 13.29 Minimal preparations for dentine-bonded crowns at UR12UL12.

4. Provision of dentine-bonded crowns at LL54, UR45 and a ceramic onlay at UR6 (Figs 13.25–13.28)
5. Provision of dentine-bonded crowns at UR12, UL12 (Figs 13.29 and 13.30).

6. Maintenance – review tooth substance loss at UR3UL3 and LL123 LR123 by way of study casts and photographs (Figs 13.31 a, b, c).

Discussion

Patients are increasingly presenting with TSL, the causes often being multifactorial, involving erosion and attrition. A management priority must be removal of the cause, and this will involve counselling the patient once the causative factors have been identified. However, in cases of erosive TSL when the patient is bulimic, counselling may be difficult, as the patient may not, at the outset, admit to the bulimic habit. In this respect, it has been considered that bulimia or other gastic reflux habits may account for a substantial proportion of cases presenting with severe TSL in which the patient does not admit to dietary factors such as excessive consumption of citrus drinks or fruits, or carbonated beverages.

Treatment of patients suffering from bulimia may be problematic, as these patients often suffer from other problems such as drug or alcohol abuse. Accordingly, there may be problems with attendance. These patients may have poor self-esteem and poor body image. The dentist may therefore play a real part in improving this. There are problems related to the retention of restorations in teeth affected by TSL, so the adhesive techniques, which are available, may be indicated. However, there is no rule which states that tooth wear must be treated by tooth-coloured restorations, and so many of this patient's mandibular teeth, which were affected by TSL and caries, were treated by placement of amalgam restorations in an undergraduate student clinic. There are other problems often associated with the treatment of teeth affected by TSL, namely the over-eruption of opposing teeth leaving reduced – or no – space for restorations. In such cases, the use of a Dahl appliance or the Dahl principle may be necessary. In this case, this did not present as a problem,

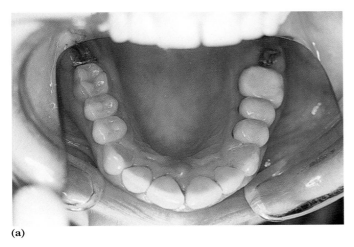

(a)

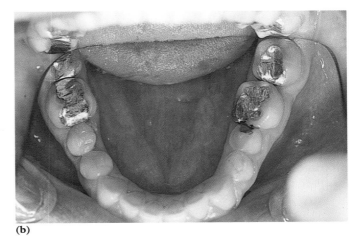

(b)

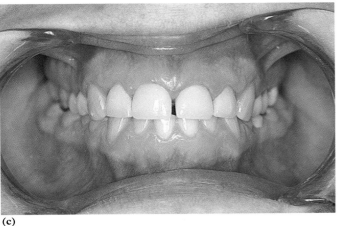

(c)

Fig. 13.31 Review of tooth substance loss at UR3UL3 and LL123LR123 by way of photographs.

which meant that treatment could be carried out without any change to the patient's occlusion.

Outcome

The patient responded well to the efforts of the dental team. She stated that she 'felt much better about herself' and eventually reduced her bulimic habit and returned to work. While this may not have been solely due to the dental treatment that the patient received, the fact that someone was prepared to care for her and treat her dentition – which also resulted in an aesthetic improvement – may have helped to improve her self-esteem. Those of the patient's teeth which have not received full coverage restorations are now checked 6-monthly for TSL. Caries appears to be under control.

Case 8

Mrs FW (63 years old)

R.F.A. The patient was referred for an implant assessment.

C.O. The main complaint was a loose lower denture.

H.P.C. The patient had been rendered edentulous over 15 years ago. An immediate denture had been provided with subsequent conventional sets over the years. The patient has always found it difficult to cope successfully with a lower denture and this has caused problems especially during eating and speaking. She is rapidly becoming a recluse as she does not accept invitations to go out to dinner with friends due to embarrassment caused by not being able to eat properly. If the dentures are worn for a long period, i.e. a few hours, then the patient suffers with ulcers.

P.M.H. There was nothing relevant.

P.D.H. The patient has had four sets of dentures made since the teeth were extracted but none of the lowers have been successful. In contrast the patient has not experienced any problems with wearing a complete upper denture.

P.H./S.H. The patient uses dentural (hypochlorite based cleaner) to soak the dentures at night time.

Extraoral. No abnormalities observed.

Intra oral. The soft tissues were healthy.

217

Denture-bearing areas

The upper edentulous ridge was well formed and the tissues were healthy. There was a good vault to the palate. The lower ridge was present and appeared healthy. However, although there was a ridge present, it was poorly defined compared to the upper ridge.

Prosthodontic assessment

The upper denture was both stable and retentive. In contrast, the lower denture was not stable or retentive. It was easily displaced by the soft tissues of the tongue and the lips.

Static/dynamic occlusion of artificial teeth

The teeth met in occlusion when the patient closed into the retruded contact position. The freeway space was measured at 3 to 4 mm. The dentures were not stable as they contacted each other in lateral or protrusive excursive movements of the mandible. During such movements the lower denture became excessively loose and was displaced away from the lower denture-bearing area.

Diagnosis

A diagnosis was made of an unstable and unretentive lower denture as a result of a poor anatomical form of the lower denture-bearing area.

Treatment plan

This patient has had a long history of difficulties with wearing a lower denture over a number of years. After a joint consultation with the oral surgery team a decision was made to provide an implant-retained lower over-denture for the patient. Two implants were placed in the anterior part of the lower mandible and these were left in situ for 3 months. After this time a small surgical procedure was undertaken to expose the underlying fixtures and two abutments with studs were placed into position (Figures 13.32–13.36).

The existing denture was adjusted in the area where the studs were positioned so that the patient could wear the old dentures during the construction of the new dentures. The major task when providing the new lower denture is the provision of gold clips which are incorporated into the denture. These precision attachments are held in the acrylic baseplate and attach onto the studs when the denture is placed into the mouth. The implant manufacturer will supply transfer impression copings which may be picked up at the final impression stage. This enables the technician to construct a replica of the studs and process the clips into the acrylic baseplate. The making of the new prosthesis follows traditional stages of complete denture construction and at the final process stage the gold clips

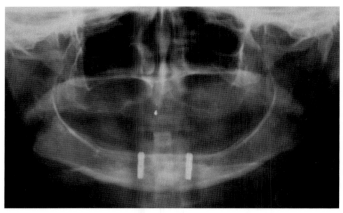

Fig. 13.32 A panoramic radiograph showing the position of two endosseous implants in the anterior part of the mandible.

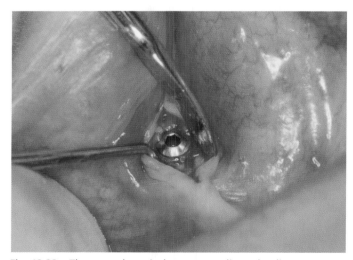

Fig. 13.33 The second surgical stage revealing a healing abutment over one of the implant fixtures.

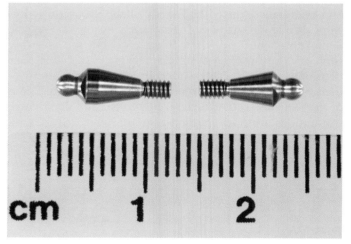

Fig. 13.34 The one-piece stud abutments which attach to the implant fixture.

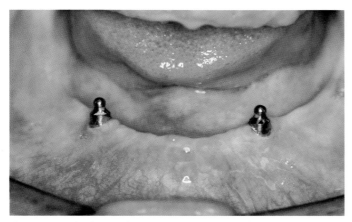

Fig. 13.35 The lower denture-bearing area with two stud attachments.

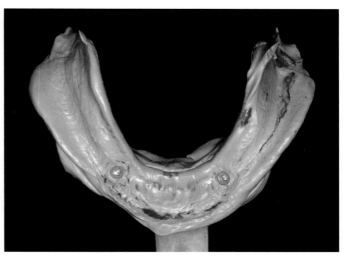

Fig. 13.37 A silicone impression which incorporates the copings.

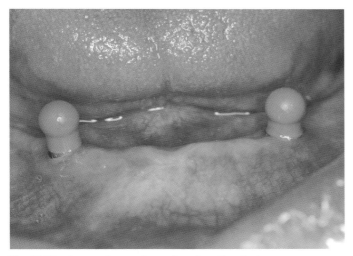

Fig. 13.36 Impression copings placed on the studs.

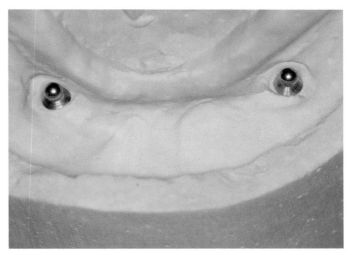

Fig. 13.38 The cast of the impression with the replica studs in position.

are processed into the denture (Figs 13.36–13.39; see also Figs 13.40 and 13.41).

The resulting denture is secured by the clips attaching themselves onto the studs. These clips are similar to press studs and can be either loosened or tightened depending on how firmly the denture is to be held on the implants.

Discussion

This is a simple overview of one particular method of using implants to secure a loose lower denture in place. Other methods of attaching the denture to the underlying implants include the use of a linked bar with clips in the denture or the use of magnets in the baseplate adhering onto keepers held on the fixtures. This form of treatment for the edentulous patient is becoming a popular method of improving the quality of life of those people who have found wearing of complete dentures to be unsatisfactory. The reader is directed to the further reading section at the

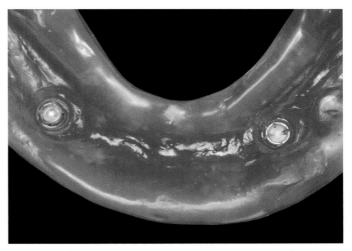

Fig. 13.39 The finished acrylic baseplate with the two clip attachments in position.

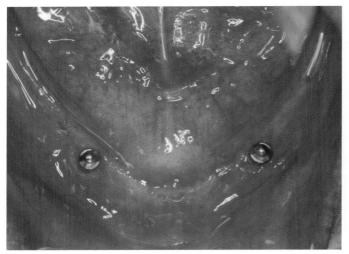

Fig. 13.40 The lower arch ready to receive the dentures.

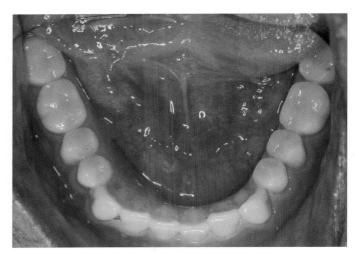

Fig. 13.41 The lower denture in position.

end of the book, where further information may be sought on this subject area.

Outcome

The outcome of treatment was a successful lower denture which provided much needed stability and retention. In such cases there is still a need to monitor the patient's oral hygiene around the implants on a regular basis. The attachments have a finite life and the continual removal and placement of the overdentures will lead to wear of the attachments with the eventual need for its replacement. This can vary from patient to patient but generally 3 to 5 years is seen as an average life for a precision attachment.

SUMMARY

It should be appreciated that there can be many different variations in the presentation of patients requiring treatment. The making of a diagnosis and then following this with an appropriate treatment plan are key factors to success in restorative dentistry. It is hoped that the above cases provide some insight into this process and allow a clearer understanding of this interesting and challenging discipline of dentistry.

References and suggested further reading

Caries

- Bjornal L, Kidd E A 2005 The treatment of deep dentine caries lesions. Dental Update 32:402–413.
- Burke F J, Wilson N H 1998 When is caries caries, and what should we do about it? Quintessence International 29:668–762.
- Kidd E A 2005 Essentials of dental caries. The disease and its management, 3rd edn. Oxford University Press, Oxford.
- Kidd E A 2004 How 'clean' must a cavity be before restoration? Caries Research 38:305–313.
- Mount G J, Hume W R 2005 Preservation and restoration of tooth structure, 2nd edn. Knowledge Books and Software, Queensland.

Complete dentures

- Basker R M, Davenport J C 2002 Prosthetic treatment of the edentulous patient, 4th edn. Blackwell Munksgaard, Oxford.
- Crawford R W, Walmsley A D 2005 A review of prosthodontic management of fibrous ridges. British Dental Journal 199:715–719.
- Gahan M J, Walmsley A D 2005 The neutral zone impression revisited. British Dental Journal 198:269–272.
- Watt D M, MacGregor A R 1986 Designing complete dentures, 2nd edn. John Wright, Bristol.

Core build-up and veneers

- Lynch C D, McConnell R J 2002. The cracked tooth syndrome. Journal of the Canadian Dental Association 68:470–475.
- Summit J B, Robbins J W, Hilton T J et al 2007 Fundamentals of operative dentistry. Quintessence Publishing, Chicago.

Endodontics

- Cohen S, Burns R 2002 Pathways of the pulp, 8th edn. Mosby, St. Louis.
- Lumley P J, Tomson P, Adams N 2006 Practical clinical endodontics (dental update). Churchill Livingstone, Edinburgh.
- Ørstavik D, Pitt Ford T R 1998 Essential endodontology, Blackwell Science, Oxford.
- Walton R E, Torabinejad M 2001 Principles and practice of endodontics, 3rd edn. Elsevier Health, Amsterdam.

Fixed prosthodontics

- Rosenstiel S F, Land M F, Fujimoto J 2006 Contemporary fixed prosthodontics, 4th edn. Elsevier Books, St Louis.
- Smith B G N, Howe L G 2006 Planning and making crowns and bridges, 4th edn. Informa Healthcare, Oxford.

Indirect tooth-coloured restorations

- Dietschi D, Spreafico R 1997 Adhesive metal-free restorations: current concepts for the esthetic treatment of posterior teeth. Quintessence Publishing Company, Berlin.

Materials

- Coombe E C, Burke F J T, Douglas W H 1999 Dental biomaterials. Kluwer Academic Press, Boston.
- McCabe J F, Walls A W G 1998 Applied dental materials, 8th edn. Blackwell Munksgaard, Oxford.
- Roeters J J, Shortall A C, Opdam N J 2005 Can a single composite resin serve all purposes? British Dental Journal 199:73–79.

Occlusion

- Klineberg I, Jagger R 2004 Occlusion and clinical practice. Elsevier Books, Edinburgh.

Osseointegrated implants

- Feine J S, Carlsson G E 2005 Implant overdentures: the standard of care for edentulous patients. Quintessence, UK.
- Hobkirk J A, Watson R, Searson L 2003 Introducing dental implants. Elsevier Books, Edinburgh.

Overdentures

- Basker R M, Harrison A, Ralph J P et al 1993 Overdentures in general dental practice, 3rd edn. British Dental Journal Books, London.
- Crum R J, Rooney J R 1978 Alveolar bone loss in overdentures: A five year study. Journal of Prosthetic Dentistry 40:610–613.

Periodontology

- Drisko C H 2000 Nonsurgical periodontal therapy. Periodontology 25:77–88.
- Lindhe J, Karring T, Lang N 2003 Clinical periodontology and implant dentistry, 4th edn. Blackwell Publishing, Oxford.
- Tonetti M S 2000 Advances in periodontology. Primary Dental Care 7:149–152.

Prevalence studies on tooth wear

- Bartlett D W, Coward P Y, Nikkah C et al 1998 The prevalence of tooth wear in a cluster sample of adolescent schoolchildren and its relationship with potential explanatory factors. British Dental Journal 184:125–129.
- Chadwick B L, White D A, Morris A J et al 2006 Non-carious tooth conditions in children in the UK, 2003. British Dental Journal 200:379–384.
- Hind K, Gregory J R 1994 National diet and nutrition survey; children to 4.5 years, volume 2: Report of the dental survey. Office of Population Census and Surveys. HMSO, London.
- Millward A, Shaw L, Smith A 1994 Dental erosion in four-year-old children from differing socioeconomic backgrounds. ASDC Journal of Dentistry for Children 61:263–266.
- Milosevic A, Young P J, Lennon M A 1994 The prevalence of tooth wear in 14-year-old school children in Liverpool. Community Dent Health 11:83–86.

Resin-bonded bridgework

- Botelho M 2000 Design principles for cantilevered resin-bonded fixed partial dentures. Quintessence International 31:613–619.

Toothwear

- Bartlett D W 2005 The role of erosion in tooth wear: aetiology, prevention and management. International Dental Journal 55(4 Suppl 1):277–284.
- Bartlett D W, Shah P 2006 A critical review of non-carious cervical (wear) lesions and the role of abfraction, erosion, and abrasion. Journal of Dental Research 85:306–312.

- Dyer K, Ibbetson R, Grey N 2001 A question of space: options for the restorative management of worn teeth. Dental Update 28:118–123.
- Lussi A 2006 Dental erosion from diagnosis to therapy. Karger AG, Basel.
- Addy M, Embery G, Edgar W M et al 2000 Tooth wear and sensitivity. Clinical advances in restorative dentistry. M Dunitz, Oxford.

Index

Note: page numbers in **bold** refer to figures or tables

DATE DUE
